CARDIOLOGY RESEARCH AND CLINICAL DEVELOPMENTS

RECENT ADVANCES IN CARDIOLOGY

Cardiology Research and Clinical Developments

Additional books in this series can be found on Nova's website under the Series tab.

Additional e-books in this series can be found on Nova's website under the e-book tab.

CARDIOLOGY RESEARCH AND CLINICAL DEVELOPMENTS

RECENT ADVANCES IN CARDIOLOGY

JOSÉ MILEI
AND
GIUSEPPE AMBROSIO
EDITORS

NOVA BIOMEDICAL
New York

For permission to use material from this book please contact us:
Telephone 631-231-7269; Fax 631-231-8175
Web Site: http://www.novapublishers.com

Library of Congress Cataloging-in-Publication Data

ISBN: 978-1-63117-282-3

Library of Congress Control Number: 2014931435

Published by Nova Science Publishers, Inc. † New York

Contents

In: Recent Advances in Cardiology
Editors: José Milei and Giuseppe Ambrosio
ISBN: 978-1-63117-282-3

Chapter 1

Endothelium and Acute Cardiovascular Events

Ricardo J. Esper,[1,2,3] Roberto A. Nordaby,[2] Jorge Curotto Grasiosi,[3] Diego Cordero[3] and Jorge O. Vilariño[4]

[1]Professor of Medicine, Universidad de Buenos Aires, Argentina
[2]Professor of Cardiology, Universidad del Salvador, Buenos Aires, Argentina
[3]Hospital Militar Central, Buenos Aires, Argentina
[4]Fundación para la Lucha contra las Enfermedades Neurológicas de la Infancia (FLENI), Buenos Aires, Argentina

Abstract

Atherosclerosis is responsible for more than 50% of deaths in adults in Western countries, and it is now expanding into underdeveloped countries as well. Atherosclerosis is closely related to risk factors, i.e., natural conditions or acquired habits that predispose to this disease. Progress in the knowledge of this disease has also identified other non-traditional risk factors, such as inflammation and activation of immunological responses.

Atherosclerotic alteration of the vessel wall is the essential condition for the occurrence of an acute vascular event, and most people over the age of 40 have evidence of coronary artery atherosclerosis. However, it is widely believed that it is necessary that other factors be involved, apart from the mere presence of atherosclerosis, for an acute vascular event to occur. They include the behavior of vascular endothelium, inflammation, thrombosis, fibrinolysis, and mechanical factors, all of which are reviewed in this chapter.

Many factors converge on the pathophysiology of acute vascular syndromes. Thus, considering just one factor is not enough to predict or account for cardiovascular events. The status of endothelium, plaque characteristics, thrombogenic potential, reduced fibrinolytic capacity, levels of inflammation, cholesterol concentration, reduced HDL cholesterol fraction, diabetes, the emotional status of the patient, and many other factors and conditions, each contribute with a small increase in the risk of acute vascular events for a given individual. This hypothesis may explain the apparent variability in the occurrence of an acute vascular event, and our difficulties in predicting events at the individual level.

Introduction

Atherosclerosis (from the Greek *atheros*: gruel and *skleros*: hard) is a disease that is characterized by the thickening, hardening and loss of elasticity of the arterial wall, due to lipid deposition in the intimal layer of the arterial wall, with infiltration of blood cells, cells from the arterial wall, blood products, lipids, and calcium, all surrounded by a layer of fibrous tissue forming the so-called atheroma plaque. This is originated by an alteration between inflow and outflow of lipids from the arterial wall that affects primarily the intima layer, and also compromises the media and adventitia. Progression of this disease leads to a partial and progressive obstruction of the artery, causing different degrees of ischemia, or thrombotic complication with total occlusion of the vessel and consequently necrosis in the corresponding territory.

Rupture of the fibrous cap of the atherosclerotic plaque releases thrombogenic material so that the vessel lumen is obstructed and acute coronary syndrome consequentely follows. Even if the plaque is not be severely obstructing the lumen, plaque rupture and thrombosis may happen at the level of relatively small lesions. In other cases, erosion of endothelium surface is sufficient for the formation of plaque thrombus; this can obstruct the artery, or detach and embolize, or organize and become part of the intimal layer thus contributing to the progressive reduction of the artery lumen [1]. According to autopsy data 65-75% of fatal myocardial infarctions are due to plaque rupture, while endothelial surface erosion causes between 20- 25% of ruptures [2]. In a much lower proportion, calcified nodules and intra plaque hemorrhage may be considered responsible.

Epidemiology

Atherosclerosis is responsible for more than 50% of deaths in adults in Western countries. This represents an enormous social burden. Atherosclerosis has long been thought to be mostly confined to affluent countries, but it is now evident that in developing countries it is going to increase and supersede the current incidence in the next decade (Figure 1). This is mostly due to the following factors [3]:

- Aging of the population.
- Patients that have suffered a cardiac, cerebral or peripheral acute vascular event now survive much longer than previously, thus increasing the number of patients with chronic ischemic heart disease, heart failure, cerebral vascular disease, and peripheral vascular disease.
- Switching to an unhealthy life style in developed countries, with diets higher in fat and salt, and cigarette smoking, with an increase of sedentary habits, diabetes, obesity, and stress.

The size of its prevalence gives atherosclerosis pandemic characteristics, and consequently increases costs in health care, which are a major burden to society [4].

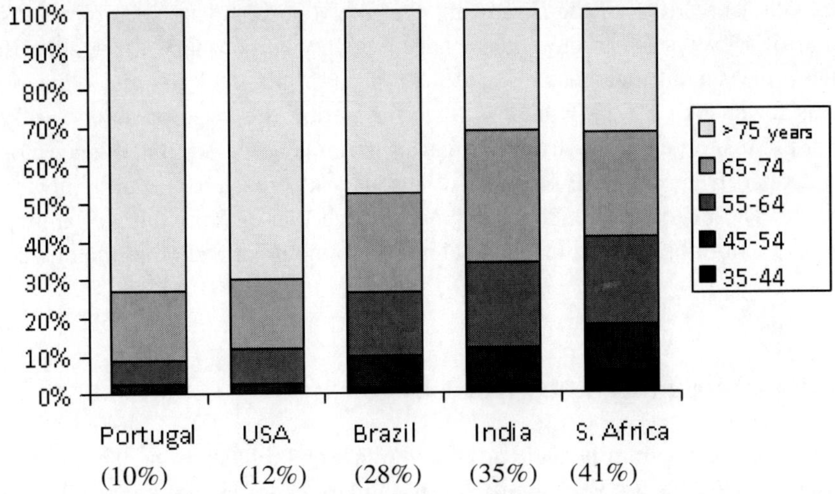

Figure 1. Projection of mortality from cardiovascular disease between the years 2000 and 2030 by age and country. Modified from Mathers CD et al. [3].

Atherosclerosis is closely related to risk factors, which are natural conditions or acquired habits that predispose to this disease. Some cannot be modified, such as age, familiarity, and gender. Others can be modified, such as hypertension, hypercholesterolemia, diabetes, cigarette smoking, obesity and sedentary life style; indeed, the last three factors should be considered eradicable because their persistence depends on the individual behavior and the support given by their medical doctor to abandon that habit [5].

Progress in the knowledge of this disease has identified other non-traditional risk factors, such as inflammation and activation of the immunological response. These mechanisms could explain how traditional risk factors can modify vascular biology and influence progression of the atheroma and its clinical complications.

Coronary Atherosclerosis

Coronary atherosclerosis is the prerequisite for an acute coronary event, except for rare situations such as coronary dissections, arteritis, myocardial bridges, thromboembolism or vasospasm without evidence of coronary artery disease.4 Nevertheless, even in some of these situations, the use of more sensitive diagnostic techniques reveals the presence of coronary artery disease [6].

Atherosclerosis starts early in childhood and even during intrauterine development [5] and progresses silently for many years until it abruptly manifests itself in the fourth or fifth decade of life, as an myocardial infarct, stroke, acute ischemia in the lower limbs or other areas [7,8]. According to its major location in different vascular beds it may have different clinical presentations [1].

Beyond age 50 the probability of presenting a cardiovascular disease is increased. Different series of autopsies performed in the USA in young adults averaging between 30 and 40 years old who died from non-natural causes, revealed coronary atherosclerosis in more than 80%, with nearly 10% of them showing obstructive lesions [9]. Therefore, most people over the age of 40 years old in our society have evidence of coronary artery atherosclerosis. Nevertheless, the annual incidence of acute coronary events, in USA and other developed countries, is fewer than 1% [9] which is low considering the large prevalence of coronary artery disease. Most observation strongly suggests that it is necessary that other factor have to be involved, apart from the mere presence of coronary atherosclerosis, for an acute vascular event to occur. These factors include the behavior of vascular endothelium, inflammation [10] thrombosis [11], fibrinolysis [12] mechanical reasons, emotional and other factors that will be discussed later.

Vascular Endothelium: Pathophysiology

The vascular endothelium is made up of a thin layer of cells that line the inner surface of blood vessels. These cells are very tightly layered in large arteries, but progressively increase their intercellular space reaching a maximum separation in capillaries, and gradually decrease the separation in the venous vessels, but to a lesser degree than in the arteries. Until a few decades ago it was thought that their only function was to prevent intravascular coagulation, whereas in recent years the discovery of its multiple functions has revealed endothelium as a true regulator of blood flow and tissue homeostasis. All endothelial cells work as central detectors and effectors that react to physical and chemical modification in their vicinities, and respond releasing appropriate molecules to maintain homeostasis [13].

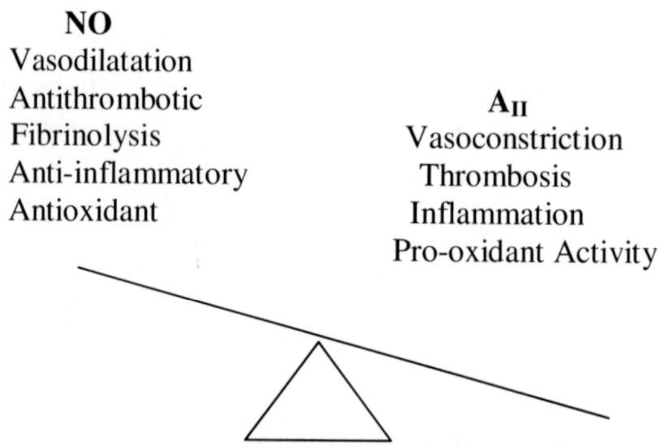

Figure 2. Intact endothelium preserves intravascular homeostasis. Endothelial dysfunction reduces its capacity to protect vascular integrity. Modified from Esper, RJ et al. [1].

Endothelial cells are capable of generating a large variety of molecules, including those with agonistic and antagonistic function on vascular tone, so it may balance its effects in both directions. In addition to vasodilators and vasoconstrictors, endothelial cells produce substances that have procoagulant and anticoagulant, fibrinolytic and antifibrinolytic, oxidizing and antioxidizing properties, and many others related to inflammation and immunity. Injury to the endothelium causes impairment of its functions, blood-cell trafficking turns unrestricted and infiltration of lipid and leukocytes (monocyte, T-lymphocyte) cause inflammation. Foam cells, the basic component of fatty streaks, are formed due to cellular uptake of oxidized LDL by activated monocytes. Thus these events drive to plaque formation. Over time, the plaques become vulnerable to rupture, favoring thrombogenesis, reducing fibrinolysis, and increasing vascular resistance and pathophysiological conditions, all leading to vascular remodeling and acute vascular occlusion (Figure 2) [14].

Nitric Oxide, Shear Stress and Endothelium

Most of the stimuli that induce vasodilatation do it through the synthesis and release of Nitric Oxide (NO), a volatile, biologically active gas. NO diffuses through endothelial cells reaching the smooth muscle cells of the arterial wall; there, through nitrosilation of the heme moiety of intracellular guanylate cyclase, it degrades cyclic guanosine tryphosphate (cGTP), releasing cyclic guanosine monophosphate (cGMP), which in turn decreases intracellular concentrations of cytosolic Ca++ causing smooth muscle cell relaxation and vasodilatation. [15]. When the effect of NO ends, a phosphodiesterase recycles cGMP to its original state, cGTP and vasodilatation ceases (Figure 3) [16, 17]. The activity of nitric oxide synthetases (NOS) on the amino acid L-arginine forms NO and L-citruline, requiring O2 and nicotinamide adenine dinucleotide phosphate/reduced phosphate (NADP/PH), a coenzyme essential in this redox process. Tetra-hydro-biopterine accelerates this process, which is also favored by other cofactors like flavin-adenine dinucleotide, and thiol group-containing molecules like cysteine and reduced glutathione.

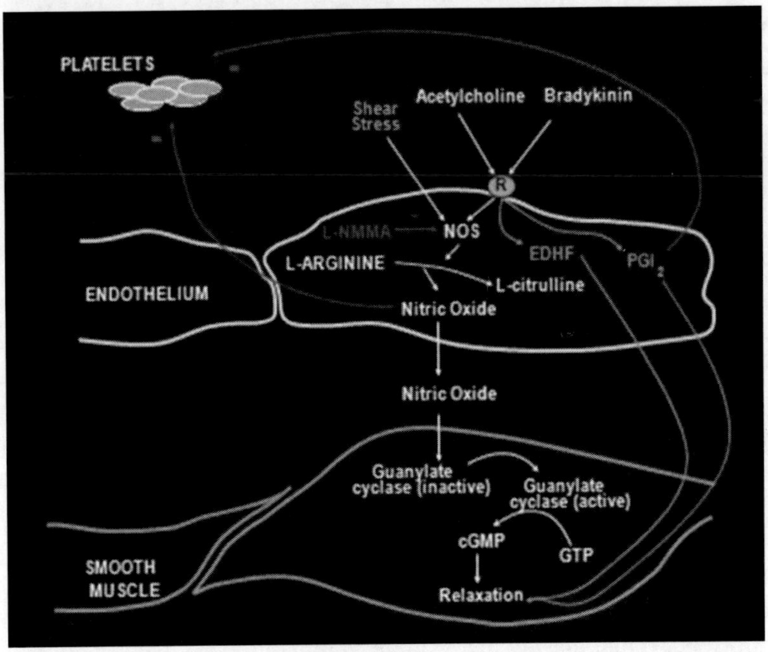

Figure 3. Nitric Oxide synthesis. Modified from Panza JA, et al. [16].

Two NOS isoenzymes, NOS-I (neurological) and NOS-III (endothelial), are constitutive forms with a low rate of production and are activated by agonists that increase intracellular Ca^{++}; a third form, NOS-II, has a high rate of production and may be induced at the transcriptional level. This latter form is expressed mostly in macrophages and endothelial cells, in response pro-inflammatory cytokines; it may release several times more NO that constitutive NOS. Both constitutive and inducible NOS are present in the endothelial cells. Constitutive NOS produces NO for short periods when it is induced by vasodilators such as acetylcholine, bradykinin or "P" substance. Inducible NOS synthesizes NO in a more sustained and prolonged manner when the stimulus comes from pro-inflammatory cytokines, such as tumor necrosis factor α (TNF α) [17].

NO can also be released from endothelial cells in response to physical stimuli, the most important being shear stress. Specifically, the increase in blood velocity within a blood vessel leads to vasodilatation, which is proportional to the amount of NO released by the endothelium, a phenomenon termed blood flow-mediated endothelium-dependent vasodilatation [18]. Shear stress induces the opening of Ca^{++} -activated K^+ channels that are present in the cell membrane, causing cellular hyper-polarization; this allows Ca^{++} entry into the cell cytoplasm that directly stimulates NOS-III (constitutive NOS) to synthetize NO [19]. Shear stress generates a persistent release of NO into the circulation that maintains a stable degree of basal vasodilatation. Nitrates are NO donors, activating guadenilcyclase directly and releasing cGMP in the smooth muscle cell and causing a vasodilatation that is not dependent of the endothelial response or blood flow [20].

Shear stress-induced NO release provides an explanation for the importance of hemodynamic factors in the location, formation and rupture of atherosclerotic plaques, which typically occur in zones of low shear stress (less than 6 dines/cm^2), where less NO release allows formation of adhesive molecules, chemotactic substances and growth factors, thus creating a pro-inflammatory environment. On the other hand, very high shear stress (greater than 70 dines/cm^2) may cause endothelial damage due to mechanical removal of endothelium and exposure of the intimal layer, which will promote local platelet aggregation and thrombosis. Thus, low shear stress allows initiation and progression of atherosclerotic lesions, whereas high shear stress allows the endothelial surface to be damaged with thrombus formation. This explains the different physiology of the thrombotic events according to the territory in which they occur; physiological protective levels of shear stress hence would be found between these two values (6 to 70 dines/cm2) [21-23].

Nitric oxide has many properties and is not only a vasodilator. Nitric oxide reduces vascular permeability, inhibits the synthesis of leukocyte adhesion molecules and reduces: platelet aggregation, oxidative processes, cellular proliferation/ migration, the expression of pro-inflammatory cytokines and inflammatory mechanisms as well. Besides NO increases fibrinolysis and production of I-κB (inhibiting factor of the nuclear factor KappaB, NF-κB) and reduces thrombogenic factors' formation. All these compounds have anti-atherogenic properties, and for this reasons NO is considered to be the most important anti-atherosclerotic molecule [22-25].

Angiotensin II is one of the antagonist of NO that the endothelium produces; it derives from the hydrolysis of angiotensin I owing to the action of the angiotensin-converting enzyme (ACE). Through AT1 receptors angiotensin II produces vasoconstriction and has thrombotic, pro-oxidative, antifibrinolitic actions; it also favors expression of leukocyte adhesion molecules, enhances cellular growth and proliferation factors, and stimulates the expression of pro-inflammatory cytokines. All of these effects promote atherosclerosis progression and complication. ATII also stimulates the activity of endothelin-converting enzyme, which degrades proendothelin (big-endothelin) into endothelin I, the most potent vasoconstrictor in the body [26,27].

According to the balance between NO and AII, the vasodilatory and anti-atherosclerotic or vasoconstrictor and pro-atherosclerotic effects will eventually prevail (Figure 2). The endothelium is in charge of maintaining homeostasis and preventing atherosclerosis, but ultimately this depends on its capacity to synthesize protective factors [27,28].

Classical cardiovascular risk factors, dyslipidemia, arterial hypertension, tobacco use, diabetes, obesity, and sedentary life style, as also bacterial or viral infection, all have a common denominator: production of a state of oxidative stress and directly, or through the heat-shock protein (HSP-60), inhibit I-κB and unblock transcription NF-κB replication, factor which regulates dozens of genes involved in inflammation that cause release of inflammatory cytokines like TNFα, Interleukin IL-1 and IL-6, leukocyte adhesive molecules, chemokines, and chemotactines, substances that inhibit the activity of NOS-III and NO release, favoring synthesis and activation of AII. At the same time, many pro-inflammatory cytokines induce expression of NF-κB, and in this way refuel the inflammation circuit [29-31].

Other mechanisms of vasodilation are not as effective as NO. The main mechanism is the prostaglandin cascade synthesis that ends in prostacyclin formation; this stimulates adenyl-cyclase that degrades cyclic adenosine-tryphosphate, releasing cyclic adenosine monophosphate that regulates cytosolic Ca^{++} as cGMP, and causes smooth muscle relaxation and vasodilatation. This is the main mechanism of vasodilatation in the cutaneous vascular bed. Other vasodilator mechanisms are the hyperpolarizing factor derived from the endothelium (EDHF), which increases intracellular potassium concentration with the help of CP_{450} cytochrome and the natriuretic C peptide. It has recently been postulated that some ACE inhibitors stimulate the endothelial hyperpolarizing factor; this may explain some of the beneficial effects these agents have which are not completely explained by the sole inhibition of ACE [32].

Blood and Tissue Oxidation

Chemical combustion of normal aerobic metabolism produces highly reactive oxidant substances, such as superoxide anion ($O2^-$), hydrogen peroxide (H2O2), hydroxy radical (HO), hypochlorous acid (HOCL), and lipid radicals (lipid hydroxiperoxide, liso-phospholipids, lipid carbonyl). To prevent oxidative damage, the organism can neutralize them with antioxidant enzymes such as superoxide dismutase, catalase, glutathione peroxidase, which catalyze degradation of the oxidizing reactive molecules into oxygen and water. Other antioxidant systems include liposoluble substances like vitamin E and beta carotene, and hydrosoluble compounds like vitamin C; they also protect plasma lipids from peroxidation and neutralize free radicals. When the capacity of controlling oxidizing substances is overcome, a state of oxidative stress ensues (Table 1). Cardiovascular risk factors generate oxidative stress [33].

A state of oxidative stress makes it easier for the LDL cholesterol molecules (especially small and dense LDL particles) to be oxidized. Native LDL are innocuous, do not cause inflammatory reaction and when internalized by macrophages through specific receptors, do not induce transformation into foam cells. In contrast, oxidized LDL are particularly immunogenic. OxLDL are found in arteriosclerotic lesions; they generate antibodies that are capable of neutralizing it [34]. Oxidized LDL have toxic effects on the endothelium, induce the activity of endothelial cell which increases the replication of pro inflammatory genes and cellular growth factor, causing endothelial dysfunction, platelet aggregation, metalloproteinase expression and favor thrombogenesis [35]. The oxidized LDL particles are located in the sub-endothelial region and contribute to the activation of monocytes that become macrophage and up-regulate their scavenger receptors, which phagocyte and internalize them. With the progressive accumulation of oxidized LDL, macrophage modulates phenotypically and becomes foam cells [36].

Oxidized LDL have toxic effects on the endothelium, induce activation of endothelial cell with increasing expression of pro-inflammatory genes and cellular growth factors, causing endothelial dysfunction, platelet aggregation, metalloproteinase expression and thrombogenesis [35]. The oxidized LDL particles are located in the sub-endothelial region and contribute to the activation of monocytes that become macrophage and up-regulate their scavenger receptors, which phagocyte and internalize them. With the progressive accumulation of oxidized LDL, macrophages modulate phenotypically, transforming into foam cells [36].

Oxidized LDL also activates TNFα and induces apoptosis of endothelial cells [37]. Indeed, the severity of acute ischemic syndromes is closely related to oxidized LDL blood concentration [38].

Table 1. Normal aerobic metabolism oxidizing and antioxidizing systems

Oxidant byproducts	**Enzymatic antioxidants**
Superoxide Anion ($O2^-$)	Superoxide dismutase
Hydrogen Peroxide (H2O2)	Glutathione peroxidase
Hydroxyl radical (HO)	Catalase
Hypoclorous acid (HOCL)	
Lipid Radicals	
Enzimatic Oxidants	**Lipid Soluble Antioxidants**
Xantin Dehydrogenase	Vitamin E
NADPH oxidase	β-Carotene
Myeloperoxidase	
Monoamine Oxidase	**Water Soluble antioxidants**
NO synthase	Vitamin C

From Esper, RJ et al. [1].

HDL cholesterol and apolipoprotein A-1 exert antioxidant effects, owing to the presence of paraoxonase, an antioxidant enzyme carried by apolipoprotein A-1 and J, normal components of the HDL particles. HDL particles also show anti-inflammatory activity, scavenge toxic phospholipids, have antithrombotic and fibrinolytic effects, help reverse cholesterol transport of the LDL particles, and attenuate endothelial dysfunction [39].

An excess of free radicals such as superoxide radicals may oxidize NO to the highly reactive peroxy nitrate (ONOO) and lead to further oxidation. Under physiological conditions, small amounts of asymmetric dimethyl-amino-Arginine (ADMA) exists in the body, which may inhibit NO synthesis by competing with L-Arginine. If ADMA concentrations increase, NO production decreases, and for that reason many investigators consider ADMA a new risk factor for atherosclerosis. ADMA blood levels are closely correlated with the concentration of LDL-oxidase and vice versa [40, 41]. On the other hand, peroxy nitrate deriving from NO oxidation, oxidizes tetra-hydro-biopterin, a critical co-factor for NOS activation [42].

Prolonged administration of NO-releasing drugs (such as nitrates) causes activation of vascular NADPH oxidase, with a consequent increase in superoxide radicals (O2) that react with NO to form peroxynitrite (NOOO) [43]. Similarly, when intracellular tetra-hydro-biopterin deposits are low, as it may happen in conditions associated with folic acid deficit, NOS-III dysfunction occurs, and superoxide radicals are generated instead of NO [44]. These actions may explain the deterioration of the endothelium-dependent vasodilatation that is observed when nitrates are given for a prolonged period of time.

Morphology of the Plaque associated to Acute Coronary Events

Two complications of the atherosclerotic plaque are classically associated with acute coronary events: rupture and erosion. A small proportion of cases, below 5%, can be attributed to a third condition, called calcified nodule [45]. In a series of 241 autopsies in people who suffered sudden cardiac death due to coronary atherosclerosis, ruptured plaque was found to be responsible for 31% of cases. [46] On the other hand, if acute thrombosis was considered, it was responsible of 60% to 75% of cases [46-47]. Denuded or eroded endothelium of the coronary arteries was found in 19% of the culprit plaque in patients who died of sudden cardiac death, and between 36% and 44% of plaques showing acute thrombosis [47]. Fresh thrombus is more frequently associated with a ruptured plaque than an eroded plaque, suggesting that rupture is more frequently associated with acute events than denudation of the endothelium [48].

High-Risk Atherosclerotic Plaque

Plaques with a greater propensity to rupture are called "vulnerable plaque" or "high-risk plaque" (Figure 4). [49-51]. They characteristically have a large lipid core, full of inflammatory cells and apoptotic remains (debris), surrounded by a thin fibrous cap containing collagen and proteoglicans generated by the smooth muscle cell of the arterial wall that phenotypically modulate from contractile to secretor cells. Vulnerable plaque are usually eccentric, nearly flat, and thin caps are prone to rupture.

Initially, the atherosclerotic plaque is only a thin fatty infiltration of the arterial wall. The inner core grows in volume owing to various mechanisms, particularly macrophage infiltration and their conversion to foam cells, deposits of apoptotic remains (debris) of these cells, intra-plaque hemorrhages and cholesterol resulting from the erythrocytes cell membranes [52-53]. The thin layer of fibrous tissue that covers the nucleus of the atheroma is subjected to the intravascular pressure of the blood stream. That is, plaque stability is influenced by the inflammation at its inside and external mechanical effects, which leads to a high probability of rupture [54]. By means of coronary angioscopy, several pathological and clinical studies have frequently documented thrombus formation at the site of ruptured plaque and less frequently at sites with erosion [55-56].

In spite of the important role played by plaque rupture in causing acute vascular events, it is now appreciated that rupture of an atheromatous plaque does not always gives rise to an occlusive thrombus [57-59]. Postmortem studies in patients who died of non-cardiac causes, show plaque rupture in 8% to 11% of cases [60-62] without history of cardiac disease, while patients who had coronary risk factors (but who still died of non-cardiac causes) showed plaque rupture in 16% to 30% [63]. Thus, plaque rupture is not synonymous with acute vascular events. Other clinical and pathology studies have also demonstrated that plaque rupture and thrombus formation are frequent in patients without symptoms [57-62]. Mann and Davis found evidence of previously ruptured plaques and thrombus formation in about 50% of stenotic lesion in arteries, although there had been no symptoms in many of those patients [64]. Finally, Rioufol et al., by intravascular ultrasound found evidence of thrombus and plaque rupture *distal* to the site of the culprit lesion in patients with stable or unstable angina [65].

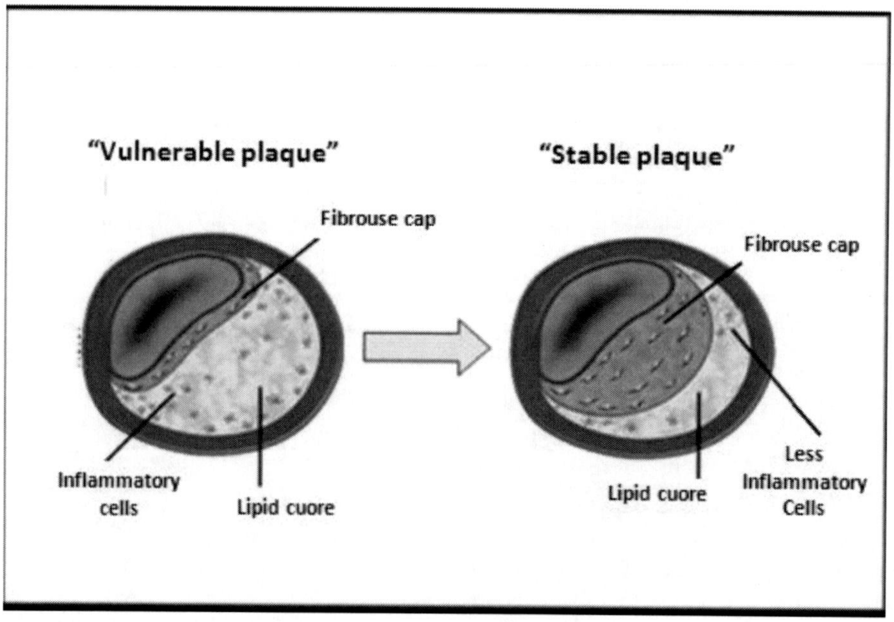

Figure 4. A stable plaque has a small lipid core, thicker fibrous cap and less inflammatory elements, which makes it more resistant to rupture. Modified from Libby P. [12].

Esper et al. observed that endothelial function was extremely impaired in unstable angina patients, with little vasodilatation indicating low NO release. This led them to postulate that endothelial dysfunction leaves the arterial wall unprotected, enhancing vascular tone and consequently vasospasm, likely resulting also in increased tissue thrombogenesis, increased platelet aggregation and less fibrinolitic potential. In the presence of a high risk plaque al these factors favour its rupture, thrombosis and occlusion of the artery (Figure 5) [66].

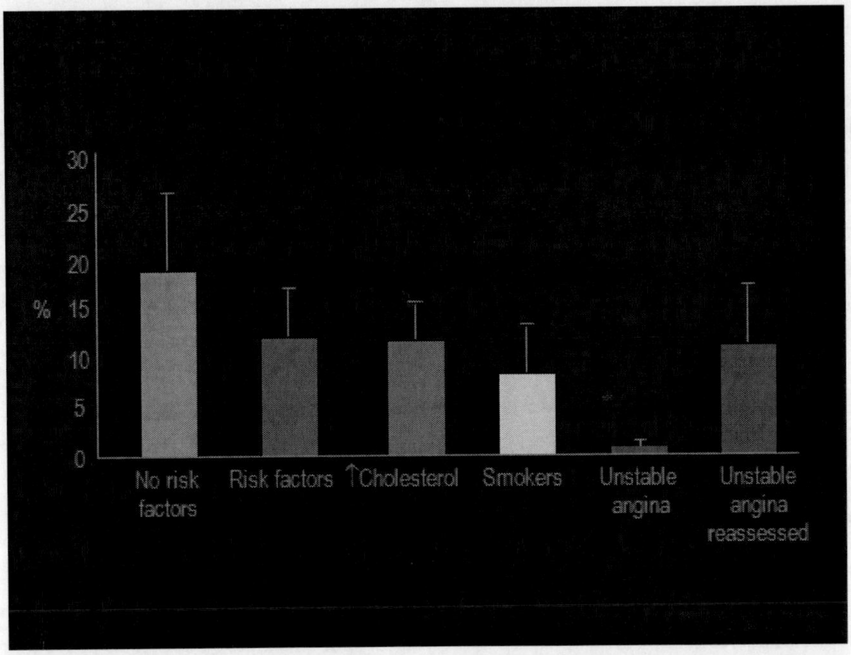

Figure 5. Impaired endothelial function in unstable angina. Esper, RJ et al. [66].

All these observations strongly suggest that acute coronary events are not necessarily a consequence of a ruptured plaque. Most plaque ruptures and erosions occur without symptoms and contribute to the progression of plaque volume. It follows that efforts aimed to identify vulnerable plaques may be less clinically relevant than it was believed [67-69].

In addition to the pathophysiological observations mentioned above, intriguing evidence has been found of temporal changes instability of plaque morphology, which may significantly alter its characteristics over time. In a clinical study with IVUS, most plaques initially showing a thin fibrous cap became thick at one year follow up [70]. On the other hand, some fibroatheromas with thick caps and some plaque described as medium-sized but with sufficiently thick fibrous cap, became fibroatheromas with thin fibrous caps over about one year. If these findings will be confirmed, a vulnerable plaque may become less vulnerable, whereas another plaque initially not vulnerable may develop vulnerable characteristics over the same time period. Thus, preliminary data suggests that coronary disease is an active process that changes constantly.

Inflammation and Mechanisms that Regulate Thrombogenesis

Plaque rupture allows Tissue Factor to come in close contact with coagulation factor VII that is found in the bloodstream, thus initiating intravascular thrombosis. The signal that induces expression of Tissue Factor by the macrophage is sent by inflammatory mediators that are found in the plaque. IL-1, TNFα and INFγ, have a slight influence on the expression of Tissue Factor by macrophages. Exogenous inflammatory factors, such as bacterial lipopolysaccharide, inborn immunological mediators through toll-like receptors (especially TLR-4), are the main stimuli of the genetic expression of Tissue Factor in mononuclear phagocytes [71]. CD40 also induce Tissue Factor expression in monocyte macrophage. All these mechanisms show how inflammation can control plaque's propensity to rupture and thrombogenicity [72].

Activated platelets can exteriorize CD40L, contributing to the perpetuation of the thrombosis vicious cycle [73]. This mechanism usually works when there is rupture of microvessels of the plaque, causing intraplaque hemorrhage and, subsequently, thrombosis. Platelet-derived CD40 can stimulate local Tissue Factor expression, increasing its effects. When superficial erosion occurs, subendothelial matrix and other components of the basal membrane that come in contact with platelets activate them and make them adhesive. CD40 expressed by platelets in these circumstances can activate Tissue Factor in the surrounding endothelial cells and contribute to the local formation of platelet thrombus. All these factors are examples of how inflammation may cause thrombosis, and vice versa.

Mechanisms of Superficial Endothelium Erosion

Superficial endothelial erosion is another mechanism that links inflammation and thrombosis. Apoptosis of endothelial cells in response to inflammatory mediators increases the risk of superficial erosion [74]. Reactive oxygen species generated in response to inflammatory stimuli promote apoptosis of endothelial cells and alter their basal membrane support. Myeloperoxidase (MPO) is released from activated granulocytes and monocytes in the atherosclerotic lesion, and it has been proposed as a useful biomarker of acute coronary events [75-78]. In areas of inflammation, myeloperoxidase can bind to the extracellular matrix and catalyze the reaction of chlorine anion with hydrogen peroxide into hypochlorous acid, a potent oxidant. Histochemical evidence shows that myeloperoxidase expression and hypochlorous acid produced by it, modify the proteins of the atheromatous plaque and those close to superficial erosion [79, 80].

Increased concentration of hypochlorous acid is found at inflammatory sites that cause programmed death of the endothelial cells. It also causes alterations of the DNA of endothelial cells, consisting in nucleosomal fragmentation, characteristic of apoptosis, and caspase-3 increase, i.e., the enzymatic mechanisms involved in the apoptosis pathway. In this way, oxidative stress, a process intimately bound to inflammation, can slough endothelial cells causing superficial erosion.

Proteinases that affect the interstitial matrix may also take part in the degradation of the basal membrane where endothelial cells attach. The proinflammatory cytokines can increase the expression of gelatinase such as MMP-2 and MMP-9, that affect a non-fibrillar form of collagen, type IV, a prominent component of the subendothelial base [81, 82].

Prototype MMP of the subendothelial membrane, the MMP-14, can convert the inactive zymogen of MMP-2 to its enzymatically active form [83]. A putative player of inflammation during atherogenesis, LDL-ox, can increase endothelial MMP-14 expression [84]. Later, inflammation promotes cellular death by inducing apoptosis and favors sloughing of the endothelium at the inflamed sites, through overexpression and activation of type IV collagenase, such as MMP-2. Proteinases have an important role in matrix degradation, in angiogenesis and vascular remodeling, including aneurisms and other types of arterial remodeling, such as compensatory enlargement of arteries; this may hide symptoms and prevent detection until the disease is advanced [85].

Plaque thrombosis: Interaction between Plaque and Blood

The outstanding characteristics of the high risk plaque include abundance of inflammatory cells, scanty collagen, high Tissue Factor expression, oxidative stress, and increased proteinase activity on the intercellular matrix. This determines the propensity of the plaque to rupture or become eroded and trigger thrombosis. Plaque rupture itself does not determine the extent of the thrombosis that occurs. Blood concentrations of fibrinogen and PAI-1 may modulate coagulation and fibrinolysis, respectively. These blood factors influence thrombus formation and stability. Inflammation may regulate the level of these factors modifying their synthesis by the liver or favoring acute phase reactant production. C-Reactive Protein (CRP) may be useful as a biomarker of plaque complication; other reactants may promote coagulation, such as fibrinogen, or plaque stability like PAI-1.

Thus, inflammation does not only modulate plaque factors making them more susceptible to rupture, but it also modulates blood factors that determine the clinical consequences of plaque alteration and may vary from a microscopic wall thrombus to lethal total occlusion of the artery.

Evolution of the Ruptured Plaque: Thrombosis, Fibrosis and Progression of the Plaque

Plaque rupture often occurs silently, not always causing occlusive thrombus progression which results in symptomatic ischemia [86, 87]. Autopsies done in non-cardiac death victims, or hearts obtained at cardiac transplant, show wall thrombus in coronary arteries although apparent clinical stability was present. Collagen synthesis by smooth muscle cells reveal that multiple mediators released at sites of thrombus formation may increase the expression of procollagen and protein production. For example, platelet-derived growth factor (PDGF) and TGF-β, both components of the activated plaque, stimulate smooth muscle cells to synthesize collagen. Local PDGF and thrombin generation recruits smooth muscle cells by migration or mitogenesis, supplying more cells capable of producing collagen. Therefore, plaque rupture and thrombus formation can occur below a recognizable clinical threshold. Apparently, plaque rupture and thrombus are a common finding for pathologists and may drive the plaque to a more fibrous aspect. Plaques that are rich in collagen have a fibrous cap less inclined to rupture and a larger proportion of extracellular matrix compared with the lipid nucleus [88].

Generally, plaques tend to stabilize with a substantial accumulation of collagen in the fibrous cap, and develop a lower probability of rupture. The fibrous process may end up in a constrictive remodeling that causes stenosis or, if the action of collagenase predominates, achieve a positive remodeling.

Psychological and emotional factors associated with an increased risk of acute coronary events.

During the earthquake in Los Angeles, USA, in 1994, Kloner et al., described a significant increase in myocardial infarcts, coupled with a comparable decrease over the subsequent 2 weeks, suggesting that the emotional factor had precipitated the vascular accident [89]. One year later, in an earthquake in Japan, the same phenomenon occurred [90].

During matches the European Football Championships and World Championship decided by penalties, a marked increase in myocardial infarcts was observed in the countries affected by those results (Figure 6) [91]. During the World Football Championship in Germany, played in 2006, myocardial infarcts increased each time the local team played [92].

Several studies done in different populations have shown that religious persons, regardless of the religion professed, but who regularly attended their places of worship, had less myocardial infarcts and arterial hypertension, a reduction of over 40% in follow up of 7 and 8 years [93-97]. In another study done in religious people a lower level of Interleukin-6 was found compared with non-religious people.98 Indeed the effect was so prominent that D. Hall fantasized in an editorial that the effectiveness of being religious was greater than being on statin therapy [99].

Depression increases 2 to 3 times the likelihood of having an acute ischemic accident, and this effect increases further with the severity of the depression [100]. On the other hand, people who are optimistic and enterprising have less acute vascular accidents [101,102]. According to Jefferson's questionnaire, diabetic patients attended by medical doctors with higher empathy have better outcomes, less complications and a better response to treatment than patients attended to by doctors with lower empathy [103].

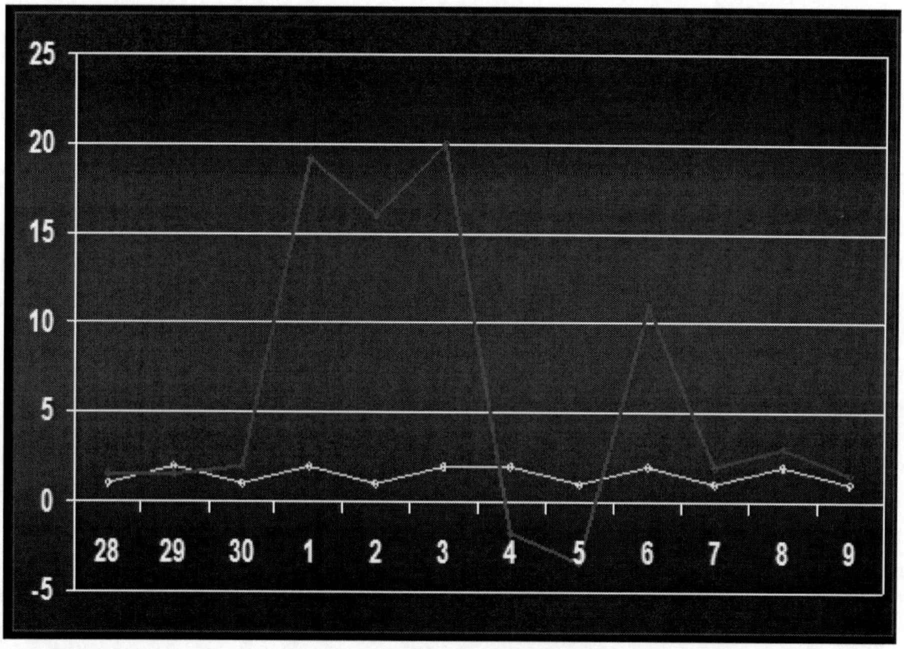

Figure 6. Increase of the levels of myocardial infarction in London, England, after the home team lost the quarter finals by penalties on the 30th of June 1998 during the World Football Championship. Taken from Esper, R.J. et al. [54].

These findings and many other observations on psychological matters and similar emotional situations, leads us to consider other factors not usually foreseen in the genesis of acute ischemic accidents, where undoubtedly autonomic nervous system influence and increased adrenal tone is present.

Conclusion

As described in this chapter, the factors that play a leading role in the pathophysiology of acute coronary syndromes are many, and it is evident that to consider only one, isolated from the rest, is insufficient to predict or justify a vascular accident. Many factors individually contribute to increase the risk of acute vascular events. Endothelium integrity and functionality, plaque characteristics, thrombogenic potential, reduced fibrinolytic capacity, intensity of the inflammatory response, LDL-cholesterol levels, reduced HDL-cholesterol levels, presence of diabetes, emotional status of the patient, etc. [104].

Given the frequency of vulnerable plaque characteristics and the many patients with evidence of plaque rupture without symptoms, it is evident that no one mechanism may entirely be responsible for triggering an acute coronary event [105]. Many components add up to cause an acute event, where probably some have more preponderance over others in each particular case, but the concomitance of factors in unfortunate conditions is always necessary [106].

Endothelial dysfunction resulting from the concurrence of risk factors and/or predisposing inmmunological conditions is crucial to drive the process [107]. If we add to this an increase in thrombogenic factors and less fibrinolytic capacity, an increase in adrenergic tone with vasospasm,and a marked emotional instability that exaggerates vasospasm, thrombogenesis, inflammation and endothelial dysfunction, this eventually leads to rupture of a vulnerable plaque with the clinical consequences of an acute vascular occlusion. Although this hypothesis is difficult to prove, it may explain the apparent variability in the presentation of an acute coronary event, and our difficulties in predicting events in individual cases [108].

Regrettably, these factors are difficult to predict and prevent. Finally it deserves to be mentioned that, although these risk factors are poor predictors of events, they still represent the best available target for prevention and treatment of this insidious disease that leads to an acute coronary event.

References

[1] Esper, RJ; Vilariño JO. La disfunción endotelial. In: Esper RJ, editor. Aterotrombosis en el tercer milenio. Barcelona: *Prous Sciences*; 2004; 49-83.

[2] Libby, P. Changing concepts of atherogenesis. *J. Intern. Med.* 2000, 247, 349–58.

[3] Mathers, CD; Loncar, D. Update projections of global mortality and burden of disease 2002-2003: data sources, methods and results. The CVD pandemic: annual incidence. World Health Organization. October 2005.

[4] Storrow, AB; Gibler, WB. Chest pain centers: diagnosis of acute coronary syndromes. *Ann. Emerg. Med. 2000*, 35, 449-61.

[5] Stary, HC; Chandler, AB; Glagov, S; Guyton, JR; Insull, W Jr.; Rosenfeld, ME; Schaffer, SA; Schwartz, CJ; Wagner, WD; Wissler, RW. A definition of initial, fatty streak, and intermediate lesions of atherosclerosis. A report from the Committee on Vascular Lesions of the Council on Arteriosclerosis, *American Heart Association. Circulation* 1994, 89, 2462-78.

[6] Castelli, WP. Epidemiology of coronary heart disease: The Framingham study. *Am. J. Med.* 1984, 76 (Suppl.2A), 4-12.

[7] Falk, E; Shah P; Fuster V. Coronary plaque disruption. *Circulation* 1995, 92, 657–71.

[8] Nemetz, PN; Roger, VL; Ransom, JE; Bailey, KR; Edwards, WD; Leibson, CL. Recent trends in the prevalence of coronary disease: a population-based autopsy study of nonnatural deaths. *Arch. Intern. Med.* 2008, 168, 264 –270.

[9] Libby, P, Folco, E, Esper, RJ. Inmunidad, Inflamación y Ateroesclerosis. In: Esper RJ, Vilariño, JO, editors. Progresos en Aterotrombosis. Buenos Aires: *Ediciones Médicas del Sur*; 2011; 21-48.

[10] Ross, R. Atherosclerosis is an inflammatory disease. Am Heart J 1999, 138, S419-20

[11] Ambrose, JA; Weinrauch, M. Thrombosis in ischemic heart disease. *Arch. Intern. Med.* 1996, 156, 1382-94.

[12] Libby, P. Molecular Bases of the Acute Coronary Syndromes. *Circulation* 1995, 91, 2844-50.

[13] Ettenson, DS; Gotlieb, AI. Role of endothelial cells in vascular integrity and repair in atherosclerosis. In: Weinstein RS, editors. Advances in Pathology and Laboratory Medicine. St. Louis (MO): Mosby-Year Book, Inc. 1993; 285-309.

[14] Esper, RJ; Nordaby, RA; Vilariño, JO; Paragano, A; Cacharrón, JL; Machado, RA. Endothelial dysfunction: A comprehensive appraisal. *Cardiovascular Diabetology* 2006, 5, 4.

[15] Loscalzo, J; Welch, G. Nitric oxide and its role in the cardiovascular system. *Prog. Cardiovasc. Dis.* 1995, 38, 87-104.

[16] Panza, JA; Cannon III, RO. Endothelium, nitric oxide, and atherosclerosis. New York: *Futura Publishing Inc;* 1999.

[17] Jones, CJH; Kuo, L; Davis, MJ; DeFily, DV; Chilian, WM. Role of nitric oxide in coronary microvascular responses to adenosine and increased metabolic demand. *Circulation* 1995, 91, 1807-1813.

[18] Cooke, JP; Tsao, PS. Go with the flow. *Circulation* 2001, 103, 2773-2775.

[19] Miura, H; Wachtel, RE; Liu, Y; Loberiza, FR Jr.; Saito, T; Miura, M; Gutterman, DD. Flow-induced dilation of human coronary arterioles: important role of $Ca^{(2+)}$-activated $K^{(+)}$ channels. *Circulation* 2001, 103, 1992-1998.

[20] Ludmer, PL; Selwyn, AP; Shook, TL; Wayne RR; Mudge, GH; Alexander, RW; Ganz P. Paradoxical vasoconstriction induced by acetylcholine in atherosclerosis coronary arteries. *N. Engl. J. Med.* 1986, 315, 1046-1051.

[21] Asakura, K; Karino, T. Flow patterns and spatial distribution of atherosclerosis lesions in human coronary arteries. *Circ. Res.* 1990, 66, 1045-1066.

[22] Makek, AM; Alper, SL; Izumo, S. Hemodynamic shear stress and its role in atherosclerosis. *JAMA* 1999, 282, 2035-2042.

[23] Jabali, S; Li, YS; Soutedeth, M. Shear stress activates p60src-Ras-MAPK signalling pathways in vascular endothelial cells. *Arterioscler. Thromb. Vasc. Biol.* 1998, 18, 227-234.

[24] Feldman, CL; Stone, PH. Intravascular hemodynamic factors responsible for progression of coronary atherosclerosis and development of vulnerable plaque. *Curr. Opin. in Cardiol.* 2000, 15, 430-440.

[25] Cooke, JP; Tsao, PS. Is NO an endogenous antiatherogenic molecule? *Arterioscler. Thromb.* 1994, 14, 753-759.

[26] Dzau, VJ. Vascular angiotensin pathways: a new therapeutic target. *J. Cardiovasc. Pharmacol.* 1987, 10, S9-S16.

[27] Johnston, CJ. Renin-angiotensin system: a dual tissue and hormonal system for cardiovascular control. *J. Cardiovasc. Pharmacol.* 1992, 20 (Suppl B), S1-S5.

[28] Esper, RJ: Interrogando al endotelio. *Rev Argent Cardiol* 2000, 68, 429-439.

[29] Baldwin, A. The transcription factor NK-kB and human disease. *J. Clin. Invest.* 2001, 107, 3-6.

[30] Tak, P; Firestein, G. NF-kB. A key role in inflammatory disease. *J. Clin. Invest.* 2001, 107, 7-11.

[31] Thurberg, B; Collins, T. The nuclear factor-kappa B/inhibitor of kappa B autoregulatory system and atherosclerosis. *Curr. Opin. Lipidol.* 1998, 9, 387-396.

[32] Esper, RJ: Detección de la placa de alto riesgo. *Intercontinental Cardiology* 2001, 10, 63-70.

[33] Givertz, MM; Sawyer, DB; Colucci, WS. Antioxidants and myocardial contractility. Illuminating the "dark side" of B-adrenergic receptor activation. *Circulation* 2001, 103, 782-783.

[34] Li, D; Mehta, JL. Antisense to LOX-1 inhibits oxidized LDL-mediated up-regulation of monocyte chemoatractant protein-1 and monocyte adhesion to human coronary artery endothelial cells. *Circulation* 2000, 101, 2889-2895.

[35] Tsimikas, S; Witzum, JL. Measuring circulating oxidized low-density lipoprotein to evaluate coronary risk. *Circulation* 2001, 103, 1930-1932.

[36] Libby P. Molecular bases of the acute coronary sindromes. *Circulation* 1995, 91, 2844-2850.

[37] Li, D; Mehta, JL. Up-regulation of endothelial receptor for oxidized LDL (LOX 1) by oxidized and implications in apoptosis of human coronary artery endothelial cells: evidence from use of antisense LOX-1 mRNA and chemical inhibitors. *Ateroscler. Thromb. Vasc. Biol. 2000*, 20, 1116-1122.

[38] Kadokami, T; Frye, C; Lemster, B; Wagner, CL; Feldman, AM; McTiernan, CF. Anti-Tumor necrosis factor-α antibody limits heart failure in a transgenic model. *Circulation* 2001, 104, 1094-1097.

[39] Shah, P; Kaul, S; Nilsson, J; Cercek, B. Exploiting the vascular protective effects of high-density lipoprotein and its apolipoproteins. An idea whose time for testing is coming. *Part I. Circulation* 2001, 104, 2376-2383.

[40] Böger, RH; Bode-Böger, SM; Szuba, A; Tsao, PS; Chan, JR; Tangphao, O; Blaschke, TF; Cooke, JP. Dimethylarginina (ADMA). A novel risk factor for endothelial Dysfunction. *Circulation* 1998, 98, 1842-1847.

[41] Ehara S; Ueda M; Naruko T; Haze K. Elevated levels of oxidated low density lipoprotein show a positive relationship with the severity of acute coronary syndrome. *Circulation* 2001, 103, 1955-1960.

[42] Landmesser U; Harrison DG. Oxidant stress and marker for cardiovascular events . Ox marks the spots. *Circulation* 2001, 104, 2638-2640

[43] Sage PR; de la Lande IS; Stafford I; Bennett CL; Phillipov G; Stubberfield J; Horowitz JD. Nitroglycerin tolerance in human vessels. Evidence for impaired nitroglycerin bioconversion. *Circulation* 2000, 102, 2810-2815.

[44] Gori T; Burstein JM; Ahmed S; Miner SES; Al-Hesayen A; Kelly S; Parker JD. Folic acid prevents nitroglycerin-induced nitric oxide synthase dysfunction and nitrate tolerance. A human in vivo study. *Circulation* 2001, 104, 1119-1123.

[45] Virmani R; Burke AP; Farb A; Kolodgie FD. Pathology of the vulnerable plaque. *J Am Coll Cardiol.* 2006, 47, C13–C18.

[46] Virmani R; Kolodgie FD; Burke AP; Farb A; Schwartz SM. Lessons from sudden coronary death: a comprehensive morphological classification scheme for atherosclerotic lesions. *Arterioscler. Thromb. Vasc. Biol.* 2000, 20, 1262–1275.

[47] Davies MJ. Anatomic features in victims of sudden coronary death: coronary artery pathology. *Circulation.* 1992, 85, I-19 –I-24.

[48] Kramer MC; Rittersma SZ; de Winter RJ; Ladich ER; Fowler DR; Liang YH; Kutys R; Carter-Monroe N; Kolodgie FD; van der Wal AC; Virmani R. Relationship of thrombus healing to underlying plaque morphology in sudden coronary death. *J. Am. Coll. Cardiol.* 2010;55: 122–132.

[49] Libby P; DiCarli M; Weissleder R. The vascular biology of atherosclerosis and imaging targets. *J. Nucl. Med.* 2010, 51, 33S–37S.

[50] Calvert PA; Obaid DR; O'Sullivan M; Shapiro LM; McNab D; Densem CG; Schofield PM; Braganza D; Clarke SC; Ray KK; West NE; Bennett MR. Association between IVUS findings and adverse outcomes in patients with coronary artery disease: the VIVA (VH-IVUS in Vulnerable Atherosclerosis) Study. *J. Am. Coll. Cardiol. Cardiovasc. Imaging* 2011,4, 894 –901.

[51] Stone GW; Maehara A; Lansky AJ; de Bruyne B; Cristea E; Mintz GS; Mehran R; McPherson J; Farhat N; Marso SP; Parise H; Templin B; White R; Zhang Z; Serruys PW; PROSPECT Investigators. A prospective natural-history study of coronary atherosclerosis. *N. Engl. J. Med.* 2011, 364, 226 –235.

[52] Libby P; Ridker PM; Hansson GK. Progress and challenges in translating the biology of atherosclerosis. *Nature* 2011, 473, 317–325.

[53] Moreno PR; Sanz J; Fuster V. Promoting mechanisms of vascular health: circulating progenitor cells, angiogenesis, and reverse cholesterol transport. *J. Am. Coll. Cardiol.* 2009, 53, 2315–2323.

[54] Esper, RJ; Vilariño, JO. La Disfunción Endotelial. Consideraciones fisiopatológicas y diagnósticas. In: Esper RJ, Vilariño JO, editors. La placa ateroesclerótica de alto riesgo. Barcelona; *Prous Sciences*; 2002; 19-42.

[55] Nesto RW; Waxman S; Mittleman MA; Sassower MA; Fitzpatrick PJ; Lewis SM; Leeman DE; Shubrooks SJ Jr; Manzo K; Zarich SW. Angioscopy of culprit coronary lesions in unstable angina pectoris and correlation of clinical presentation with plaque morphology. *Am. J. Cardiol.* 1998, 81, 225–228.

[56] Takano M; Inami S; Ishibashi F; Okamatsu K; Seimiya K; Ohba T; Sakai S; Mizuno K. Angioscopic follow-up study of coronary ruptured plaques in nonculprit lesions. *J. Am. Coll. Cardiol.* 2005, 45, 652–658.

[57] Davies MJ. The contribution of thrombosis to the clinical expression of coronary atherosclerosis. *Thromb. Res.* 1996, 82,1–32.

[58] Finn AV; Nakano M; Narula J; Kolodgie FD; Virmani R. Concept of vulnerable/unstable plaque. *Arterioscler. Thromb. Vasc. Biol.* 2010;30: 1282–1292.

[59] Hudson J; McCaughey WT. Mural thrombosis and atherogenesis in coronary arteries and aorta: an investigation using antifibrin and antiplatelet sera. *Atherosclerosis* 1974, 19,543–553.
[60] Arbustini E; Grasso M; Diegoli M; Pucci A; Bramerio M; Ardissino D; Angoli L; de Servi S; Bramucci E; Mussini A. Coronary atherosclerotic plaques with and without thrombus in ischemic heart syndromes: a morphologic, immunohistochemical, and biochemical study. *Am. J. Cardiol.* 1991, 68: 36B–50B.
[61] Davies MJ; Bland JM; Hangartner JR; Angelini A; Thomas AC. Factors influencing the presence or absence of acute coronary artery thrombi in sudden ischaemic death. *Eur. Heart J.* 1989, 10:203–208.
[62] Falk E. Plaque rupture with severe pre-existing stenosis precipitating coronary thrombosis: characteristics of coronary atherosclerotic plaques underlying fatal occlusive thrombi. *Br. Heart J.* 1983,50,127–134.
[63] Cheruvu PK; Finn AV; Gardner C; Caplan J; Goldstein J; Stone GW; Virmani R; Muller JE. Frequency and distribution of thin-cap fibroatheroma and ruptured plaques in human coronary arteries: a pathologic study. *J. Am. Coll. Cardiol.* 2007, 50, 940 – 949.
[64] Mann J; Davies MJ. Mechanisms of progression in native coronary artery disease: role of healed plaque disruption. *Heart* 1999, 82, 265–268.
[65] Rioufol G; Finet G; Ginon I; Andre-Fouet X; Rossi R; Vialle E; Desjoyaux E; Convert G; Huret JF; Tabib A. Multiple atherosclerotic plaque rupture in acute coronary syndrome: a three-vessel intravascular ultrasound study. *Circulation.* 2002, 106, 804–808.
[66] Esper RJ; Vilariño J; Cacharrón JL; Machado R; Ingino CA; García Guiñazú CA; Bereziuk E; Bolaño AL; Suarez DH; Kura M. Impaired endothelial function in patients with rapidly stabilized unstable angina: assessment by noninvasive brachial artery ultrasonography. *Clin. Cardiol.* 1999, 22, 699-703.
[67] Stone GW; Maehara A; Lansky AJ; de Bruyne B; Cristea E; Mintz GS; Mehran R; McPherson J; Farhat N; Marso SP; Parise H; Templin B; White R; Zhang Z; Serruys PW; PROSPECT Investigators. A prospective natural-history study of coronary atherosclerosis. *N. Engl. J. Med.* 2011;364:226 –235.
[68] Libby P; Ridker PM; Hansson GK. Progress and challenges in translating the biology of atherosclerosis. Nature 2011, 473, 317–325.
[69] Moreno PR; Sanz J; Fuster V. Promoting mechanisms of vascular health: circulating progenitor cells, angiogenesis, and reverse cholesterol transport. *J. Am. Coll. Cardiol.* 2009, 53, 2315–2323.
[70] Kubo T; Maehara A; Mintz GS; Doi H; Tsujita K; Choi SY; Katoh O; Nasu K; Koenig A; Pieper M; Rogers JH; Wijns W; Bose D; Margolis MP; Moses JW; Stone GW; Leon MB. The dynamic nature of coronary artery lesion morphology assessed by serial virtual histology intravascular ultrasound tissue characterization. *J. Am. Coll. Cardiol.* 2010, 55, 1590–1597.
[71] Mackman N; Brand K; Edgington TS. Lipopolysaccharide-mediated transcriptional activation of the human tissue factor gene in THP-1 monocytic cells requires both activator protein 1 and nuclear factor kappa B binding sites. *J. Exp. Med.* 1991, 174, 1517–26.

[72] Mach F; Schoenbeck U; Bonnefoy J-Y; Pober J; Libby P. Activation of monocyte / macrophage functions related to acute atheroma complication by ligation of CD40. Induction of collagenase, stromelysin, and tissue factor. *Circulation* 1997, 96, 396–9

[73] Henn, V; Slupsky, JR; Gräfe, M; Anagnostopoulos, I; Förster, R; Müller-Berghaus, G; Kroczek, RA. CD40 ligand on activated platelets triggers an inflammatory reaction of endothelial cells. *Nature* 1998, 391, 591–4.

[74] Libby P; Ganz P; Schoen FJ; Lee RT. The vascular biology of the acute coronary syndromes. In: Topol EJ, ed. Acute Coronary Syndromes. New York: Marcel Dekker, Inc., 2000; 33–57.

[75] Sugiyama S; Okada Y; Sukhova GK; Virmani R; Heinecke JW; Libby P. Macrophage myeloperoxidase regulation by granulocyte macrophage colony-stimulating factor in human atherosclerosis and implications in acute coronary syndromes. *Am. J. Pathol.* 2001, 158, 879–91.

[76] Baldus, S; Heeschen, C; Meinertz, T; Zeiher, AM; Eiserich, JP; Münzel, T; Simoons, ML; Hamm, CW; CAPTURE Investigators. Myeloperoxidase serum levels predict risk in patients with acute coronary syndromes. *Circulation* 2003, 108, 1440–5.

[77] Brennan ML; Penn MS; Van Lente F; Nambi V; Shishehbor MH; Aviles RJ; Goormastic M; Pepoy ML; McErlean ES; Topol EJ; Nissen SE; Hazen SL. Prognostic value of myeloperoxidase in patients with chest pain. *N. Engl. J. Med.* 2003, 349, 1595–604.

[78] Meuwese MC; Stroes ES; Hazen SL et al. Serum myeloperoxidase levels are associated with the future risk of coronary artery disease in apparently healthy individuals: the EPIC-Norfolk Prospective Population Study. *J. Am. Coll. Cardiol.* 2007; 50: 159–65

[79] Daugherty A; Dunn JL; Rateri DL; Heinecke JW. Myeloperoxidase, a catalyst for lipoprotein oxidation, is expressed in human atherosclerotic lesions. *J. Clin. Invest.* 1994; 94: 437–44.

[80] Sugiyama S; Kugiyama K; Aikawa M; Nakamura S; Ogawa H; Libby P. Hypochlorous acid, a macrophage product, induces endothelial apoptosis and tissue factor expression: involvement of myeloperoxidase-mediated oxidant in plaque erosion and thrombogenesis. *Arterioscler. Thromb. Vasc. Biol.* 2004, 24, 1309–14.

[81] Galis, Z; Muszynski, M; Sukhova, G; Simon-Morrissey, E; Unemori, EN; Lark, MW; Amento, E; Libby P. Cytokine-stimulated human vascular smooth muscle cells synthesize a complement of enzymes required for extracellular matrix digestion. *Circ. Res.* 1994, 75, 181–9.

[82] Saren, P; Welgus, HG; Kovanen, PT. TNF-alpha and IL-1beta selectively induce expression of 92-kDa gelatinase by human macrophages. *J. Immunol.* 1996; 157: 4159–65.

[83] Sato, H; Takino, T; Okada, Y; Cao, J; Shinagawa, A; Yamamoto, E; Seiki, M. A matrix metalloproteinase expressed on the surface of invasive tumour cells. *Nature* 1994, 370, 61–5.

[84] Rajavashisth, TB; Liao, JK; Galis, ZS; Tripathi, S; Laufs, U; Tripathi, J; Chai, NN; Xu, XP; Jovinge, S; Shah, PK; Libby, P. Inflammatory cytokines and oxidized low density lipoproteins increase endothelial cell expression of membrane type 1-matrix metalloproteinase. *J. Biol. Chem.* 1999, 274, 11924–9.

[85] Dollery, CM; Libby P. Atherosclerosis and proteinase activation. *Cardiovasc. Res.* 2006, 69, 625–35.

[86] Thomas, AC; Knapman, PA; Krikler, DM; Davies, MJ. Community study of the causes of ''natural'' sudden death. *Brit. Med. J.* 1988, 297, 1453–6.

[87] Davies, MJ; Woolf, N; Rowles ,PM; Pepper, J. Morphology of the endothelium over atherosclerotic plaques in human coronary arteries. *Br. Heart J.* 1988, 60, 459–64.

[88] Arad, Y; Goodman, KJ; Roth, M; Newstein, D; Guerci, AD. Coronary calcification, coronary disease risk factors, C reactive protein, and atherosclerotic cardiovascular disease events: the St. Francis Heart Study. *J. Am. Coll. Cardiol.* 2005, 46: 158-65.

[89] Kloner, RA; Leor, J; Poole, WK; Perrit,t R. Population-based analysis of the effect of the Northridge Earthquake on cardiac death in Los Angeles County, California. *J. Am. Coll. Cardiol.* 1997, 30, 1174-1180.

[90] Minami, J; Kawano, Y; Ishimitsu, T; Yoshimi, H; Takishita, S. Effect of the Hanhin-Awaji earthquake on home blood pressure in patients with essential hypertension *Am. J. Hypertens* 1997, 10, 222-225.

[91] Carrol, D; Shah, E; Tilling, K; Macleod, J; Smith, GD. Admissions for myocardial infarction and World Cup football: database survey. *BMJ* 2002, 325, 1439–1442.

[92] Wilbert-Lampen U; Leistner D; Greven S; Pohl T; Sper S; Völker C; Güthlin D; Plasse A; Knez A; Küchenhoff H; Steinbeck G. Cardiovascular Events during World Cup Soccer. *N. Engl. J. Med.* 2008, 358, 475-83.

[93] Hill DT; Angel JL; Ellison CG; Angel RJ. Religious attendance and mortality: a 8 years follow-up in older mexican, *J. Gerontol. B Psychol. Sci. Soc. Sci.* 2005, 60, S102-9.

[94] Music MA; House JS; Williams DR. Attendance at religious services and mortality in a national sample. *J. Health Soc. Behav.* 2004, 45, 198-213.

[95] Hummer RA; Rogans RG; Nam CB; Ellison CG. Religious involvement & US mortality. *Demography* 1999, 36, 273-85.

[96] Miller L; Wickramaratne P; Gameroff MJ; Sage M; Tenke CR; Weissman MH. Religiosity and Major Depression in Adults at High Risk: A Ten-Year Prospective Study. *Am. J. Psychiatry* 2012, 169, 89-94.

[97] Blazer D. Religion/Spirituality and Depression: What Can We Learn From Empirical Studies? *Am. J. Psychiatry* 2012, 169, 10-12.

[98] Lutgendorf SK; Russell D; Ullrich P; Wallace R. Religious participation, Interleukin-6, and mortality in older adults. *Health Psychol.* 2004, 23, 465-75.

[99] Hall D. Religious attendance: more cost-effective than lipitor? *J. Am. Board Fam. Med.* 2006, 19, 103-9.

[100] Lichtman JH; Bigger JT Jr; Blumenthal JA; Frasure-Smith N; Kaufmann PG; Lespérance F; Mark DB; Sheps DS; Taylor CB; Froelicher ES. Depression and coronary artery disease. *Circulation* 2008, 118, 1768-75.

[101] Tajer CD. Joy of the heart. Positive emotions and cardiovascular health. *Rev. Argent. Cardiol.* 2012, 80, 1-8.

[102] Kubzansky, LD; Sparrow, D; Vokonas, P; Kawachi, I. Veterans Affairs Normative Aging Study Minnesota Multiphasic Personality Inventory Bipolar Revised Optimism-Pessimism Scale. *Psychosom. Med.* 2001, 63, 910-6.

[103] Del Canale S, Louis DZ, Maio V, Wang X, Rossi G, Hojat M, Gonnella JS. The relationship between physician empathy and disease complications: an empirical study of primary care physicians and their diabetic patients in Parma, Italy. *Acad. Med.* 2012, 87, 1243-9.

[104] Stone GW; Maehara A; Lansky AJ; de Bruyne B; Cristea E; Mintz GS; Mehran R; McPherson J; Farhat N; Marso SP; Parise H; Templin B; White R; Zhang Z; Serruys PW; PROSPECT Investigators. A prospective natural-history study of coronary atherosclerosis. *N. Engl. J. Med.* 2011, 364, 226 –235.

[105] Motoyama S; Sarai M; Harigaya H; Anno H; Inoue K; Hara T; Naruse H; Ishii J; Hishida H; Wong ND; Virmani R; Kondo T; Ozaki Y; Narula J. Computed tomographic angiography characteristics of atherosclerotic plaques subsequently resulting in acute coronary syndrome. *J. Am. Coll. Cardiol.* 2009, 54, 49–57.

[106] Emerging Risk Factors Collaboration; Kaptoge, S; Di Angelantonio, E; Lowe, G; Pepys, MB; Thompson, SG; Collins, R; Danesh, J. C-reactive protein concentration and risk of coronary heart disease, stroke, and mortality: an individual participant meta-analysis. *Lancet* 2010, 375, 132–140.

[107] Wilson, PW; D'Agostino, RB; Levy, D; Belanger, AM; Silbershatz, H; Kannel, WB. Prediction of coronary heart disease using risk factor categories. *Circulation* 1998, 97, 1837–1847.

[108] Ierodiakonou, K; Vandenbroucke, JP. Medicine as a stochastic art. *Lancet* 1993, 341, 542–543.

In: Recent Advances in Cardiology
Editors: José Milei and Giuseppe Ambrosio
ISBN: 978-1-63117-282-3

Chapter 2

Non-Pharmacological Treatment of Hypercholesterolemia

***Roberto Volpe*[1,*] *and Arrigo F. G. Cicero*[2,†]**
[1] Italian National Council of Research (CNR), Rome, Italy
[2] Atherosclerosis and Metabolic Diseases Research Unit, University of Bologna, Bologna, Italy

Abstract

Hypercholesterolemia is a major risk factor for the premature development of cardiovascular diseases (CVD). Many controlled studies undertaken with dietary or pharmacological interventions have demonstrated that reduced plasma levels of total and LDL cholesterol (LDL-C) result in a decreased incidence of CV events. Between the dietary and pharmacological treatment, the non-pharmacological treatment could be considered to be an important alternative for patients in primary prevention with mild-moderate hypercholesterolemia at low-moderate global risk of CVD. However, only some functional food and nutraceutical (i.e., soluble fibers, phytosterols, soy proteins, monacolines of red yeast rice, policosanols, berberine and omega-3 fatty acids) have shown be efficacious, safe and well tolerated, and some (monacolines and omega-3 fatty acids) have been largely studied in long-term randomized clinical trials showing a reduction of CV events (morbidity, mortality).

Keywords: Hypercholesterolemia, functional foods, nutraceuticals, cardiovascular prevention

Introduction

Hypercholesterolemia is a major risk factor for the premature development of coronary heart disease (CHD) [1, 2] and, in general, cardiovascular diseases (CVD) [3]. Many

* roberto.volpe@cnr.it.
† Email: afgcicero@cardionet.it.

controlled studies undertaken with dietary or pharmacological interventions have demonstrated that reduce plasma levels of total cholesterol (TC) and LDL cholesterol (LDL-C) result in a decreased incidence of such events. The risk reduction is strongly related to the magnitude of the decline in LDL-C. In general, a 1% decrease in plasma levels of TC or LDL-C is followed, on average, by a 1% risk-reduction. Moreover, the effect on cardiovascular risk appears to be independent of the methods used to achieve a lower plasma cholesterol level [4].

Dietary modification, being very cost-effective approach in delaying or preventing the onset of CVD, is the first step in all lipid-lowering regimens, often useful for lowering TC and LDL-C in patients with mild hypercholesterolemia (TC levels between 200 and 239 mg/dL) [5]. On the other hand, in patients with moderate hypercholesterolemia (TC levels between 240 and 299 mg/dL) or, above all, with severe hypercholesterolemia (TC levels >300 mg/dL), dietary therapy is often not adequate on its own and requires drug therapy for optimal reduction [6]. Various drugs traditionally used to reduce concentrations of TC and LDL-C, both in primary prevention studies such as resins [7], fibrates [8-10] and statins [11] and secondary prevention studies as statins [11], have exerted significant reductions of the incidence of coronary events in primary and secondary prevention studies. However, drug treatment may be associated with adverse effects and may also be costly. In primary prevention furthermore, evidence of the reduction of total mortality in long-term studies is often missing [6, 7, 12]. Moreover, the benefit of long-term treatment with statins in hypercholesterolemic premenopausal women is not well documented, and those patients of childbearing potential age may be at risk of faetal malformations [13]. Therefore, in primary prevention, non-pharmacological treatment could be considered to be an important alternative for many patients, as: those with mild-moderate hypercholesterolemia but without other cardiovascular risks and than at low-moderate global risk of CVD; hypercholesterolemic premenopausal women; hypercholesterolemic children of parents with premature CVD; hypercholesterolemic patients with liver or renal failure; hypercholesterolemic patients not yet adequately corrected with available drugs; hypercholesterolemic patients intolerant to pharmaceutical drugs; hypercholesterolemic patients consuming multiple drugs.

A relatively large number of functional foods or dietary supplements (foods that contains substances that provide medical or health benefits including the prevention and treatment of disease) and nutraceuticals (extracts of foods that provide medical or health benefits, including the prevention and treatment of disease) have been studied for their ability to reduce hypercholesterolemia in humans and for some positive effects on other CVD risk factors (i.e., hypertriglycerides, hyperglycemia/diabetes, arterial hypertension), on biomarkers of CVD risk (i.e., insulin-resistance, systemic inflammation, prothrombotic conditions), or on the risk to develop CV events. The National Cholesterol Educational Program suggests to integrate dietary supplements such as soluble fibres, omega-3 polyunsaturated fatty acids (PUFA), plant sterols and soy protein in everyday diet in order to achieve an optimal LDL-cholesterolemia [14]. These suggestions have also been supported by the recent European guidelines of the management of dyslipidemias [15] and that cite some nutraceuticals (monacolins, policosanols, berberine) as potentially useful lipid-lowering substances. Since CVD prevention needs a life-course approach, both the tolerability and safety of dietary supplements/nutraceuticals used to control plasma cholesterol levels has to be adequately defined as well as the risk/benefit ratio of their assumption.

Modulators of Cholesterol Absorption

Soluble Fibers

Soluble fibers are edible parts of plants or similar carbohydrates resistant to digestion and absorption in the human small intestine with complete or partial fermentation in the large intestine. Among fibers the ones that appear to have a significant metabolic effect are soluble and gel forming: beta-glucan, glucomannan, guar, pectin, psyllium for which the dietary sources are cereals, such as barley and oat, and legumes [14-16].

Beta-glucans of barley and oat, glucomannan and Psyllium husk (comes from the plant *Plantago pysllium),* have the largest scientific evidence of efficacy and the US Food and Drug Administration (FDA) allowed the claim of a 'reduction of cardiovascular risk' (within a low-cholesterol and saturated fat diet) [16].

Soluble fibers lower LDL-C by decreasing bowel (ileum) cholesterol absorption (and increasing fecal excretion) and increasing the fractional turnover of both chenodeoxycholic acid and cholic acids. Animal studies also suggest that psyllium and glucomannan increases activity of cholesterol 7-alpha hydroxylase, which is the rate limiting enzyme for bile acid synthesis.

Different meta-analyses suggest that fibers supplementation has a mild but significant dose- and time-dependent cholesterol lowering effect in hypercholesterolemic patients, with a final effect of mean decrease of LDL-C by 5 to 7% for 5-10 gr/day of supplemented fiber, without significant effect on HDL-cholesterol and triglycerides [14]. A meta-analysis [17] concluded that each gram of soluble fiber reduces TC levels by ~2 mg/dl and plasma LDL-C levels by ~2.5 mg/dl, with small variations due to study groups and doses.

Psyllium also increases the efficacy of bile acid sequestrant drugs (even reducing their bowel side effects) [18], phytosterols [19, 20] and statins [21].

Although long-term data from trials focusing on specifical dietary fiber are lacking, several international guidelines [14, 15, 22] recommend an increased consumption of fiber-rich food to achieve a daily intake of 25-30 g based on a diet rich in whole grains, fruits and legumes. This diet could decrease the risk of obesity, metabolic syndrome and type 2 diabetes mellitus (related also to low glycemic index of food rich in soluble fibers) and through the satiating effect of bulky food with low caloric load) [23]. Some guidelines suggested that such a target amount could be reached using fiber supplements in doses that range from 5 to 10 g/day. However, it is not completely clear if the same effect could be achieved by fiber supplementation: if several studies considering hypertensive, overweight patients show that a supplementation with fibers significantly improved body mass index, fasting plasma glucose, fasting plasma insulin, and glycosilated-hemoglobin, as well as systolic and diastolic blood pressure [24], some did not observe any improvements in blood pressure or vascular function in overweight and obese individuals with fiber supplementation [25]. In conclusion, based on current data, consumption of whole foods is preferable over the use of purified fiber.

All available trials and meta-analysis confirm the overall safety of soluble fibers, either as a component of the normal diet or supplemented [26]. However, they could have transient gastrointestinal side effects which are usually not severe and only mildly decrease compliance to the treatment, especially when micronized fibers are used. Entire seeds, used for the treatment of constipation, did not demonstrate lipid-lowering action, but they could exacerbate diverticulitis in patients affected by chronic diverticulosis.

A main safety concern regarding soluble fibers used as cholesterol lowering agents is the risk of interaction with oral antidiabetic drugs, digoxin, iron, lithium, oral steroids, tricyclic antidepressants, carbamazepin, warfarin, and other molecules [27].

Overall a large number of epidemiological observation and clinical trials support the middle-term safe use of this dietary supplement in adults, the elderly and children.

Glucomannan

Glucomannan is an unabsorbable polysachharide, composed of glucose and mannose in 1:1.6 ratio derived from tubers of the Amorphophallus konjac plant. It is grown primarily in the tropical, sub-tropical and temperate zones of Asia. Glucomannan is [28]. It has been consumed in the Orient, especially in Japan, for at least 1000 years. Due to the high fiber content, it was tested in diabetes, postprandial hypoglycaemia, obesity, gastrointestinal problems, some cancers and hyperlipidemia [29].

Like other gel forming fibers, it interferes with the motility and absorption of nutrients from the gut, slowing absorption of fats and glucose and interfering with gut hormones [30]. Moreover, it appears to inhibit the active transport of cholesterol in the jejunum and the absorption of bile acids in the ileum, yielding improvements in plasma LDL and apolipoprotein B levels [31]. As mentioned, it has also been suggested that glucomannan increases the activity of 7-alpha-hydroxylase, an enzyme required for cholesterol conversion to bile acids [32].

A meta-analysis evaluating 14 randomized clinical trials including a total of 531 patients concluded that glucomannan significantly reduces TC levels -19 mg/dL, LDL-C -16 mg/dL, and triglycerides (TG) -11 mg/dL when compared to the placebo. However, it has no effect on HDL-C and blood pressure [33].

Glucomannan's cholesterol-lowering effects have also been evaluated in children at doses 1 to 1.5 g twice daily. Treatment with glucomannan caused a significant reduction in LDL-C values from baseline compared with the control group. Specifically, significant reductions were noted in favour of girls compared with boys (LDL-C: -30% vs -9%, P= 0.046) [34]. This gender-related effect has also been observed with other fibers and seems to be mediated by an interaction between sexual hormones and lipoprotein metabolism, although this has yet to be fully clarified [35].

Glucomannan may reduce fat-soluble vitamin absorption while removing bile acids in humans. Moreover, in one study measuring the effect of unavailable carbohydrates on the gastrointestinal absorption of calcium in rats during a 7 to 8 week period, calcium absorption was also compromised by nearly 20%, partially by calcium-binding protein caused by the gastrointestinal transit of large amounts of undigested food [36]. As for psyllium, glucomannan may reduce the bioavailability of some oral medications, as well. Thus, it is recommended to take other medications 1 hour before or 4 hours after glucomannan administration [26].

Overall a relatively large body of clinical evidence supports the short-term safe use of this dietary supplement in adults and children. However, long-term data is lacking.

Phytosterol-Enriched Food Products

Phytosterols (or plant sterols and stanols, saturated sterols) are hydrophobic molecules that are structurally similar to that of cholesterol (Figure 1). The most commonly found plant sterols are β-sitosterol, campesterol and stigmasterol [37]. They occur naturally in vegetable oils and, in smaller amounts, in vegetables, fresh fruits, nuts, grains, and legumes. The dietary intake of plant sterols does not usually exceed 250–300 mg/day in Northern European countries, whereas it appears to be higher (up to 500–600 mg/day) in Mediterranean countries [38].

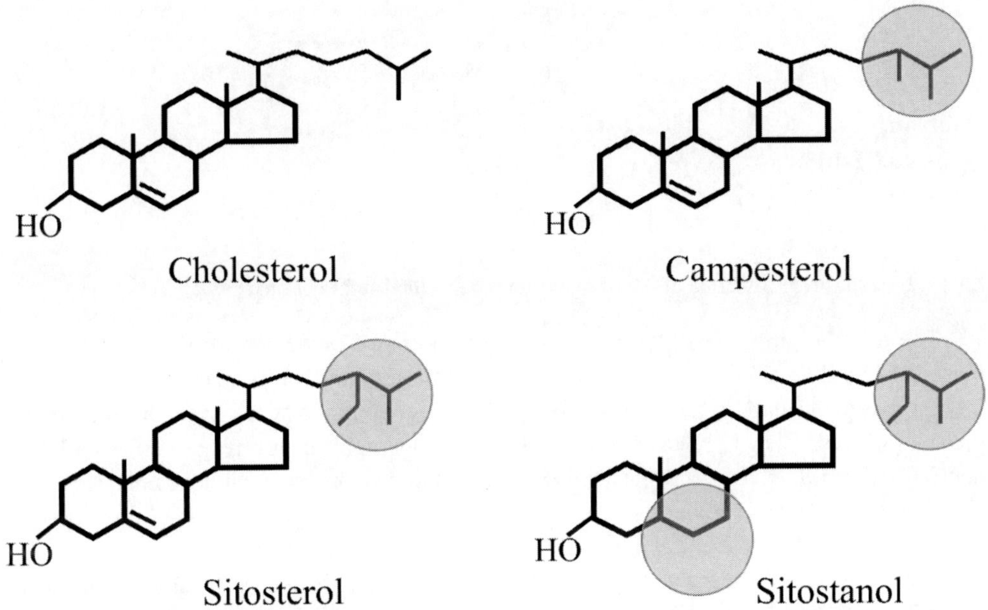

Figure 1. Plant sterols: naturally occurring compounds structurally similar to cholesterol.

Plant sterols are not synthesized in the human body, but are being derived from the diet through intestinal absorption. Despite their significant initial absorption from the intestinal tract via the same efficient pathway that mediates cholesterol absorption, phytosterols are almost completely returned to the intestinal lumen through specific transporters. As a result, their net absorption is much lower than that of cholesterol (0.02–3.5% vs 35–70%) and their plasma total levels in humans are very low, in the range from 1 to 2 mg/dL [39].

The interest in phytosterols lies in their ability to compete with cholesterol for intestinal absorption, through their interference with biliary and food-derived cholesterol for micelle formation in the gut displacing cholesterol from micelles and thus reducing absorption [40] (Figure 2). Besides inhibition of bowel cholesterol absorption, they indirectly increase de novo hepatic synthesis of cholesterol, decrease hepatic and lipoprotein lipase activities and increase serum lechitin:cholesterol acyl transferase activity. However, the ability of phytosterols to modulate dietary cholesterol absorption entails a decrease in plasma cholesterol levels, in particular the LDL-bound fraction, through a partially dose-dependent mechanism [41].

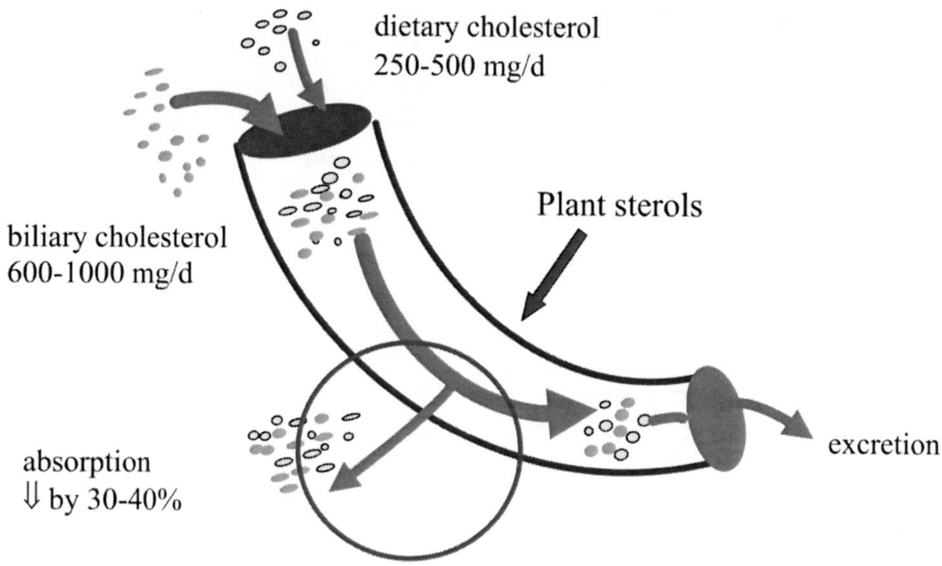

Figure 2. Cholesterol-lowering effect of plant sterols: mechanism of action.

The correlation between the use of different doses of phytosterols and the reduction of plasma LDL-C levels was examined in several studies and meta-analysis that show that incorporation of food products that contain 1,5-2 g of phytosterols into the diet reduces plasma total and LDL-C levels by about 10% (without significant effects on plasma HDL-C and TG) [42-43]. Even if some studies have demonstrated that phytostanols were more effective as cholesterol lowering agents than phytosterols, a recent meta-analysis concluded that they are more or less equal in their cholesterol lowering ability [44].

The cholesterol-lowering effect seems to be associated also with an improvement in arterial elasticity and endothelial function, proportional to the achieved reduction in cholesterolemia [45].

Available data suggest that if plasma LDL-C reductions increase with phytosterol doses, at least in the range from 0.7 to 2.0–2.5 g/day. The use of higher doses provides no so important additional benefits in terms of plasma cholesterol reduction, and because may reduce serum levels of fat soluble vitamins [46, 47] and very high doses of plant sterols may affect reproduction in animals [48, 49], is therefore not advisable [50, 51].

It seems that the efficacy of plant sterols is highly variable from patient to patient in relationship with the rate of intestinal absorption [52].

Food matrices appear to affect the cholesterol-lowering efficacy of phytosterols at equivalent doses, and milk and yoghurt appear more effective than cereals [41]. Phytosterols do not appear to be more effective if ingested in several daily doses during meals, whereas linking the time of ingestion to a principal meal is markedly more effective than consumption not linked to meals [41].

It has previously been suggested that plant sterols are ineffective if the diet is low in cholesterol [53]. However, the cholesterol reduction to plant sterol treatment was obtained also in patients on a low-fat, low-cholesterol diet [43]. These results confirm the hypothesis [52, 54] that plant sterols can inhibit the absorption not only of dietary but also of biliary cholesterol in the gut. Moreover, if saturated fatty acid intake was very low, this may improve the effect of plant sterol treatment, because saturated fatty acids increase cholesterol synthesis in the liver and may thus impair the cholesterol-lowering effect of plant sterols. Furthermore, their effect on the lipid profile is additive to that of lipid-lowering diets and does not change in subjects treated with statins and/or fibrates, which thereby reduces the plasma LDL-C levels achieved with pharmacological treatment by a further 8–10%, as evaluated in a meta-analysis of 8 randomized clinical trials [55].

Plant sterols are usually well tolerated also in children [56,57]. However, in some studies, a few patients have complained of mild gastrointestinal symptoms such as constipation [52] or a decrease in appetite [58].

Since phytosterols mainly act on inhibition of lipid absorption and they are not totally specific to cholesterol, they may also reduce absorption of carotenoids and fat soluble vitamins. A number of studies have shown that at suggested doses of phytosterols changes in the plasma levels of several lipophilic vitamins are insignificant. By contrast, a 7–17% decline in the plasma levels of ß-carotene after adjustment for LDL reduction was observed, although this may be controlled by increasing the intake of fresh high-carotenoid vegetables [59]. Therefore, people using phytosterols may be advised to use adequate dosages (no more than 2 g/day) and to increase their diet intake of carotene-rich vegetables.

The main concern about phytosterols is its use in patients with very rare genetic phytosterolemia where the phytosterols are abnormally absorbed in the bowel. Based on the elevated coronary disease risk in the very few patients with phytosterolemia caused by mutations in the ABC G5/G8 transporters, some Authors have raised the possibility that the modest increase in the plasma concentration of phytosterols in subjects treated with 2 g/day may be atherogenic. The three published case-control studies that compare subjects with and without a history of coronary disease, however, are not consistent (the risk increased in one study, remained unchanged in the second, and decreased in the third) and, therefore, do not support this hypothesis [60].

Based on the available information, it is thus reasonable to concur with the Nutrition Foundation of IItaly Document published in 2008 [61], which recommend a daily intake of 2 g/day of phytosterols and/or phytostanols in patients with primary hypercholesterolemia to achieve an additional plasma LDL-C reduction when dietary interventions are not successful.

Modulators of Cholesterol Synthesis at Hepatic Level

Soybean Proteins

Soybeans contain high-quality proteins and have been consumed for approximately 5000 years in Asian countries. The role of soy products to be effective cholesterol-lowering agents were found in the last three to four decades. The most effective cholesterol-lowering soy component are proteins, whereas isoflavones do not appear to contribute significantly to the effects on lipid metabolism. Several mechanisms for the lipid-lowering action of soy protein have been proposed and included decreased cholesterol synthesis, increased bile acid synthesis (or fecal bile acid excretion), increased apolipoprotein B or E receptor activity and decreased hepatic lipoprotein secretion and cholesterol content, both associated with an increased clearance of cholesterol from the blood [62]. Soy protein also reduces the insulin/glucagon ratio, which in turn down-regulates the expression of the hepatic transcription factor sterol regulatory element binding protein (SREBP)-1. The SREBP-1 reduction in turn decreases the expression of several lipogenic enzymes, thus reducing serum and hepatic triglycerides [63]. Additionally, soy components also induce the SREBP-2 regulated gene expression, which increases serum cholesterol clearance [64]. However, the most important cholesterol-lowering effect may be attributable to the ability of soy protein to upregulate the expression of apo-B receptors [65,66].

The soybean protein cholesterol lowering effect is clearly dose-related [67]. In a meta-analysis of 38 randomized clinical trials carried out by Anderson et al., it was estimated that, after adjustments for initial serum cholesterol concentrations and other variables were made, the ingestion of 25 gr or 50 gr (mean 47 g/day) of soy protein per day decreases serum cholesterol by 9 mg/dL or 17 mg/dL respectively [68].

The observed reduction was related to the initial plasma cholesterol concentrations, that is it was greater in subjects with established hypercholesterolemia and minor or negligible in those with baseline cholesterolemia below 230 mg/dl. This set of data has been reconfirmed by a new meta-analysis published recently [69] (Figure 3).

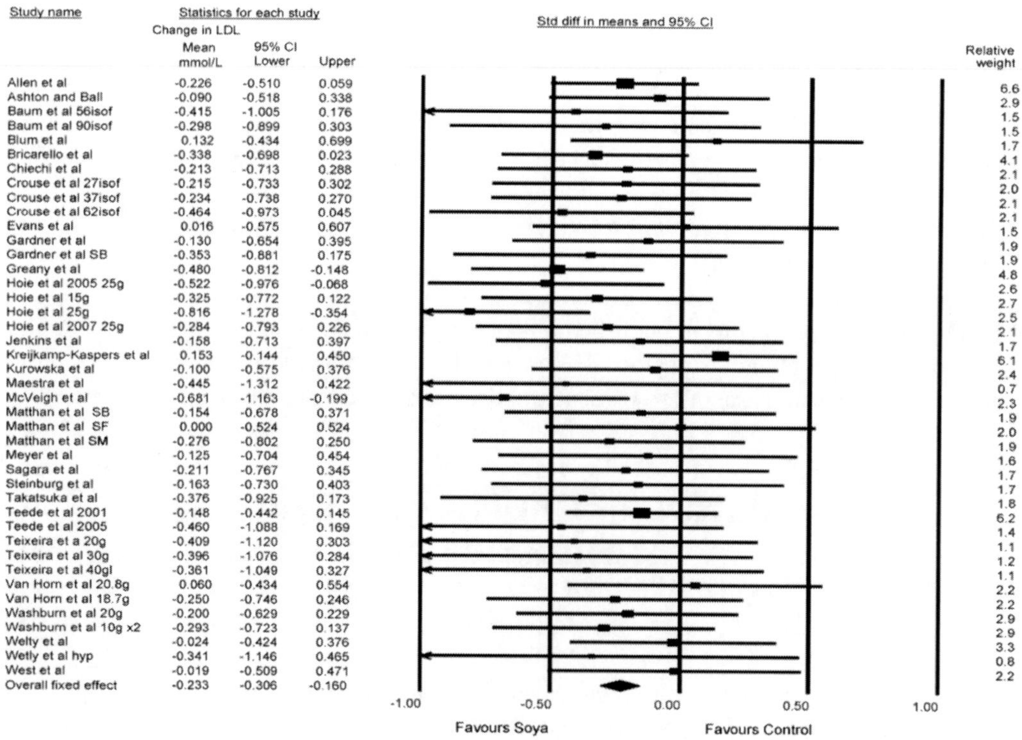

Figure 3. Meta analysis of LDL cholesterol lowering effect of soy protein. Modified by Harland JI, Haffner TA. Atherosclerosis 2008;200:13-27

Although one trial reported no effect of intakes of soy isoflavones on wave reflections, evidence from other 4 trials suggested a benefit of intakes of soy and related isoflavones on arterial stiffness measured through pulse-wave velocity and arterial compliance.[70] The beneficial effect of soy intake on arterial stiffness may partly explain why populations that consume high amounts of soy have a low incidence of CHD [71]. Moreover, soy may have an inhibitory effect on adipose tissue enlargement [72].

Based on the available scientific evidence, in 1999 the US (food and Drug Administration (FDA) released a claim that a daily dietary supplementation with four soy-protein servings (6.25 g each) may significantly reduce the risk of CVD [73]. At these doses, the average fall in plasma cholesterol levels is about 10%, depending on the baseline cholesterolemia (as noted above) and is mostly accounted for by the reduction in LDL-C, whereas HDL-C and TG levels are essentially unchanged after treatment.

Also the US National Cholesterol Education Program Adult Treatment Panel III recommends including four servings of at least 6.25g each (25g/day) of soy protein into a low saturated fat and cholesterol diet to reduce the risk of CHD [74].

Meta-analyses conclude that soy protein can be safely used for cholesterol reduction. Moreover, soy proteins with 0.25-0.5 g/kg body weight dosage were also safely tested in children.adolescents [75] and hemodialysis patients [76]. The main risk associated with the use of a high dosage of isolated soy protein is the dietary unbalance due to excessive protein intake. If the overall protein intake is not adequately controlled, some patients, such as those with advanced chronic renal failure, may have excessive dietary protein load. Although the thyramine content of soy protein is not higher than 0.6 mg per serving, it should be considered in patients using monoamine oxidase inhibitor antidepressant medications [77]. Only one report suggests an interaction between soy milk and warfarin [78]. In vitro, unhydrolyzed soy extract produces very little inhibition of CYP1A2, CYP2A6, and CYP2D6 and a trend of activation of CYP3A4, while hydrolyzed soy extract shows mild inhibition of CYP2C9 and CYP3A4, but the clinical relevance of these observations doesn't appear relevant [79].

Soy-foods or soy dietary supplements containing not only proteins but also isoflavones merit closer attention. In fact, on one hand it seems that isoflavones could slightly increase the cholesterol lowering effect of soy proteins [80] and increase the HDL-C plasma level [81]. On the other hand, isoflavones are phytoestrogens with a heterocyclic phenol structure similar to 17-β estradiol. However, the concentrations of estrone sulfate, estrone, estradiol, testosterone, androstendione, dihydrotestosterone, dehydroepiandrosterone, and dehydroepiandrosterone sulfate are not altered for consumption of soy protein (25 g) containing isoflavones (50 mg) in elderly women, when compared with animal proteins [82]. Moreover, epidemiologic and clinical data on isoflavones consumption shows no increased risk of hormone related cancers, while it appears that pharmacologic unopposed oestrogen exposure in postmenopausal women is associated with a lower breast cancer risk [83]. In fact, isoflavones have partial agonist/antagonists effects on oestrogen receptors, most likely related to this protective effect.

Overall there is much clinical literature supporting the middle-term safe use of this dietary supplement, but long-term data of soy consumption in the Western population is lacking.

Monacolins

Monacolins, molecules derived by the mycotic fermentation of yeast rice from *Monascus purpureus*, inhibit HMGCoA reductase [84]. Monacolin K is in fact lovastatin. Among all the Chinese herbal medicine with lipid-lowering activity, it is the one with the largest literature support [85]. The lipid-lowering efficacy of monacolins was tested in different clinical settings, from relatively healthy subjects in a general practice setting [86] to high-risk patients, such as those under antiretroviral therapy [87] or with chronic kidney disease [88]. In a meta-analysis evaluating 93 randomized clinical trials including 9625 subjects, red yeast rice preparations showed short-time cholesterol-lowering effects similar to those of low-dose statins [89]. Miming statin action, we could expect that red yeast rice has also similar effects on systemic microinflammation and on vascular function. A number of evidence confirms this hypothesis. In particular, treatment with red yeast rice in CHD patients was associated to an improvement in flow-mediated dilation (FMD) proportional to the reduction in serum hsCRP level [90]. Moreover, together with n-3 PUFAs, red yeast rice is the only nutraceutical for which some evidence exist of effects on hard outcomes such as morbidity and mortality [91]. In fact in the large Chinese Coronary Secondary Prevention Study, involving nearly 5000 patients affected by coronary artery disease, the group of patients treated with red yeast rice extracts vs placebo experienced a significant reduction in CV event and total mortality risk with a low number needed to treat (NNT) to avoid a new coronary event, above all in elderly patients [92] (Figure 4).

In the same meta-analysis of 93 trials no relevant side effects were highlighted. It is well tolerated also in statin intolerant subjects, at the dosage of 0.6-1.2-2.4 g/day red yeast rice form, with a 0.2% monakolin K content [93].

Acting through a direct inhibition of the 3-hydroxy-3-methyl-glutaryl-coenzyme A (HMGCoA) reductase, red yeast extract could potentially have the same side effects as the statins: myopathy, rhabdomyolysis and hepatotoxiciy. In fact some cases reported occurrences of symptomatic myopathy, rhabdomyolisis in a renal transplant patient and acute toxic hepatitis [94]. A single report of anaphylaxis [95] is also available.. Other more common and relatively mild adverse reactions associated with red yeast rice consumption are headache, abdominal discomfort, heartburn, gas, bloating, muscle pain or damage, dizziness, and asthma. Those with liver damage and kidney problems, pregnant or lactating women, children, and people with bleeding tendency should avoid monakolines, due to lack of safety data. It also recommended that co-administration with gemfibrozil, cyclosporine, azole-antifungals, erythromycin, clarithromycin, and protease inhibitors be avoided [96], since monakolins are mostly metabolized by the cytochrome P3A4. The majority of these effects appear with the use of high red yeast rice dosages. Finally, issues with long-term safety, the wide variability of active ingredients in available formulations, and the potential toxic products such as mycotoxin citrinin in some cultivation conditions, suggest a strict control in its long-term use in treating hyperlipidemia [97-99].

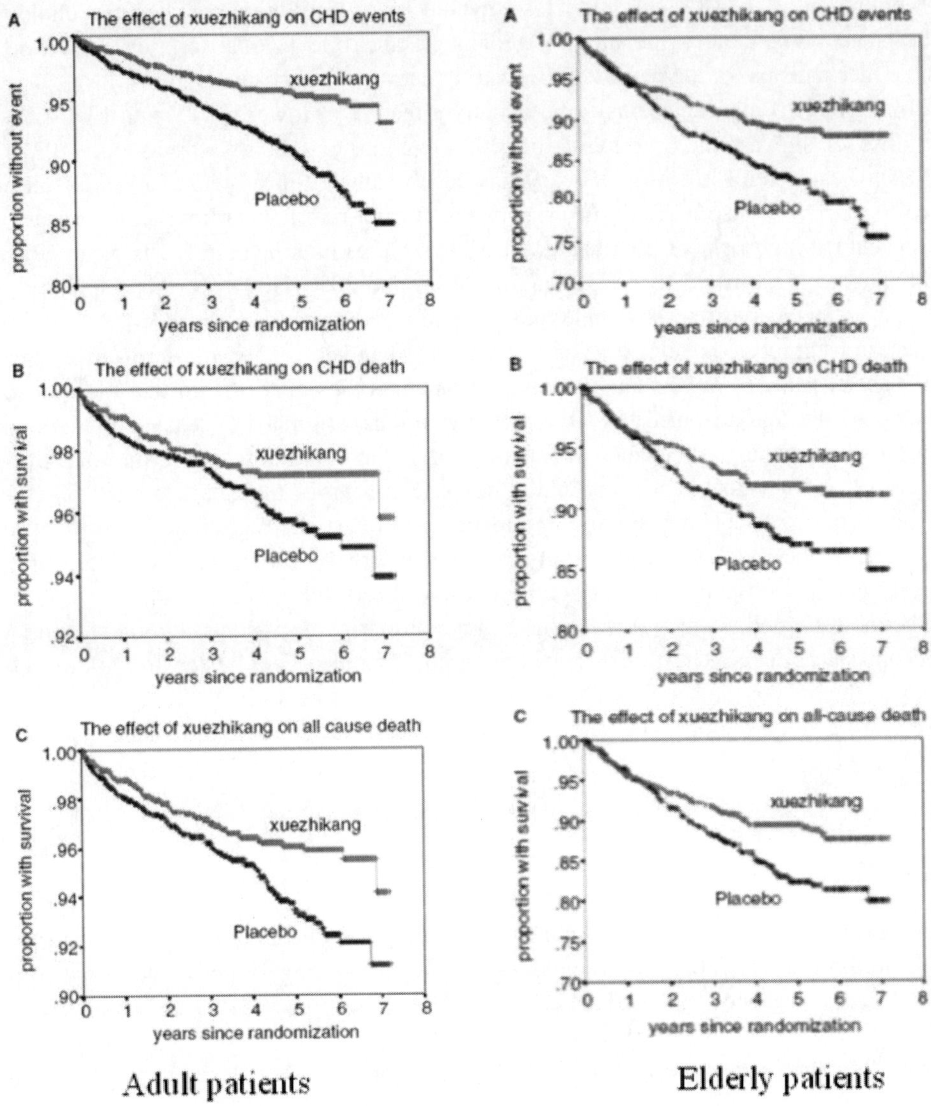

Figure 4. China Coronary Secondary Prevention Study: 4780 patients in secondary prevention, 1445 aged 65 to 75. 7 years follow-up. Modified by Ye P, et al. J Am Geriatr Soc 2007.

Policosanols

Policosanols are aliphatic primary alcohols mainly extracted from sugarcane (*Saccharum officinarum* L) wax. Its main components are octacosanol (62.9%), triacontanol (12.6%), and hexacosanol (6.2%). Cuban studies claim that 1 to 20 mg/day of the original policosanol supplement are effective reducing TC and LDL-C. These studies also show that policosanol supplements are potent antioxidants, promote proper arterial endothelial cell function, inhibit platelet aggregation and thrombosis, and serve as effective treatments for intermittent claudication [100].

Modulation of HMGCoA reductase synthesis or inhibition of hepatic cholesterol synthesis at a step before mevalonate generation and bile acid absorption inhibition are possible mechanisms for the cholesterol-lowering action of policosanols [101].

Policosanol 10 mg/day seems to be equally effective in lowering TV and LDL-C at the same dose of simvastatin or pravastatin [102], but not at that of atorvastatin [103]. The policosanol cholesterol-lowering efficacy has been evaluated in a meta-analysis of different clinical trials [104], also carried out on subjects at high risk for cardiovascular disease like diabetics and at high risk for pharmacological interactions like the elderly. Its mean effect on LDL-C has been estimated to be a reduction of around 20%. However, this relatively large effect has not been confirmed by some recent randomized controlled trials [101].

Research groups outside of Cuba failed to validate the cholesterol-lowering and antioxidant efficacy of policosanols. Cuban researchers, however, affirm that the efficacy is attributed to the unique purity and composition of the original policosanol preparation, a mixture not found in policosanol products used by external research groups [105]. The absence of independent and external studies confirming the therapeutic benefits of policosanol in disease prevention and treatment raises questions regarding their true efficacy [101]. One of the reasons is most likely due to the largely variant ability of the different components of policosanols to reduce cholesterol synthesis in liver cell [106].

The above cited studies involving a large number of patients did not report any significant side effects. The policosanol tolerability has also been tested in children [107]. Moreover, the policosanols seem to have no interaction with warfarin [108].

Overall a large number of clinical trials support the middle-term safe use of this nutraceutical.

Berberine

Berberine is a natural alkaloid with lipid-lowering, antidiabetic, anti-inflammatory, and antiproliferative effects [109]. A three month treatment of 400 mg of berberine extracted from *Coptis chinensis* reduced plasma LDL-C by 25% and TG by 35% in a preliminary clinical trial carried out on 91 mixed hyperlipidaemic subjects (110). The supposed mechanism of action is the increased expression of the liver receptor for LDL. Besides its up regulation effect on the LDL receptor, berberine could also reduce TG by AMP kinase activation and MAPK/ERK pathway blocking [111]. Due to its peculiar mechanism of action not directly involving the HMCGCoA reductase, berberine has been observed to increase the cholesterol-lowering action of both simvastatin and monakolines [110].

Apart from its antihyperlipidemic effect, numerous preclinical studies and some well-carried out clinical trials strongly support berberine as a powerful insulin-sensitizing agent [112]. An anti-inflammatory action of berberine was described in acute coronary syndrome patients following percutaneous coronary intervention (berberine 300 mg, t.i.d., for 30 days in addition to standard therapy) [113]. Another recent study demonstrated that berberine treatment contributed to the amelioration of endothelial function through a partially reducing oxidative stress of vascular endothelium induced by circulating CD31+/CD42- microparticles in humans [114]. Moreover it could have a vascular protective action, by positively affecting flow mediated dilatation (FMD) and endothelial cell progenitors [115] and metalloproteinases 2 and 9 serum levels [116] all markers of improvement in vascular health.

Standard lipid-lowering doses of berberine (500-100 mg/die) are usually well-tolerated and adverse reactions are rare and mild. On the contrary, high doses have been associated to arterial hypotension, dyspnoea, cardiac damage, flu-like symptoms, gastrointestinal discomfort and constipation. It has been shown that berberine in fact delays small intestinal transit time. This may account for part of its gastrointestinal side effects (but also of its and antidiarrhoel one) [117].

The main safety issue of berberine involves the risk of some pharmacological interaction. In fact, berberine displaces bilirubin from the albumin about ten-fold more than phenylbutazone. Thus any herb containing large amounts of berberine should be avoided in jaundiced infants and pregnant woman [118]. Berberine displaces warfarin, thiopental, and tolbutamide from their protein binding sites, thus increasing their plasma levels [119].

Berberine can also markedly increase blood levels of cyclosporine A due to CYP3A4 and P-glycoprotein inhibition in the liver and gut wall respectively and because of an increase in gastric emptying time, thus causing increased cyclosporine A bioavailability and reduced metabolism. In renal transplant recipients taking cyclosporine 3 mg/kg twice daily, the co-administration of berberine (0.2 g/day for three times a day for three months) increases the mean cyclosporine A AUC by 34.5% and its mean half-life by 2.7 hours [120].

Although the main mechanism of pharmacological interaction of berberine involves CYP3A4 and intestinal P-glycoprotein, it also inhibits CYP1A1, therefore potentially interacting with drugs metabolized by this cytochrome isoform as well [121]. The impact of this observation in clinical practise has to yet to be evaluated since the CYP1A1 metabolized drugs are relatively rare.

Modulator of Triglycerides Synthesis

Omega-3 Polyunsaturated Fatty Acids: Docosahexaenoic Acid (DHA)/Eicosapentaenoic Acid (EPA)

Polyunsaturated fatty acids (PUFAs), organic acids naturally containing more than one double bond in the aliphatic chain, are named according to the number, position, and configuration of such double bonds, which also largely determines their physical and biological properties. PUFAs are essential for mammals that lack the enzyme to insert the double bond in the n–6 or n–3 position. While n-6 PUFAs are relatively abundant in a regular diet and while there is no substantial evidence of their therapeutic potential when supplemented in a diet, n-3 PUFA are found in nuts and vegetables as alpha-linolenic acid (ALA) and in marine products as eicosapentaenoic acid (EPA), and docosahexaenoic acid (DHA), supplementation is being studied as a potential treatment or preventive agent for numerous diseases.

In hyperlipemia they mainly affect triglyceride-rich lipoproteins (very low density lipoproteins, VLDLs), whose synthesis and hepatic excretion are reduced by fatty acids. Consequently, n-3 fatty acid intake tends to decrease plasma TG levels. This effect is more pronounced in patients with elevated basal plasma TG levels [122-124]. The effects n-3 fatty acids have on VLDL metabolism, which occur through different mechanisms, include the reduction of VLDL secretion and TG transport, with the formation of smaller VLDLs and, likely, an increased VLDL clearance. The main mechanism of action is the reduced availability of fatty acids for incorporation into TG because of the increased beta-oxidation, reduced synthesis through the inhibition of key enzymes, and the modulation of membrane composition.

Some studies showed a positive effect of n-3 fatty acids, such as fish oil, on plasma HDL-C levels, namely via increased HDL_2 (larger and richer in cholesterol) and reduced HDL_3 levels. However, the results are not consistent and other studies reported limited or no effects of n-3 fatty acids on these parameters [125].

Similarly, most studies concur that the effects of n-3 fatty acids on total and plasma LDL cholesterol levels are negligible (Figure 5). Qualitatively, supplementation with EPA and DHA leads to the formation of larger (hence less atherogenic) LDLs, possibly through the inhibition of cholesteryl ester transfer protein (CETP) [126].

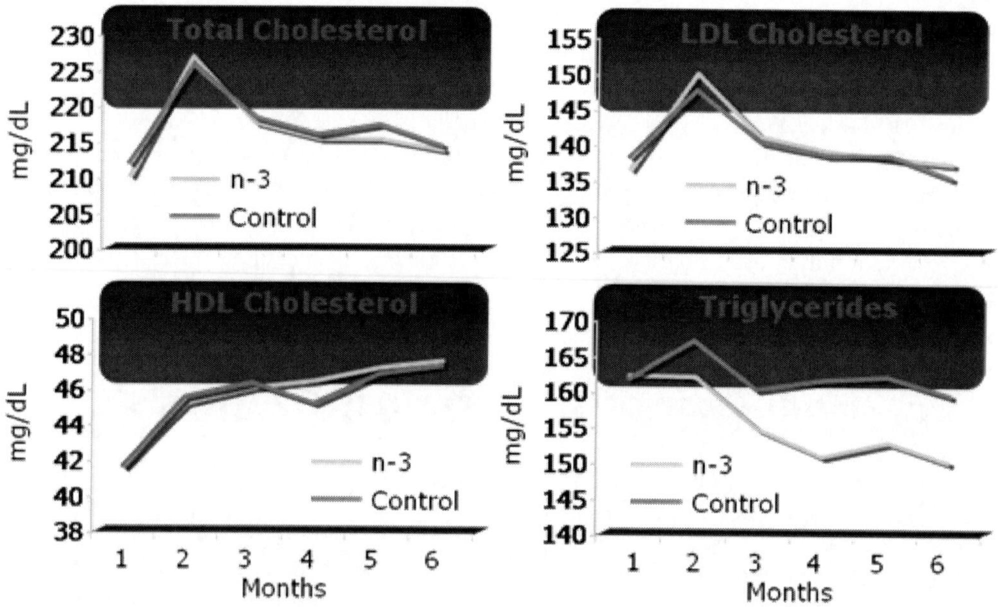

Figure 5. GISSI-Prevenzione: effects of 850 mg/die of EPA+DHA on serum lipids. Modified by Marchioli R, et al. Circulation 2002;105:1897-1903.

Various studies show that omega (n)-3 polyunsaturated fatty acids (n-3 PUFAs) at doses >3 g/day can improve other CV risk factors, including reducing blood pressure, platelet aggregation, and inflammation, along with improving vascular reactivity. A recent systematic review on the effect of n-3 PUFAs in fish oil on blood pressure (BP), which examined 17 studies, with a total of 1524 participants, concluded that n-3 PUFAs supplementation was associated with mild but significant reduction in both systolic and diastolic BP, particularly in hypertensive subjects [127]. Current evidence from several small studies suggests that n-3 supplementation provides an effective means of reducing arterial stiffness, independently of blood pressure: a recent meta-analysis of randomized clinical trials revealed that n-3 was statistically significant in effectively improving both pulse wave variability and arterial compliance [128]. The endothelium protective effect of n-3 PUFAs has been clinically confirmed by a randomized controlled trial of patients awaiting carotid endarterectomy indicated that n-3 PUFAs from fish oil enhanced the stability of atherosclerotic plaques [129].

Some prospective cohort studies and randomized control trials in secondary prevention have found that fish or fish oil containing eicosapentaenoic acid (EPA) and docosahexaenoic acid (DHA) consuming was associated with a decreased CV death rate [130]. The GISSI Prevenzione trial, which examined 11,323 patients who had experienced myocardial infarction within 3 months, showed that daily intake of 1 g n-3 PUFA supplementation was associated with a significant reduction in all-cause and CV mortality, especially the risk of sudden cardiac death [131] (Figure 6). These data have been recently confirmed by a large metanalysis of 21 randomized clinical trials: in subjects with high CV risk the dietary supplementation with n-3 PUFAs lead to a decrease of risk of suffering a cardiovascular event of any kind of 10%, a 9 % decrease of risk of cardiac death, and a decrease of coronary events (fatal and non-fatal) of 18 % [132].

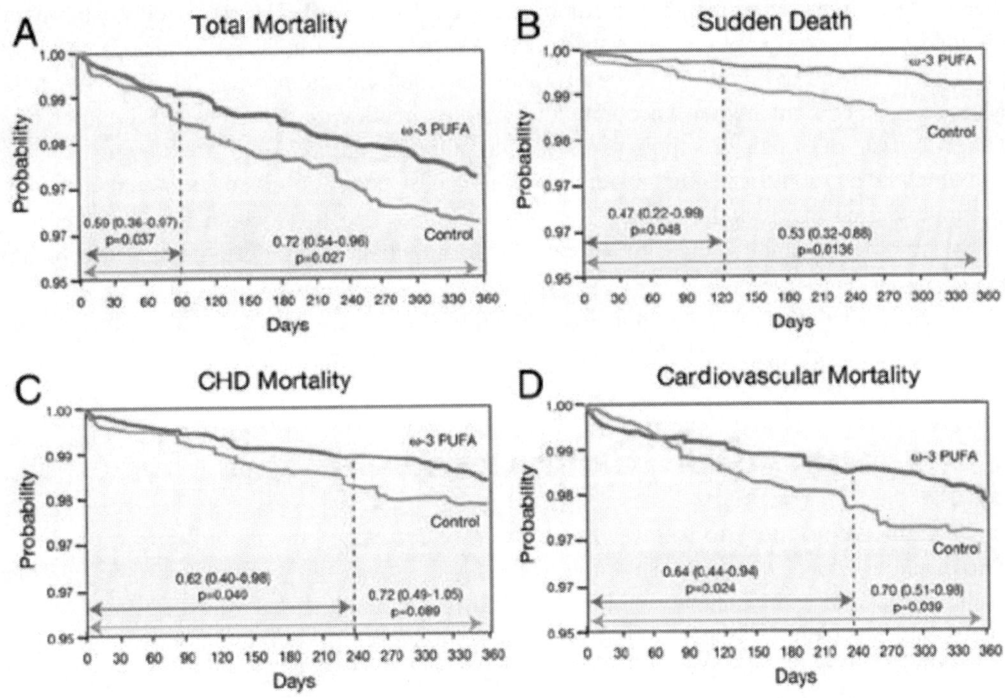

Figure 6. Data from the GISSI-Prevenzione trial : effects of 850 mg/die of EPA+DHA on morbidity and mortality events. Modified by Marchioli R, et al. Circulation 2002;105:1897-1903.

On the basis of these currently available evidence, the American Heart Association (AHA) has recommended that all adults eat fish (particularly fatty fish) at least twice a week, as well as vegetables containing plant-derived n–3 fatty acids. The AHA also suggests that patients with documented CHD consume approximately 1 g of EPA and DHA (combined) per day either from oily fish or fish-oil capsules (after consultation with a physician). The AHA recommendations also state that EPA/DHA supplements may be useful in patients with severe hypertriglyceridemia (>500 mg of TG per deciliter) for whom effective doses are higher (2 to

4 g of EPA/DHA per day to lower TG levels by 20-40%) [133]. Their efficacy and safety have also be tested when associated with statins and fibrates, during pregnancy, and in a large sample of patients affected by psychiatric, neurological, rheumatological, infective, dermatological and autoimmune diseases [134].

Side effects such as fishy aftertaste are uncommon and gastrointestinal complaints, reduced when esterified n-3 is used, are infrequent for moderate intakes. . Data from the Woman Health Initiative shows that PUFA intake higher than 2 gr/day is associated with a significant increase in incidences of type 2 diabetes [135]. Moreover, some reports show that fish oil may worsen glycemic control in diabetes, but recent data excludes that this adverse effect is common when diabetics are inadequately treated [136]. PUFAs could also mildly increase the LDL-C plasma level and LDL oxidation, but data is contradictory. Overall, apparent cardiac benefits of n-3 PUFAs outweigh these effects [137]. Meanwhile, n-3 PUFAs may exert a mild dose-related effect on bleeding time. However, clinical relevance of this has yet to be clearly assessed [138].

More specific concerns regarding dietary fish relate to environmental contaminants and mercury in fish may diminish their cardioprotective effects [139]. The risk-benefit analysis of population fish consumption suggests to restrict fish intake in specific groups, such as pregnant women and children, due to possible contamination or pollutants [140,141]. Moreover, since contaminants accumulate in larger, predatory fish, the consumption of a variety of fish (or of fish oil supplements) should minimize any possible adverse effects.

Finally, no significant negative interaction has been observed between the most commonly used drugs and PUFAs. The only exemption to this, which has been recently discovered, is the small increasing effect of anticoagulant drugs during large dose intake [138].

Overall a large number of clinical trials support the long-term safe use of this dietary supplement as a lipid-lowering agent in adults, the elderly and children.

Nutraceuticals in Combined Therapy

The market responds to safety requirements by decreasing the daily dose of the drugs. This usually achieves an improved tolerability and safety, but also reduces the possible usefulness of these products. On the other hand, some studies are evaluating the eventual synergistic or (more simply) additive effects of different compounds with different mechanisms of action when administered at the minimal efficacious dosages. Of particular interest in this field and in the area of no pharmacological treatment are recent studies evaluating the association of berberine 500 mg and monacolines 3 mg 10 mg [142,143]. This combined therapy reduces the possibility of gastrointestinal side effects from berberine and muscular side effects from monacolines at a minimal level, all the while obtaining a lipid-lowering action similar to that of a full-dosed weak statin.

In addition, also the simultaneous use of no pharmacological treatment and statin could be encouraged, because the combination seems to be more effective than statin alone. The two approaches are complementary, and could together represent a co-ordinated strategy for reducing the risk of CVD.

Physical Activity

The epidemiological studies observations clearly indicate that physical inactivity increases the CVD. On the contrary, regular physical activity, improving plasma lipid profile and also overweight, hyperglicemia and hypertension control, reduce CVD [144,145]. Observational studies indicate that the impact of physical activity on lipid fractions is greatest for HDL-C, which tends to increase, and for TG, which tend to fall in active individuals as compared with inactive controls. The increase in HDL-C levels observed in active with respect to sedentary subjects varies from 9 to 50% and TG reduction ranges from 19 to 50% [146)] while changes in plasma TC and LDL-C values are not consistent.

Most observational studies show a relationship between total quantity of physical activity and the changes in plasma lipid parameters. The threshold is around 1.500 Kcal /week. This means that aerobic physical activity, such as walking, jogging, cycling, or swimming, with total energy expenditure of 1500 kcal/week (which corresponds to about 24 km of brisk walking or jogging per week) may increase plasma HDL-C levels by 3.5–6 mg/dL and lower plasma triglyceride levels by 7–20 mg/dL. A further 16 km/week would trigger an additional 3 mg/dL increase in plasma HDL-C levels and an additional 3–8 mg/dL drop in plasma TG concentrations [147-149].

Conversely, resistance exercise programs do not significantly modify plasma lipids [146], but may increase lean muscle mass and insulin sensitivity, and reduce the gain in waist circumference associated with aging [150].

Key Points

- Cardiovascular disease remains the first cause of death and one of the first causes of invalidity in the industrialized countries.
- Dyslipidemia is one of the main cardiovascular disease risk factors.
- Several compounds marketed as functional foods or nutraceuticals (soluble fibers, phytosterols, soy proteins,, monakolines, policosanols, berberine and omega-3 fatty acids) have demonstrated ability to improve dyslipidemia, to have cardiometabolic benefits beyond lipids, and some (monacolines of red yeast rice and omega-3 fatty acids) have been largely studied in long-term randomized clinical trials showing a reduction of cardiovascular events (morbidity, mortality) (Tables 1 and 2).
- Soluble fibers, phytosterols, soy proteins, monacolines, policosanols, berberine and omega-3 fatty acids tolerability and safety are supported by clinical evidence (Table 1).

Conclusion

Recently international guidelines on CVD prevention have recognized that, at least at therapeutic doses, some functional foods and nutraceuticals (soluble fibers, phytosterols, soy proteins, monacolines, policosanols, berberine and omega-3 fatty acids) are efficacious, safe and well tolerated.

Table 1. Effects, documentation level, side effects and clinical risks of evidence-based functional foods and nutraceuticals used for hyperlipidemia

Substance	Effect on lipids	Available clinical data	Main side effects	Side effects intensity	Mechanism of damage	Known pharmacological interactions	Clinical risk
Berberine	↓ LDL and ↓ TG via increased expression of the liver receptor for LDL, AMP kinase activation and MAPK/ERK pathway block	Randomized clinical trials	Gastrointestinal discomfort, constipation, rarely arterial hypotension, dyspnoea, flu-like symptoms, and cardiac damage with high doses; jaundice risk in newborns	Mild-to-moderate	Impairment of bowel microflora, displacement of bilirubin from albumin	Warfarin, thiopental, tolbutamide, cyclosporine	Mild
Glucomannan	↓ LDL by inhibition of the active transport of cholesterol in the jejunum and the absorption of bile acids in the ileum	Randomized clinical trials	Decrease fat soluble vitamin absorption, Esophageal obstruction and perforation, cholestatic hepatitis	Mild-to-moderate	Antagonism of liposoluble vitamins absorption, Excessive hydroscopic expansion	Oral antidiabetics, insulin	Mild
Monascus	↓ LDL and ↓ TG direct inhibition of the HMG-CoA reductase	Randomized clinical trials, meta-analyses	Myalgia, more rarely headache, abdominal discomfort, heartburn, gas, bloating, dizziness, and asthma	Mild-to-moderate	Statin-like myotoxicity	Gemfibrozil, cyclosporine, azole-antifungals, erythromycin, clarithromycin, and protease inhibitors	Mild-to-moderate, very rarely severe

Substance	Effect on lipids	Available clinical data	Main side effects	Side effects intensity	Mechanism of damage	Known pharmacological interactions	Clinical risk
Omega-3 PUFA	↓ TG via competition with omega-6 PUFAs, PPAR mediated lipogenesis downregulation, ↑HDL proportional to TG decrease	Randomized clinical trials, meta-analyses	Fishy aftertaste, gastrointestinal complaints, LDL increase, hyperglycemia, Increased bleeding risk	Mild	Direct stomach or bowel irritation, mild antiplatelet effect	Sirolimus, anti-retrovirals	Mild
Phytosterols	↓ LDL by decreasing cholesterol absorption and increasing bile acid turnover	Randomized clinical trials, meta-analyses	Sitosterolemia, carotenoid and liposoluble vitamins malabsorption	Mild-to-moderate	Abnormal phytosterol absorption; Antagonism of liposoluble vitamins absorption	Liposoluble vitamins	High for sitosterolemia (very rare), low for malabsorption
Policosanols	↓ LDL via modulation of HMG-CoA reductase synthesis , inhibition of hepatic cholesterol synthesis at a step before mevalonate generation, bile acid absorption inhibition	Randomized clinical trials, meta-analyses	Not reported	NA	NA	Not reported	NA

Table 1. (Continued)

Substance	Effect on lipids	Available clinical data	Main side effects	Side effects intensity	Mechanism of damage	Known pharmacological interactions	Clinical risk
Psyllium	↓ LDL by decreasing cholesterol absorption and increasing bile acid turnover, probable effect on cholesterol 7-alpha hydroxylase	Randomized clinical trials, meta-analyses	GI side effects	Mild-to-moderate		Oral antidiabetics, digoxin, warfarin, lithium, iron, oral steroids, tricyclic antidepressants, carbamazepin	Mild
Soybean proteins	↓ LDL and ↓ TG via decreasing cholesterol synthesis, increasing bile acid synthesis (or fecal bile acid excretion), increasing apolipoprotein B or E receptor activity and decreased hepatic lipoprotein secretion	Randomized clinical trials, meta-analyses	Dietary unbalance, very doubtful oncological risk	Mild	Unbalanced dietary protein Intake, Estrogenic effects of isoflavones	Monoamine oxidase inhibitors, drugs metabolized by CYP2C9 and CYP3A4 .	Mild

NA= Not applicable.

Table 2. Lipid lowering functional foods and nutraceuticals: cardiometabolic benefits beyond lipids in human trials

	Fibers	Phytosterols	Soybean proteins	Monacolins	Policosanols	Berberine	N-3 PUFAs
Blood pressure reduction	+	0	+/-	0	0	0	+
Insulin-sensitizing effect	+	0	0	0	0	+	+/-
Antithrombotic effect	0	0	0	0	+/-	0	+
Inflammation parameters	+/-	+/-	+/-	+	0	+	+
Vascular health improvement	0	+/-	+	+	+/-	+/-	+
Cardiovascular disease event prevention	+/-*	0	+/-*	+	0	0	+

*= Epidemiological (non interventional) evidence

+/-= Conflicting results or non confirmed evidence

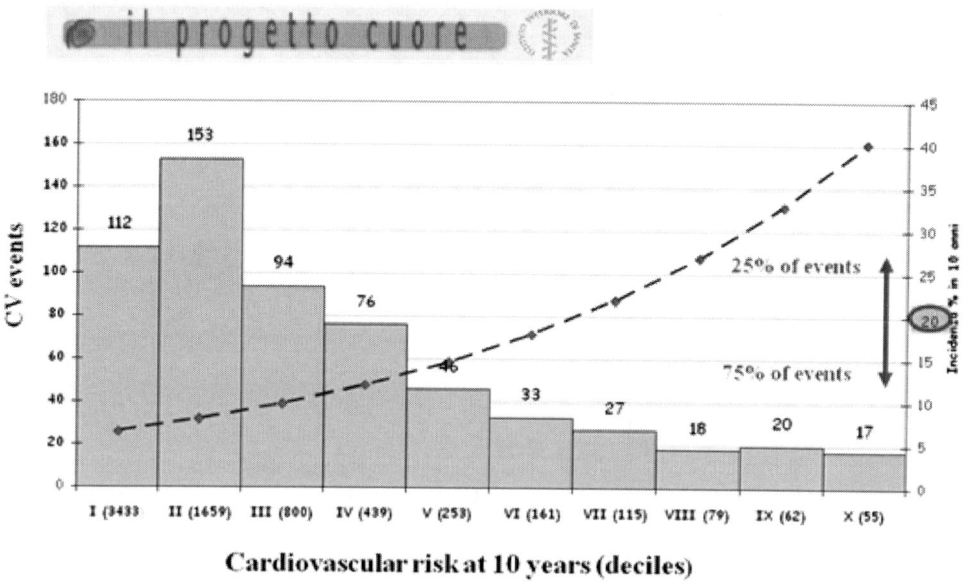

Figure 7. Cardiovascular events (bars) in relation to the calculated cardiovascular risk at 10 years (line), Men 35-69 years old. Modified by Giampaoli S, et al. Ital Heart J 2004;5(Suppl):S122S-S35.

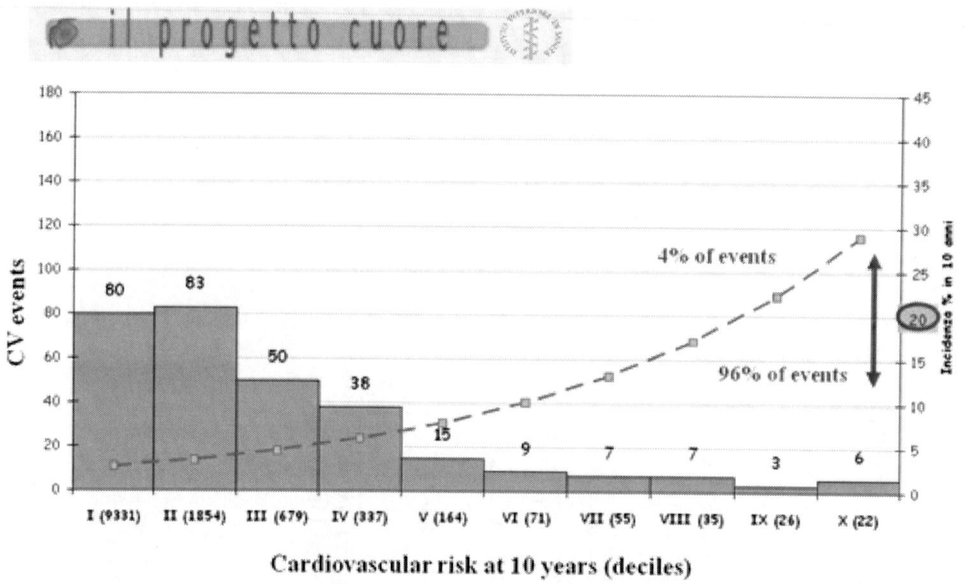

Figure 8. Cardiovascular events (bars) in relation to the calculated cardiovascular risk at 10 years (line), Women 35-69 years old. Modified by Giampaoli S, et al. Ital Heart J 2004;5(Suppl):S122S-S35.

Their use can be done in primary prevention in the treatment of hypercholesterolemia (and, for omega-3 fatty acids and berberine, of hypertriglyceridemia) in whom not yet candidates for statin therapy, with the aim to delay pharmacological treatment, but in the same time, treating the hypercholesterolemia (and hypertriglyceridemia), reduce CV risk in these patients always at risk, also if are not classified as high-risk. Therefore, non-pharmacological treatment could be considered to be an important alternative for many patients, as: those with mild-moderate hypercholesterolemia but without other cardiovascular risks and than at low-moderate global risk of CVD; hypercholesterolemic premenopausal women; hypercholesterolemic children of parents with premature CVD, hypercholesterolemic patients with liver or renal failure; hypercholesterolemic patients not yet adequately corrected with available drugs; hypercholesterolemic patients intolerant to pharmaceutical drugs; hypercholesterolemic patients consuming multiple drugs.

We already suggested that no pharmacological therapy could be effective in reducing CV risk in those patients who are not classified as high-risk because their risk at 10-years is <20%. By the way, data from "Progetto Cuore" ("The Italian Heart Project" of the Italian Institute of Health) demonstrated that men and women with a 10-year CV risk ≥20%, generate 25% and 4%, respectively, of the overall number of yearly CV events, whereas men and women with a 10-year risk <20% generate 75% and 96% of all events, respectively (151) (Figures 7 and 8). Therefore, the intervention targeted at those patients deemed at not high CV risk, would bring to a significant reduction in CV events occurring in the population, effectively improving the CV profile of our patients in primary prevention. By the way, some molecules discussed in this review, namely omega-3 fatty acids and monacolines of red yeast rice, have been largely studied in long-term randomized clinical trials with definitive outcomes (morbidity, mortality).

Beyond the ones described, there are many other dietary supplements and nutraceuticals that are used for their supposed lipid lowering effect but without adequate scientific support. The clinical trials available in these cases are more focused on detection of short-term lipid-lowering effects in healthy or nearly healthy subjects during monotherapy. However, a more in-depth understanding of specific health risks and pharmacological interactions of the single compounds is needed for the management of frail patients (children, elderlies, patients with liver or renal failure, and patients undergoing multiple drug treatment). Since these products are actually distributed not only in pharmacies, but also in supermarkets and drug shops, information regarding safety and precautions must be communicated compared to chemical drugs, whose use is more strictly monitored by physicians. Therefore FDA and the European Food Safety Agency, as well as other Scientific Societies, are working to regulate and to monitor their use.

References

[1] Anderson KM, Castelli WP, Levy. Cholesterol and mortality. 30 years of follow-up from the Framingham Study. *J Am Med Assoc* 1987;257:2176-80.

[2] Stamler J, Wentworth D, Neaton JD for MRFIT Research Group. Is relationship between serum cholesterol and risk of premature death from coronary heart disease continuous or graded? Findings in 356222 primary screenees of the Multiple Risk Factor Intervention Trial (MRFIT). *J Am Med Assoc* 1986;256:2823-8.

[3] Grundy SM. Cholesterol and coronary heart disease. Future directions, *J Am Med Assoc* 1990;264:3053-9.

[4] Lichtenstein AH. Thematic review series: patient-oriented research. Dietary fat, carbohydrate, and protein: effects on plasma lipoprotein patterns. *J Lipid Res* 2006;47:1661-7.

[5] Consensus Development Conferences: Lowering blood cholesterol to prevent heart disease. *J Am Med Assoc* 1085; 263:2080-6.

[6] Volpe R, Angelico F, Arca M, et al. Effects of simple dietary advice on serum lipids in severe and moderate primary hypercholesterolemia. In: Gotto AMr, Mancini M, Richter WO, Schwandt P. *Treatment of severe dyslipoproteinemia in the prevention of coronary heart disease.* Basel, Switzerland: Karger, 1992:226-30.

[7] Lipid Research Clinics Program. The Lipid Research Clinics Coronary Primary Prevention Trial Results: I and II. *JAMA* 1984;251:351-74.

[8] Frick MH, Eb O, Haapa K, et al. Helsinki Heart Study: Primary prevention trial with gemfibrozil in middle-aged men with dyslipidemia. *N Engl J Med* 1987;317:1237-45.

[9] Secondary prevention by raising HDL cholesterol and reducing triglycerides in patients with coronary artery disease: the Bezafibrate Infarction Prevention (BIP] study. *Circulation* 2000;102:21-7.

[10] Robins SJ, Collins D, Wittes JT, et al: Relation of Gemfibrozil Treatment and Lipid Levels With Major Coronary Events VA-HIT: A Randomized Controlled Trial. *J Am Med Assoc* 2001;285:1585-91.

[11] Baigent C, Blackwell L, Emberson J, et al. Cholesterol Treatment Trialists' (CTT] Collaboration. Efficacy and safety of more intensive lowering of LDL cholesterol: a meta-analysis of data from 170 000 participants in 26 randomised trials. *Lancet* 2010;376:1670–81.

[12] Shepherd J, Cobbe SM, Ford I, et al. Prevention of coronary heart disease with Pravastatin in men with hypercholesterolemia. N Engl J Med 1985;333:1301-07.

[13] Ghidini A, Sicherer S, Willner J. Congenital abnormalities (VATER] in baby born to mother using lovastatin. *Lancet* 1992; 339: 1416-17.

[14] NCEP expert panel. Expert Panel on detection, evaluation and treatment of high blood cholesterol in adults. Executive summary of the third report of the National Cholesterol Education Program (NCEP](Adult Treatment Panel III). *J Am Med Assoc* 200;:285:2486-97.

[15] Catapano AL, Reiner Z, De Backer G, et al. European Society of Cardiology (ESC); European Atherosclerosis Society (EAS). ESC/EAS Guidelines for the management of dyslipidaemias The Task Force for the management of dyslipidaemias of the European Society of Cardiology (ESC) and the European Atherosclerosis Society (EAS). *Atherosclerosis* 2011;217:3-46.

[16] Poli A, Marangoni, F, Paoletti R, et al. Non-pharmacological control of plasma cholesterol levels. *Nutr Metab Cardiovasc Dis* 2008;18:S1-S16.

[17] Brown L, Rosner B, Willet W and Sacks SM. Cholesterol-lowering effects of dietary fiber: a meta-analysis. *Am J Clin Nutr* 1999;69:30–42.

[18] Maciejko JJ, Brazg R, Shah A, et al. Psyllium for the reduction of cholestyramine-associated gastrointestinal symptoms in the treatment of primary hypercholesterolemia. *Arch Fam Med* 1994;3:955-60.

[19] Yoshida M, Vanstone CA, Parsons WD, et al. Effect of plant sterols and glucomannan on lipids in individuals with and without type 2 diabetes. *Eur J Clin Nutr* 2006;60:529-37.

[20] Shrestha S, Freake HC, McGrane MM, et al. A combination of psyllium and plant sterols alters lipoprotein metabolism in hypercholesterolemic subjects by modifying the intravascular processing of lipoproteins and increasing LDL uptake. *J Nutr* 2007;137:1165-70.

[21] Moreyra AE, Wilson AC, Koraym A. Effect of combining psyllium fiber with simvastatin in lowering cholesterol. *Arch Intern Med* 2005;165:1161-6.

[22] Lichtenstein AH, Appel LJ, Brands M, et al. Diet and lifestyle recommendations revision 2006: a scientific statement from the American Heart Association Nutrition Committee. *Circulation* 2006;114:82-96.

[23] Finks SW, Airee A, Chow SL, et al. Key articles of dietary interventions that influence cardiovascular mortality. Pharmacotherapy 2012;32:54-87.

[24] Cicero AF, Derosa G, Manca M, et al. Different effect of psyllium and guar dietary supplementation on blood pressure control in hypertensive overweight patients: a six-month, randomized clinical trial. *Clin Exp Hypertens* 2007;29:383-94.

[25] Pal S, Khossousi A, Binns C, et al. The effects of 12-week psyllium fibre supplementation or healthy diet on blood pressure and arterial stiffness in overweight and obese individuals. *Br J Nutr* 2012;107:725-34.

[26] Cicero AFG, Ferroni A, Ertek S. Tolerability and safety of commonly used dietary supplements and nutraceuticals with lipid-lowering effects. *Expert Opin Drug Saf 2012* Jul 13 [*Epub ahead of print*].

[27] Mechanick JI, Brett EM, Chausmer AB, et al. AACE Nutrition Guidelines Taskforce. American Association of Clinical Endocrinologists Medical Guidelines for the clinical use of dietary supplements and nutraceuticals. *Endocrine Pract* 2003;9:417-70.

[28] Keithley J, Swanson B. Glucomannan and obesity: a critical review. Altern Ther Health Med 2005;11:30-4.

[29] Yoshida M, Vanstone CA, Parsons WD, et al. Effect of plant sterols and glucomannan on lipids in individuals with and without type 2 diabetes. *Eur J Clin Nutr* 2006;60:529-37.

[30] Morgan LM, Tredger JA, Wright J, Marks V. The effect of soluble- and insoluble-fibre supplementation on post-prandial glucose tolerance, insulin and gastric inhibitory polypeptide secretion in healthy subjects. *Br J Nutr* 1990;64:103-10.

[31] Vuksan V, Sievenpiper JL, Xu Z, et al. Konjac-Mannan and American ginsing: emerging alternative therapies for type 2 diabetes mellitus. *J Am Coll Nutr* 2001;20(S5):S370-S380.

[32] McCarty MF. Glucomannan minimizes the postprandial insulin surge: a potential adjuvant for hepatothermic therapy. *Med Hypotheses* 2002;58:487-90.

[33] Sood N, Baker WL, Coleman CI. Effect of glucomannan on plasma lipid and glucose concentrations, body weight, and blood pressure: systematic review and meta-analysis. *Am J Clin Nutr* 2008;88:1167-75.

[34] Martino F, Martino E, Morrone F, et al. Effect of dietary supplementation with glucomannan on plasma total cholesterol and low density lipoprotein cholesterol in hypercholesterolemic children. *Nutr Metab Cardiovasc Dis* 2005;15:174-80.

[35)Vega-López S, Freake HC, Fernandez ML. Sex and hormonal status modulate the effects of psyllium on plasma lipids and monocyte gene expression in humans. *J Nutr* 2003;133:67-70.

[36] Chua M, Baldwin TC, Hocking TJ, Chan K. Traditional uses and potential health benefits of Amorphophallus konjac K. Koch ex N.E.Br. J Ethnopharmacol 2010;128:268-278.

[37] Pollak OJ. Reduction of blood cholesterol in man. *Circulation* 1953;7:702-6.

[38] Plat J, Mensink RP. Plant stanol and sterol esters in the control of blood cholesterol levels: mechanism and safety aspects, *Am J Cardiol* 2005;96:15D–22D.

[39] A. de Jong, J. Plat and R.P. Mensink, Metabolic effects of plant sterols and stanols, *J Nutr Biochem* 2003;14:362-9.

[40] Ikeda I, Tanabe Y, Sugano M. Effects of sitosterol and sitostanol on micellar solubility of cholesetrol. *Journal of Nutrition Scienceand Vitaminology* 35, 361-369.

[41] Ostlund REjr. Phytosterols and cholesterol metabolism. *Curr Opin Lipidol* 2004;15:37-41.

[42] Moruisi, W. Oosthuizen W, Opperman AM. Phytosterols/stanols lower cholesterol concentrations in familial hypercholesterolemic subjects: a systematic review with meta-analysis. *J Am Coll Nutr* 2006;25;41-8.

[43] Volpe R, Niittynen L, Korpela R, et al. Effects of yoghurt enriched with plant sterols on serum lipids in patients with moderate hypercholesterolemia. *Br J Nutr* 2001;86:233-9.

[44] Talati R, Sobieraj DM, Makanji SS, et al. The comparative efficacy of plant sterols and stanols on serum lipids: a systematic review and meta-analysis. *J Am Diet Assoc* 2010;110:719-26.

[45] Plant stanol ester consumption and arterial elasticity and endothelial function. *Br J Nutr* 2008;100:603-8.

[46] Gylling H, Puska P, Vartiainen P, Miettinen TA. Serum retinol, α-tocopherol, carotenes and lipid peroxide production during serum cholesterol lowering by sitostanol ester margarine in a mildly hypercholesterolemic population. *Circulation* 1996;94, Suppl1:578.

[47] Westrate JA, Meijer QW. Plant sterol-enriched margarines and reduction of plasma total- and LDL-cholesterol concentrations in normocholesterolaemic and mildly hypercholesterolaemic subjects. *Eur J Clin Nutr* 1998;52:334-43.

[48] Malini T, Vanithakumari G. Effect of β-sitosterol on uterine biochemistry: A comparative study with estradiol and progesterone. *Biochem Molec Biol Intern* 1993;31:659-68.

[49] MacLatchy DL, Van der Kraak GJ. The phytoestrogen beta-sitosterol alters the reproductive endocrine status of coldfish. *Toxicol Appl Pharmacol* 1995;134:305-12.

[50] Becker M, Staab D, von Bergmann K. Treatment of severe familiar hypercholesterolemia in children: effect of sitosterol and bezafibrate. *Pediatrics* 1992;89:138-42.

[51] Pelletier X, Belbraouet S, Mirabel D, et al. A diet moderate enriched in phytosterols lowers plasma cholesterol concentrations in normocholesterolemic humans. *Ann Nutr Metabol* 1995;39:291-5.

[52] Lees AM, Mok HYI, Lees RS, et al. Plant sterols as cholesterol-lowering agents: clinical trials in patients with hypercholesterolemia and studies of sterol balance. Atherosclerosis 1977;28:325-38.

[53] Denke MA. Lack of efficacy of low-dose sitostanol sterapy as an adjunct cholesterol-lowering diet in men with moderate hypercholesterolemia. *Am J Clin Nutr* 1994;61:392-6.

[54] Gylling H, Radhakrishnan R, Miettinen TA. Reduction of serum cholesterol in postmenopausal women with previous myocardial infarction and cholesterol malabsorption induced by dietary sitostanol ester margarine. *Circulation* 1997;96:4226-31.

[55] Scholle JM, Baker WL, Talati R, Coleman CI. The effect of adding plant sterols or stanols to statin therapy in hypercholesterolemic patients: systematic review and meta-analysis. *J Am Coll Nutr* 2009;28:517-24.

[56] Guardamagna O, Abello F, Baracco V, et al. Primary hyperlipidemias in children: effect of plant sterol supplementation on plasma lipids and markers of cholesterol synthesis and absorption. *Acta Diabetol* 2011:48:127-33.

[57] Becker M, Staab D, von Bergmann K. Treatment of severe familiar hypercholesterolemia in children: effect of sitosterol and bezafibrate. *Pediatrics* 1992;89:138-42.

[58] Gylling H, Hallikainen M, Nissinen MJ, Miettinen TA. The effect of a very high daily plant stanol ester intake on serum lipids, carotenoids, and fat soluble vitamins. *Clin Nutr* 2010;29;112-8.

[59] Lea LJ, Hepburn PA. Safety evaluation of phytosterol-esters. Part 9: Results of a European post-launch monitoring programme, Food Chem Toxicol 2006;44:1213-22.

[60] Tikkanen MJ. Plant sterols and stanols. *Handb Exp Pharmacol* 2005;170:215-30.

[61] Poli A, Marangoni, F, Paoletti R, et al: Non-pharmacological control of plasma cholesterol levels. *Nutr Metab Cardiovasc Dis* 2008;18:S1-S16.

[62] Potter SM. Overview of proposed mechanisms for the hypocholesterolemic effect of soy. *J Nutr* 1995;125(3 Suppl):S606-S11.

[63] Torres N, Torre-Villalvazo I, Tovar AR. Regulation of lipid metabolism by soyprotein and its implication in diseases mediated by lipid disorders. *J Nutr Biochem* 2006;17:365-373.

[64] Mullen E, Brown RM, Osborne TF, Shay NF. Soy isoflavones affect sterol regulatory element binding proteins (SREBPs] and SREBP-regulated genes in HepG2 cells. *J Nutr* 2004;134:2942-7.

[65] Descovich GC, Ceredi C, Gaddi A, et al. Multicentre study of soybean protein diet for outpatient hyper-cholesterolaemic patients. *Lancet* 1980;2:709–12.

[66] Zhan S, Ho SC. Meta-analysis of the effects of soy protein containing isoflavones on the lipid profile. *Am J Clin Nutr* 2005;81:397-408.

[67] Sirtori CR, Lovati MR. Soy proteins and cardiovascular disease. *Curr Atheroscler Rep* 2001;3:47-53.

[68] Anderson JW, Johnstone BM, Cook-Newell ME. Meta-analysis of the effects of soy protein intake on serum lipids. *N Engl J Med* 1995;333;276-82.

[69] Sirtori CR, Eberini I, Arnoldi A, Hypocholesterolaemic effects of soya proteins: results of recent studies are predictable from the Anderson meta-analysis data, *Br J Nutr* 2007;97:816–22.

[70] Pase MP, Grima NA, Sarris J. The effects of dietary and nutrient interventions on arterial stiffness: a systematic review. *Am J Clin Nutr* 2011;93:446-54.

[71] Adlercreutz H. Epidemiology of phytoestrogens. *Baillieres Clin Endocrinol Metab* 1998;12:605-23.

[72] Ørgaard A, Jensen L. The effects of soy isoflavones on obesity. *Exp Biol Med* 2008;233:1066-80.

[73] AHA Science Advisory. Soy protein and cardiovascular disease: A statement for healthcare professionals from the Nutrition Committee of the AHA. *Circulation* 2002;102:2555-9.

[74] Lenz TL. Therapeutic lifestyle changes and pharmaceutical care in the treatment of dyslipidemias in adults. *J Am Pharm Assoc* 2005;45:492-9.

[75] Weghuber D, Widhalm K. Effect of 3 month treatment of children and adolescents with familial and polygenic hypercholesterolemia with a soy-substituted diet. *Br J Nutr* 2008;99:281-6.

[76] Chen ST, Ferng SH, Yang CS, et al. Variable effects of soy protein on plasma lipids in hyperlipidemic and normolipidemic hemodialysis patients. *Am J Kidney Dis* 2005;46:1099-106.

[77] Hutchins AM, McIver IE, Johnston CS. Hypertensive crisis associated with high dose soy isoflovane supplementation in a post-menopausal woman; a case report. *BMC Women's Health* 2005;5:9.

[78] Cambria-Kiely JA. Effect of soy milk on warfarin. *Ann Pharmacother* 2002;36:1893-6.

[79] Anderson GD, Rosito G, Mohustsy MA, Elmer GW. Drug interaction potential of soy extract and Panax ginseng. *J Clin Pharmacol* 2003;43:643-8.

[80] Taku K, Umegaki K, Sato Y, et al. Soy isoflovanes lower serum total and LDL cholesterol in humans: a meta-analysis of 11 randomized controlled trials. *Am J Clin Nutr* 2007;85:1148-56.

[81] Zhan S, Ho SC. Meta-analysis of the effects of soy protein containing isoflavones on the lipid profile. *Am J Clin Nutr* 2005;81:397-408.

[82] Goldin BR, Brauner E, Adlercreutz H, et al. Hormonal response to diets high in soy or animal protein without and with isoflavones in moderately hypercholesterolemic patients. *Nutr Cancer* 2005;51:1-6.

[83] Messina MJ, Wood CE. Soy isoflavones, estrogen therapy, and breast cancer risk: analysis and commentary. *Nutr J* 2008;7:17.

[84] Monograph. monascus purpureus (red yeast rice). *Alternative Medicine Review* 2004;9:208-10.

[85] Liu ZL, Liu JP, Zhang AL, et al. Chinese herbal medicines for hypercholesterolemia. *Cochrane Database Syst Rev* 2011;6:CD008305.

[86] Cicero AFG, Brancaleoni M, Laghi L, et al. Antihyperlipidaemic effect of a Monascus purpureus brand dietary supplement on a large sample of subjects at low risk for cardiovascular disease: a pilot study. *Complem Ther Med* 2005;13:273-8.

[87] Keithley JK, Swanson B, Sha BE, et al. A pilot study of the safety and efficacy of cholestin in treating HIV-related dyslipidemia. *Nutrition* 2002;18:201-4.

[88] Gheit O, Sheashaa H, Abdelsalam M, et al. Efficacy and safety of Monascus purpureus Went rice in subjects with secondary hyperlipidemia. *Eur J Intern Med* 2009;20:e57-61.

[89] Liu J, Zhang J, Shi YI, et al. Chinese red yeast rice (monascus purpureus) for primary hyperlipidemia: a meta-analysis of randomized controlled trials. Chin. Medicine 2006;1:4.

[90] Zhao SP, Liu L, Cheng YC, et al. Xuezhikang, an extract of cholestin, protects endothelial function through antiinflammatory and lipid-lowering mechanisms in patients with coronary heart disease. *Circulation* 2004;110: 915-20.

[91] Lu Z, Kou W, Du B, et al. Chinese Coronary Secondary Prevention Study Group. Effect of Xuezhikang, an extract from red yeast Chinese rice, on coronary events in a Chinese population with previous myocardial infarction. *Am J Cardiol* 2008;101:1689-93.

[92] Ye P, Lu ZL, Du BM, et al. CCSPS Investigators. Effect of xuezhikang on cardiovascular events and mortality in elderly patients with a history of myocardial infarction: a subgroup analysis of elderly subjects from the China Coronary Secondary Prevention Study. *J Am Geriatr Soc* 2007;55:1015-22.

[93] Halbert SC, French B, Gordon RY, et al. Tolerability of red yeast rice (2,400 mg twice daily) versus pravastatin (20 mg twice daily] in patients with previous statin intolerance. *Am J Cardiol* 2010;105:198-204.

[94] Nijjar PS, Burke FM, Bloesch A, Rader DJ. Role of dietary supplements in lowering low-density lipoprotein cholesterol: a review. *J Clin Lipidol* 2010;4:248-58.

[95] Grieco A, Miele L, Pompili M, et al. A cute hepatitis caused by a natural lipid-lowering product: when "alternative" medicine is no "alternative" at all. *J Hepatol* 2009;50:1273-7.

[96] Wigger-Alberti W, Bauer A, Hipler UC, Elsner P. Anaphylaxis due to Monascus Purpureus fermented rice (red yeast rice). *Allergy* 1999;54:1330-1.

[97] In YL, Wang TH, Lee MH, Su NW. Biologically active components and nutraceuticals in Monascus-fermented rice: a review. *Appl Microbiol Biotechnol* 2008;77:965-73.

[98] Eisenbrand G. Toxicological evaluation of red mould rice. *Mol Nutr Food Res* 2006;50:322-7.

[99] Gordon RY, Becker DJ, The role of red yeast rice for the physician. Curr Atheroscler Rep 2011;13:73-80.

[100] Monogram: *Alternative Medicine Review* 2004;9:208-10.

[101] Marinangeli CP, Jones PJ, Kassis AN, Eskin MN. Policosanols as nutraceuticals: fact or fiction. *Crit Rev Food Sci Nutr* 2010;50:259-67.

[102] Gouni-Berthold I, Berthold HK. Policosanol: clinical pharmacology and therapeutic significance of a new lipid-lowering agent. *Am Heart J* 2002;143:356-65.

[103] Castaño G, Mas R, Fernández L, et al. Comparison of the efficacy and tolerability of policosanol with atorvastatin in elderly patients with type II hypercholesterolemia. *Drugs Aging* 2003;20:153-63.

[104] Berthold HK, Unverdorben S, Degenhardt R, et al. Effect of policosanol on lipid levels among patients with hypercholesterolemia or combined hyperlipidemia: a randomized, controlled trial. *J Am Med Assoc* 2006;95:2262-9.

[105] Sirtori CR, Galli C, Anderson JW, Sirtori E, Arnoldi A. Functional foods for dyslipidaemia and cardiovascular risk prevention. *Nutr Res Rev.*2009;22:244-61.

[106] Singh DK, Li L, Porter TD. Policosanol inhibits cholesterol synthesis in hepatoma cells by activation of AMP-kinase. *J Pharmacol Exp Ther* 2006;318:1020-6.

[107] Guardamagna O, Abello F, Baracco V, et al. The treatment of hypercholesterolemic children: efficacy and safety of a combination of red yeast rice extract and policosanols. *Nutr Metab Cardiovasc Dis* 2011;21:424-9.

[108] Abdul MI, Jiang X, Williams KM, et al. Pharmacokinetic and pharmacodynamic interactions of echinacea and policosanol with warfarin in healthy subjects. *Br J Clin Pharmacol* 2010;69:508-15.

[109] Cicero AFG, Ertek S. Berberine: metabolic and cardiovascular effects in preclinical and clinical trials. *Nutr Diet Suppl* 2009;1:1-10.

[110] Kong W, Wei J, Abidi P, et al. Berberine is a novel cholesterol-lowering drug working through a unique mechanism distinct from statins. *Nature Med* 2004;10:1344-51.

[111] Yin J, Xing H, Ye J. Efficacy of berberine in patients with type 2 diabetes mellitus. *Metabolism* 2008;57:712-7.

[112] Cicero AFG, Tartagni E. Antidiabetic properties of berberine: from cellular pharmacology to clinical effects. *Hosp Pract* 2012;40:56-63.

[113] Meng S, Wang LS, Huang ZQ, et al. Berberine ameliorates inflammation in patients with acute coronary syndrome following percutaneous coronary intervention. *Clin Exp Pharmacol Physiol* 2012;39:406-11.

[114] Cheng F, Wang Y, Li J, et al. Berberine improves endothelial function by reducing endothelial microparticles-mediated oxidative stress in humans. *Int J Cardiol* 2012 Mar 30 [Epub ahead of print].

[115] Xu MG, Wang JM, Chen L, et al. Berberine-induced mobilization of circulating endothelial progenitor cells improves human small artery elasticity. *J Hum Hypertens* 2008;22:389-93.

[116] Cicero AFG, Tartagni E, Ferroni A, et al. Combined nutraceutical approach to postmenopausal syndrome and vascular remodeling biomarkers. *J Alt Compl Med* 2013 Jan 11 [Epub ahead of print].

[117] Kupeli E, Kosar M, Yesilada E, et al. A comparative study on the anti-inflammatory , antinociceptive and antipyretic effects of isoquinoline alkaloids from the roots of Turkish berberis species. *Life Sci* 2002;72:645-57.

[118] Affuso F, Mercurio V, Fazio V, Fazio S. Cardiovascular and metabolic effects of Berberine. *World J Cardiol* 2010;2:71-7.

[119] Chan E. Displacement of bilirubin from albumin by berberine. *Biol Neonat* 1993;63:201-8.

[120] Xin HW, Wu XC, Li Q, et al. The effects of berberine on the pharmacokinetics of cyclosporine A in healthy volunteers. *Methods Find Exp Clin Pharmacol* 2006;28:25-9.

[121] Lin HL, Liu TY, Wu CW, Chi CW. Berberine modulates expression of mdr1 gene product and the responses of the digestive tract cancers to Paclitaxel. *Br J Cancer* 1999;81:416-22.

[122] Connor WE, De Francesco CA, Connor SL. Nn-3 fatty acids from fish oil. Effects on plasma lipoproteins and hypertriglyceridemic patients. *Ann NY Acad Sci* 1993;683:16-34.

[123- Rubenfire M, Brooke RD, Rosenson RS. Treating mixed hyperlipidemia and the atherogenic lipid phenotype for prevention of cardiovascular events. *Am J Med* 2010;123:892-8.

[124)Mozaffarian D, Wu JH. Omega-3 fatty acids and cardiovascular disease: effects on risk factors, molecular pathways, and clinical events. *J Am Coll Cardiol* 2011;58:2047-67.

[125] Harris WS. N-3 fatty acids and serum lipoproteins: human studies. *Am J Clin Nutr* 1997;65:1645S-54S.

[126] Zock PL, Mensink RP, Dietary trans-fatty acids and serum lipoproteins in humans. *Curr Opin Lipidol* 1996;7:34-7.

[127] Campbell F, Dickinson HO, Critchley JA, et al. A systematic review of fish-oil supplements for the prevention and treatment of hypertension. *Eur J Prev Cardiol* 2012 Jan 30 [Epub ahead of print].

[128] Pase MP, Grima NA, Sarris J. Do long-chain n-3 fatty acids reduce arterial stiffness? A meta-analysis of randomised controlled trials. *Br J Nutr* 2011;106:974-80.

[129] Thies F, Garry JM, Yaqoob P, et al. Association of n-3 polyunsaturated fatty acids with stability of atherosclerotic plaques: a randomised controlled trial. *Lancet* 2003;361:477-85.

[130] Cicero AFG, Ertek S, Borghi C. Omega-3 polyunsaturated fatty acids: their potential role in blood pressure prevention and management. *Curr Vasc Pharmacol* 2009;7:330-7.

[131] Valagussa F, Franzosi MG, Geraci E, et al. Dietary supplementation with n-3 polyunsaturated fatty acids and vitamin E after myocardial infarction: results of the GISSI Prevenzione trial. *Lancet* 1999;354:447-55.

[132] Delgado-Lista J, Perez-Martinez P, Lopez-Miranda J, Perez-Jimenez F. Long chain omega-3 fatty acids and cardiovascular disease: a systematic review. *Br J Nutr* 2012;107(Suppl2):S201-S13.

[133] Kris-Etherton PM, Harris WS, Appel LJ. Omega-3 fatty acids and cardiovascular disease: new recommendations from the American Heart Association. *Arterioscler Thromb Vasc Biol* 2003;23:151-2.

[134] Cicero AFG, De Sando V, Parini A, Borghi C. Polyunsaturated Fatty Acids application in Internal Medicine: beyond the established cardiovascular effects. *Arch Med Sci* 2012;9:784-93.

[135] Djoussé L, Gaziano JM, Buring JE, Lee IM. Dietary omega-3 fatty acids and fish consumption and risk of type 2 diabetes. *Am J Clin Nutr* 2011;93:143-50.

[136] Nettleton JA, Katz R. N-3 long-chain polyunsaturated fatty acids in type 2 diabetes: a review. *J Am Diet Assoc* 2005;105:428-40.

[137] Hooper L, Thompson RL, Harrison RA, et al. Risks and benefits of omega 3 fats for mortality, cardiovascular disease, and cancer: systematic review. *Brit Med J* 2006;332:752-60.

[138] Harris WS. Expert opinion: omega-3 fatty acids and bleeding-cause for concern? *Am J Cardiol* 2007;99:44C-6C.

[139] Guallar E, Sanz-Gallardo MI, van't Veer P, et al. Mercury, fish oils, and the risk of myocardial infarction. Heavy Metals and Myocardial Infarction Study Group. *N Engl J Med* 2002;347:1747-54.

[140] Eliat-Adar S, Goldbourt U. Nutritional recommendations for preventing coronary heart disease in women: evidence concerning whole foods and supplements. *Nutr Metab Cardiovasc Dis* 2010;20:459-66.

[141] Cohen JT, Bellinger DC, Connor WE, et al. A quantitative risk-benefit analysis of changes in population fish consumption. *Am J Prev Med* 2005;29:325-34.

[142)Trimarco B, Benvenuti C, Rozza F, et al. Clinical evidence of efficacy of red yeast rice and berberine in a large controlled study versus diet. *Med J Nutrition Metab* 2011;4:133-9.

[143] Affuso F, Ruvolo A, Micillo F, et al. Effects of a nutraceutical combination (berberine, red yeast rice and policosanols) on lipid levels and endothelial function randomized, double-blind, placebo-controlled study. *Nutr Metab Cardiovasc Dis* 2010;20:656-61.

[144] Myers J. Exercise and cardiovascular health. *Circulation* 3003;107:E2-E5.

[145] Astrup A, The role of dietary fat in the prevention and treatment of obesity. Efficacy and safety of low-fat diets. *Int J Obes Relat Metab Disord* 2001;25:S46–S5.

[146] Durstine LJ, Granjean PW, Davis PG, et al. Blood lipid and lipoprotein adaptations to exercise. A quantitative analysis. *Sports Med* 2001;31:1033-62.

[147] Panagiotakos DB, Pitsavos C, Chrysohoou C, et al. Effect of leisure time physical activity on blood lipid levels: the ATTICA study. *Coron Artery Dis* 2003;14:533-9.

[148] Kokkinos P, Holland J, Narayan P, et al. Miles run per week and high density lipoprotein cholesterol levels in healthy middle aged men: a dose–response relationship. *Arch Intern Med* 1995;155:415-20.

[149] Kraus We, Houmard JA, Duscha BD, et al. Effects of the amount and intensity of exercise on plasma lipoproteins. *N Engl J Med* 2002;347:1483-92.

[150] Koh-Banerjee, P, Chu NF, Spiegelman D, et al. Prospective study of the association of changes in dietary intake, physical activity, alcohol consumption, and smoking with 9-y gain in waist circumference among 16,587 US men. *Am J Clin Nutr* 2003;78:719-27.

[151] Giampaoli S, Palmieri L, Chiodini P, et al. The Italian charter of the global cardiovascular risk. *It Heart J* 2004;5(Suppl):S177-S85.

In: Recent Advances in Cardiology
Editors: José Milei and Giuseppe Ambrosio
ISBN: 978-1-63117-282-3

Chapter 3

Angina Pectoris in Women

Cinzia Zuchi, Isabella Tritto and Giuseppe Ambrosio*
Division of Cardiology,
University of Perugia School of Medicine,
Perugia, Italy

Abstract

Ischemic heart disease (IHD) is the leading cause of death among women in Western countries, and it is associated with higher morbidity and mortality than in men. Nevertheless, the misperception that females are "protected" against cardiovascular disease leads to underestimation of their cardiovascular risk and IHD in women remains underdiagnosed and undertreated. Women suffering from angina pectoris have a higher prevalence of non-significant coronary artery disease compared to men. Angina in women is more commonly microvascular in origin than in men, and therefore standard diagnostic algorithms may be suboptimal for women. This different pathophysiology impacts clinical management of IHD in women. Women are scarcely represented in clinical trials, but response to medical therapy may differ in this group. Therefore, solid data in terms of gender efficacy of antianginal drugs are lacking, and particularly when angina is microvascular in origin women often continue to be symptomatic despite maximal therapy with classical antianginal drugs. Recently, new molecules have shown promising results in women. In conclusion, women with angina are a group of patients in whom it seems appropriate to concentrate efforts aimed at reducing morbidity and improving quality of life.

* Address for correspondence: Prof. Giuseppe Ambrosio, Cardiologia e Fisiopatologia Cardiovascolare, Ospedale S. Maria della Misericordia, Piazzale Menghini, 1, 06132, Perugia, Italy. Phone: +39 075 5782394, Fax: +39 0755271244. E-mail: giuseppe.ambrosio@ospedale.perugia.it.

Introduction

It is a widely-held tenet that coronary artery disease affects mainly men. However, contrary to this common perception, more women than men die from coronary artery disease in Western countries [1, 2]. Furthermore, in addition to being a major cause of death, IHD is also a major cause of morbidity. In fact, stable angina is a very common condition, with a prevalence around 5% of general population [3], which impacts quality of life and ability to work, and with significant economic consequences. In a recent meta-analysis of both cross-sectional and prospective studies from 31 countries world-wide, encompassing almost 25,000 cases of patients with angina of either sex, a statistically significant 20% female excess was consistently shown [3].

Features of Women with Ischemic Heart Disease

Women suffering from angina pectoris differ substantially from men with the same disease. Women with IHD are older, tend to have a greater burden of comorbidities as well as more functional disability than men [4-5]; IHD is less prevalent in premenopausal women, its incidence lagging 10-15 years behind that of men until approximately the seventh decade of life.

From a pathophysiological point of view, about 50% of all women referred for elective coronary angiography because of angina actually do not show evidence of significant coronary artery stenosis [4, 6-11]. In that very large cohort of >300,000 patients referred for angiographic evaluation of stable angina at 388 US hospitals, the risk-adjusted OR for significant coronary artery stenosis was only 0.34 for women compared to men ($P<0.0001$) [4, 8]. Lower prevalence of obstructive coronary artery disease (CAD) in women with angina holds true across all age groups [8]; however, it becomes astonishingly low at relatively young ages, as almost 80% of <60 years old women referred for elective, diagnostic coronary angiography with suspected stable angina had no significant coronary artery stenosis [8].

One problem with correctly diagnosing and managing IHD in women is due to the fact that physicians tend to equate angina pectoris with underlying significant coronary stenoses. However, chest discomfort due to myocardial ischemia can also occur in other conditions. Women show structural and functional differences in the coronary circulation [12]. Indeed, coronary arteries in women are smaller than men, independent of body size [13]; this might be of some relevance, since it has been shown that even in the absence of discrete stenosis diffuse narrowing of vessel lumen by atherosclerosis may result in abnormal resistance, limiting myocardial flow [14]. Of greater relevance is the finding that angina in women is less likely to be associated with angiographically significant coronary artery stenosis than in men, microvascular disease of coronary arteries being more common in women than men.

As already mentioned, substantial amount of observational and registry data indicate that a majority of women (from 51% to 65%) referred for a diagnostic cath for evaluation of angina actually has no significant coronary artery stenosis [4, 6-11]. Furthermore, growing evidences suggests that coronary microvascular dysfunction can be an etiological factor for IHD, and it frequently explains the presence of chest pain in the absence of significant coronary obstruction, configuring the so called “microvascular angina”, or cardiac “syndrome

X" [15-28]. In this regard, studies that specifically looked into patients with microvascular angina consistently report a large female excess (ranging from 54% to 100%) of enrolled patients [10, 15-16, 22, 24, 28-29]. A recent systematic review on this topic [20] of 47 studies on microvascular angina (accruing 1,934 patients), found a significantly higher proportion of women, with a pooled relative female frequency of 56%.

One important question is whether chest pain in those patients with microvascular angina is indeed due to true myocardial ischemia. Women with angina and non-significant coronary artery stenosis may show impaired cardiac energy metabolism by nuclear magnetic resonance spectroscopy, unequivocally documenting exercise-induced ischemia [30-31]. Furthermore, evidence of blunted coronary vasodilator reserve, which can be assessed by means of various techniques [21, 32], has been documented in patients (mostly women) with angiographically normal coronary arteries and microvascular angina [21-28], thus providing evidence of coronary microvascular dysfunction in patients with otherwise angiographically normal coronary arteries.

These peculiar demographic and angiographic findings may influence clinical presentation and diagnosis of IHD in women. These differences may actually lead to substantially underdiagnosing IHD in women, due to the following several major factors

Inappropriate perception of cardiovascular risk. There is widespread underappreciation of cardiovascular risk in women, not just among lay people but among physicians as well. In the Euro Heart Survey of Stable Angina, women with anginal pain were less likely to undergo an exercise electrocardiogram, and less likely to be referred for coronary angiography [33]. Interestingly, there are reasons for this misconception which partly stem from the use of risk algorithms originally derived from predominantly male populations. Indeed, by this approach, even up to age 80, three quarters of women would have a 10-year Framingham Risk Score of <10% [34]. However, the assessment may change if one uses a more refined strategy. A novel, specifically tailored risk score was tested in 24,558 women involved in the Women Health Study [35]; this new algorithm, the Reynolds Risk Score, which includes age, systolic blood pressure, haemoglobin A1c if diabetic, current smoking, total and HDL-C, hsCRP, and parental history of myocardial infarction before age 60, reclassified 15% of women predicted to be at intermediate risk (according to Adult Treatment Panel III criteria) into high-risk category [35]. Among the new risk factors examined in the Reynolds Risk Scores, hsCRP, a marker of inflammation, seems to be of particular importance. Indeed, among postmenopausal hypertensive women, a high peripheral neutrophil count has recently been shown to be an independent predictor of cardiovascular events [36], highlighting that inflammation may be of relevance in identifying women at increased risk of cardiovascular disease.

Inappropriate evaluation of symptoms. Definition of what constitutes "typical" anginal symptoms is largely derived from observations made in predominantly male populations; thus, an issue could be made as to whether symptoms in women should also be judged by the same criteria used to diagnose stable IHD in men. In this respect, the very recently-issued NICE guidelines on stable angina state that differences in symptomatic presentation between men and women are small and it is the pre-test likelihood of coronary atherosclerosis which should influence management, not gender alone [37]. This recommendation is in line with current understanding and treatment of IHD, which is typically based on the "significant stenosis" approach, and undoubtedly it is appropriate for a large number of women with stable angina due to coronary artery disease.

However, it is of interest to consider that possible gender differences in presenting symptoms may still exist with respect to characteristics, frequency, and quality of symptoms noted during chest pain [38-41], which at times may make it difficult to properly evaluate chest pain in women. These differences on the one hand hinge around description of symptoms, which may be influenced by the characteristics of the population investigated, while on the other hand the "trigger" of symptoms sometimes may differ between genders.

With respect to clinical characteristics, if one looks at patients with documented coronary artery stenosis, as reviewed in NICE guidelines [37], typical effort angina is indeed the main symptom referred by both women and men. Pepine et al. studied 5125 outpatients with chronic stable angina and documented coronary artery disease (53% female); angina with physical activity was present in 90% of these patients, with no significant differences between men and women [39]. In another cohort of patients with coronary artery stenosis, Kimble et al. [40] reported similar physical limitation related to angina in women compared to men by Seattle Angina Questionnaire (SAQ). On the other hand, however, if one considers all patients who complain of angina symptoms -regardless of coronary anatomy- most women actually refer atypical symptoms, more so than men. In a caucasian population (2676 women and 2929 men) Zaman et al. found a significant difference between genders in presenting symptoms, 53.6% of women reporting atypical chest pain [38]. This may have substantial practical implications, since as mentioned significant coronary artery stenosis is often absent in women.

On the trigger side, women complain more often than men of mental-stress evoked angina [39, 41], as well as of episodes of angina not clearly related to physical exercise [39]. Women with chronic stable angina and documented coronary artery disease are more likely than men to report chest pain during rest, sleep, or episodes of mental stress [39]; indeed, female sex has been associated with significant excess risk for mental stress angina (RR 1,28), and rest angina (RR 1,09) [39]. Similarly, in 196 patients with documented CAD Sheps et al. found that women refer angina episodes during mental stress more frequently than men (19% vs 3.6%, $p<0,01$) [41]. It is also worth noting that microvascular angina -which is much more common in women [10,15-16, 20, 22, 24, 28-29] (see below)- may have atypical features, such as pain at rest, prolonged duration of attacks, poor response to sublingual nitrates [15].

Together, these various findings suggest that mechanisms other than classical demand-vs-supply imbalance due to stenosis of a large vessel may at times be involved in angina of women with IHD, and therefore in women episodes of chest pain not clearly related to exercise, or presence of symptoms during exertion other than typical angina, while less likely to accompany significant coronary artery stenosis, should not allow the physician to rule out IHD altogether. As summarized in 2010 NICE guidelines on Chest Pain [42], when discussing possible gender differences in symptoms "Cardiovascular risk factors are at least as important in women as in men, if not more so, [i.e., compared to symptoms] in determining the likelihood of women having coronary events".

Inappropriate assessment. According to Bayes theorem, the predictive value of a diagnostic test depends on the prevalence of disease in the population tested, and on sensitivity and specificity of the test itself. Non-invasive tools currently used to diagnose IHD, namely exercise stress test, perfusion imaging, stress-echo, all rely on the possibility of inducing and detecting regional ischemia. While this approach is useful for the purpose of revealing discrete flow-limiting stenoses, it may be ill-suited to detect ischemia in the absence of a significant stenosis. So, the lower prevalence of obstructive coronary artery disease in women makes diagnostic testing designed to detect focal areas of relative underperfusion less sensitive and specific in this population [5]. Similarly, the interpretation of results of an exercise ECG stress test as "false positive" when there is no angiographic evidence of significant CAD has to be made with caution in women, as it may derive from microvascular alterations. Also, sensitivity and specificity of exercise stress testing are not in favour of women. Indeed, in a meta-analysis of exercise testing in women, sensitivity and specificity of ST-segment depression in symptomatic, intermediate risk women were just 61% and 70%, respectively [43]. ECG changes during exercise have been reported to be of diminished accuracy in women as a result of more frequent resting ST-T wave changes, lower ECG voltage, and hormonal factors such as endogenous estrogens in premenopausal women and hormone replacement therapy in postmenopausal women [44-48]. Handberg et al, analyzing data from 190 women enrolled in the National Heart, Lung, and Blood Institute (NHLBI)-sponsored Women's Ischemia Syndrome Evaluation (WISE) study, showed that women with reduced coronary flow reserve were significantly more likely to have reduced functional capacity [49]. A Consensus Statement indicates that the diagnostic and prognostic accuracy of exercise ECG stress test in symptomatic women with suspected IHD can be enhanced by the inclusion of additional parameters (e.g., functional capacity, treadmill scores) to the interpretation of the ST-segment response to exercise [48].

Treatment of Stable Angina in Women

More complex pathophysiology of angina in women may also lead to lower response to therapy. Angina pectoris is also considerably undertreated in women [33]. In the Euro Heart Survey of Stable Angina, antiplatelet and statin therapies were used significantly less in women than in men, even when there was direct documentation of coronary artery disease [33]. Women with confirmed coronary disease were less likely to be revascularized than men, and were twice as likely to suffer death or nonfatal myocardial infarction during follow-up, even after multivariable adjustment for age, abnormal ventricular function, severity of coronary artery disease, and diabetes [33].

More extensive use of revascularization procedures, however, may reduce the burden of ischemic symptoms in women only to some extent, since: a) PCI or CABG do not eradicate symptoms in many such patients, as a sizable number of women remain symptomatic in spite of successful revascularization [57-60]; b) as already pointed out, angina in the absence of significant stenosis of native coronary arteries (i.e., microvascular dysfunction) is particularly prevalent in women [8, 10, 15-16, 20, 22, 24, 28-29], and women in this latter group quite frequently continue to have symptoms in spite of therapy with classical antianginal drugs [52, 61]; c) drugs currently available tend to be less effective in women, due to specific pathophysiology which may not favor treatment of angina following the traditional "supply-vs-demand" approach [62]. Indeed, consistent with the notion that women with angina tend to have symptoms less linked to degree of physical activity [40, 63], exercise stress test in women is a less sensitive indicator of treatment efficacy than angina frequency or nitroglycerin consumption [64].

Response to medical therapy may differ in women when compared with men because there may be gender-specific physiological differences [65], and differences in the activity of drug-metabolizing enzymes [65]. For example, significantly lower therapeutic effect on stress-induced angina pectoris was reported in women with coronary artery disease treated with metoprolol compared with men [62], in spite of the fact that greater plasma concentrations of metoprolol are achieved in women [66].

1) Classical Antianginal Drugs

Besides small studies, women are poorly represented in large randomized clinical trials on stable angina [67-68], and data on gender differences on the effect of anti-ischemic drugs are lacking. A metanalysis of 90 studies on stable angina treatment with "classical antianginal" drugs (beta-blockers, calcium antagonists, and nitrates) shows that less than 20% of enrolled patients were women [68].

The picture becomes even fuzzier when ischemia, although documented by chest pain and ST-segment depression during exercise stress test, is not accompanied by evidence of obstructive coronary artery disease at angiography. Regrettably, intervention studies with antianginal drugs in patients affected by microvascular angina (summarized in Table 1) tend to be small, and too short, to firmly establish whether the benefit observed remains stable over time. Among classical anti-anginal drugs, only β-blockers have been consistently shown to effectively reduce chest pain episodes during daily life in this condition [69-71]. Ca++ antagonists seem to do little to prevent chest pain in patients with "normal" angiograms [69, 72-73], and they fail to ameliorate the diminished coronary blood flow reserve of these patients [72]. Nitrates are anedoctally reported to be of help in some patients but not in others [15], but randomized, placebo-controlled trials on nitrates are lacking. Interestingly, benefits on various parameters of exercise tolerance have been obtained in patients with microvascular angina through a substantially different approach, namely trying to influence microcirculation function, either via potentiation of endogenous adenosine (by aminophylline [74-75]), or secondary to a putative increase in the activity of nitric oxide with ACE-inhibitors [76-79], or statins [80-81]. However, none of these studies went past the "proof-of-concept" stage, with only a handful women treated for a few weeks. Recently, the NICE guidelines on stable angina reviewed the interventional studies on Cardiac Syndrome X [37]. They state that only evidence for limited outcomes over short periods of time is available and the evidence does not support use of standard antianginal drugs for long term benefit [37], and concluded that drug treatment for stable angina in patients already on treatment should be continued only if it improves symptoms [37].

2) Newer Drugs

Ranolazine is a novel molecule approved in the USA and Europe for treatment of stable angina[82]. Unlike classical antianginal drugs, it shows anti-ischemic actions at concentrations that have negligible effect on heart rate, blood pressure, or O_2 consumption [83]. During ischemia there is an elevation in intracellular Na^+ in myocytes [84-86] secondary to increase in the late Na^+ inward current (I_{Na}) [84, 86]; this condition induces intracellular Ca^{++} overload

[86], which in turn increases actin/myosin filament interaction and LV diastolic tension [87]. As a consequence, on the one hand there is abnormal increase in contractile work and O_2 consumption, and on the other hand compression of vasculature, both leading to further ischemia. By inhibiting myocyte I_{Na}; ranolazine would reduce $[Na^+]$i-dependent Ca^{++} overload induced by ischemia. Consistent with this mechanism, in patients with IHD ranolazine causes a downward shift of LV pressure-volume relationship, increases peak filling rate and wall lengthening of ischemic regions of LV [88-89]. Recently, a small mechanistic study on ranolazine has been performed in women with microvascular angina, no obstructive coronary artery disease, and evidence of ischemia as perfusion abnormalities on adenosine stress cardiac magnetic resonance imaging [90]. Compared with placebo, women on ranolazine scored significantly better on SAQ, including physical functioning (p=0.046), angina stability (p=0.008), and quality of life (p=0.021); interestingly, in women with reduced baseline CFR (i.e., reduced microvascular perfusion) ranolazine significantly improved myocardial perfusion reserve index.

Ranolazine has been tested overall in 1,737 patients with stable angina enrolled in 4 randomized clinical trials (MARISA; CARISA; ERICA; RAN080) [91-94], showing effective anti-anginal activity. Kass-Wenger et al. [95] have recently performed gender comparison of efficacy and safety of ranolazine in patients with stable angina and a similar gender distribution of concomitant treatment with ACE-inhibitors, α- and β-blockers, and statins. The effect of ranolazine on exercise tolerance was less pronounced in women, whereas it afforded comparable reduction of angina frequency and nitroglycerin consumption in women and men. Patients who completed the MARISA or CARISA trials were then enrolled in The Ranolazine Open Label Experience (ROLE) [96], where the safety of ranolazine was assessed.

In MERLIN-TIMI36 trial, the efficacy and safety of ranolazine was tested during long-term treatment of patients with non-ST elevation acute coronary syndrome [97]. Women were more represented than in other trials, comprising 35% of study population (n=2291) [98]; again, women were less likely to have significant epicardial coronary artery disease. Interestingly, incidence of worsening angina did not differ between women with and without obstructive epicardial disease; women treated with ranolazine reported less angina and required less intensification of their antianginal medical regimen during follow up [98].

Ivabradine is an inhibitor of the If current in the sinus node and as such capable of slowing heart rate, particularly during exercise, without detrimental effects on contractility [99]. In randomized clinical trials on patients with effort angina and documented CAD, ivabradine showed a significant reduction in heart rate, as expected, and a better exercise performance [100-103]. The drug resulted non-inferior to atenolol, and conferred additional benefit when added on top of beta-blockers [101-102]. Moreover, ivabradine showed comparable efficacy to amlodipine in improving exercise tolerance with a superior effect on the reduction of rate-pressure product (a surrogate marker of myocardial oxygen consumption) [103]. Regrettably, presence of women in these trials was low (10-15%) [100-102], nor was subgroup analysis for gender performed. A large observational prospective study showed effective treatment of angina pectoris by ivabradine in a population of patients mainly not taking beta-blockers due to contraindications or intolerance [104]; of 4954 patients, 41% of whom were women, and therefore those findings could be translated to a female population [104]; However, because of its open-label design and absence of a placebo-controlled group, those data are not definitive.

Table 1. Clinical studies on treatment of microvascular angina

Author	Year	N	Women	Drug	Study design	Length
Lanza GA [70]	1999	10	6	Atenolol 100 mg/day; Amlodipine 10 mg/day, ISMN 50 mg/day	Cross-over, double blind, randomized	4 weeks each treatment
Fragasso G [71]	1997	22	16	Atenolol 100 mg/day	Single-blind, randomised, crossover trial, placebo-controlled	10 days
Cannon RO [107]	1985	26	15	Verapamil 40-160 mg x4/day or nifedipine 10-30 mg x4/day	Randomized, double-blind, placebo-controlled outpatient study	4 weeks
Sutsch G [72]	1995	16	7	Diltiazem 10 mg iv	Case-control	Acute study
Montorsi P [108]	1990	18	12	Nifedipine 10 mg sl; Nifedipine 10 to 20 mg x4/day	Double blind, placebo controlled	Acute and 4 weeks
Cannon RO [109]	1990	22	12	Lidoflazine 240 or 360 mg/day	Randomized, double blind, placebo controlled	7 weeks
Bugiardini R [69]	1989	16		Verapamil 320 mg/day; Propranolol 120-160 mg/day	Randomized double-blind crossover placebo-controlled trial	7 days each treatment
Lanza GA [110]	1994	51	22	ISDN 5 mg sl	Case-control	Acute study
Radice M [111]	1996	20	19	Nitroglycerin 0.3 mg sl Aminophylline 400 mg os	Randomized	3 exercise tests
Yoshio [74]	1995	12	10	Aminophylline 6 mg/kg iv	Single-blind, placebo-controlled	Acute study
Elliot PM [75]	1997	13	11	Aminophylline 350 or 225 mg x2/day	Randomized, double-blind, cross-over, placebo-controlled	3 weeks
Kaski JC [77]	1994	10	7	Enalapril 10 mg/day	Randomized, single-blind, crossover, placebo-controlled study	2 weeks
Chen [78]	2002	20	5	Enalapril 20 mg x2/day	Randomized, double-blind, placebo controlled	8 weeks
Nalbantgil I [79]	1998	18	15	Cilazapril 5 mg /day	Randomized double-blind crossover placebo-controlled trial	3 weeks

Author	Year	N	Women	Drug	Study design	Length
Russel SJ [112]	2007	28	25	Irbesartan 150 mg daily300 mg daily	Double-blind, randomised, placebo-controlled, two periods crossover	1 week
Pizzi C [76]	2004	45	40	Ramipril 10 mg/day + Atorvastatin 40 mg/day	Randomized, placebo-controlled	24 weeks
Fabian E [80]	2004	40 C	15	Simvastatin 20 mg/day	Randomized, placebo controlled	12 weeks
Kayikcioglu [81]	2003	40	22	Pravastatin 40 mg/day	Single-blind, randomized, placebo-controlled	12 weeks
Rosano GM [113]	1996	25 MI	25	17-β-estradiol cutaneous patches 100 μg/day	Double-blind, placebo-controlled, cross-over	8 weeks
Lerman [114]	1998	26	13	L-Arg 3g x3/day	Double-blind, randomized, placebo-controlled	24 weeks
Botker HE [115]	1998	16	14	Doxazosin 1- 4 mg/day	Double-blind, placebo controlled, crossover study	10 weeks
Jadhav S [29]	2006	33 ND	33	Metformin 500 mg x2/day	Double-blind, randomized, placebo-controlled	8 weeks

Conclusion

Ischemic heart disease is a major cause of death in women, and it is largely underrecognized and undertreated; indeed, greater awareness of possible differences in presentation and pathophysiology of angina in women is in order. Appropriate therapeutic strategies need to be properly evaluated, as solid data for classical antianginal drugs do not exist in terms of gender efficacy. Of equal or greater importance, the approach to ischemic heart disease in women should change, the aim being at identifying patients at high risk for cardiovascular events, rather than patients with obstructive coronary artery disease. In this context, postmenopausal women with angina are a group of patients in whom it seems appropriate to concentrate efforts aimed at reducing morbidity and improving quality of life. This can be considered a major unmet need in terms of modern-day cardiovascular therapy. The current focus of randomized trials and clinical guidelines in angina on male patients ignores the substantial burden of this disease in women.

References

[1] Rosamond W, Flegal K, Friday G, Furie K, Go A, Greenlund K, et al. Heart disease and stroke statistics--2007 update: a report from the American Heart Association Statistics Committee and Stroke Statistics Subcommittee. *Circulation* 2007;115:e69-171.

[2] Peterson S PV, Rayner M, Luengo-Fernandez R, Gray A. European Cardiovascular Disease Statistics. 2end ed. *London: British Heart Foundation* 2005.

[3] Hemingway H, Langenberg C, Damant J, Frost C, Pyorala K, Barrett-Connor E. Prevalence of angina in women versus men: a systematic review and meta-analysis of international variations across 31 countries. *Circulation* 2008;117:1526-36.

[4] Bairey Merz CN, Shaw LJ, Reis SE, Bittner V, Kelsey SF, Olson M, et al. Insights from the NHLBI-Sponsored Women's Ischemia Syndrome Evaluation (WISE) Study: Part II: gender differences in presentation, diagnosis, and outcome with regard to gender-based pathophysiology of atherosclerosis and macrovascular and microvascular coronary disease. *J. Am. Coll. Cardiol.* 2006;47:S21-9.

[5] Shaw LJ, Bairey Merz CN, Pepine CJ, Reis SE, Bittner V, Kelsey SF, et al. Insights from the NHLBI-Sponsored Women's Ischemia Syndrome Evaluation (WISE) Study: Part I: gender differences in traditional and novel risk factors, symptom evaluation, and gender-optimized diagnostic strategies. *J. Am. Coll. Cardiol.* 2006;47:S4-S20.

[6] Sharaf BL, Pepine CJ, Kerensky RA, Reis SE, Reichek N, Rogers WJ, et al. Detailed angiographic analysis of women with suspected ischemic chest pain (pilot phase data from the NHLBI-sponsored Women's Ischemia Syndrome Evaluation [WISE] Study Angiographic Core Laboratory). *Am. J. Cardiol.* 2001;87:937-41; A3.

[7] Likoff W, Segal BL, Kasparian H. Paradox of normal selective coronary arteriograms in patients considered to have unmistakable coronary heart disease. *N. Engl. J. Med.* 1967;276:1063-6.

[8] Shaw LJ, Shaw RE, Merz CN, Brindis RG, Klein LW, Nallamothu B, et al. Impact of ethnicity and gender differences on angiographic coronary artery disease prevalence

and in-hospital mortality in the American College of Cardiology-National Cardiovascular Data Registry. *Circulation* 2008;117:1787-801.

[9] Shaw LJ, Merz CN, Pepine CJ, Reis SE, Bittner V, Kip KE, et al. The economic burden of angina in women with suspected ischemic heart disease: results from the National Institutes of Health--National Heart, Lung, and Blood Institute--sponsored Women's Ischemia Syndrome Evaluation. *Circulation* 2006;114:894-904.

[10] Ong P, Athanasiadis A, Borgulya G, Mahrholdt H, Kaski JC, Sechtem U. High Prevalence of a Pathological Response to Acetylcholine Testing in Patients With Stable Angina Pectoris and Unobstructed Coronary Arteries The ACOVA Study (Abnormal COronary VAsomotion in patients with stable angina and unobstructed coronary arteries). *J. Am. Coll. Cardiol.* 2012;59:655-62.

[11] Jespersen L, Hvelplund A, Abildstrom SZ, Pedersen F, Galatius S, Madsen JK, et al. Stable angina pectoris with no obstructive coronary artery disease is associated with increased risks of major adverse cardiovascular events. *Eur. Heart J.* 20011.

[12] Pepine CJ, Kerensky RA, Lambert CR, Smith KM, von Mering GO, Sopko G, et al. Some thoughts on the vasculopathy of women with ischemic heart disease. *J. Am. Coll. Cardiol.* 2006;47:S30-5.

[13] Sheifer SE, Canos MR, Weinfurt KP, Arora UK, Mendelsohn FO, Gersh BJ, et al. Sex differences in coronary artery size assessed by intravascular ultrasound. *Am. Heart J.* 2000;139:649-53.

[14] De Bruyne B, Hersbach F, Pijls NH, Bartunek J, Bech JW, Heyndrickx GR, et al. Abnormal epicardial coronary resistance in patients with diffuse atherosclerosis but "Normal" coronary angiography. *Circulation* 2001;104:2401-6.

[15] Kaski JC, Rosano GM, Collins P, Nihoyannopoulos P, Maseri A, Poole-Wilson PA. Cardiac syndrome X: clinical characteristics and left ventricular function. Long-term follow-up study. *J. Am. Coll. Cardiol.* 1995;25:807-14.

[16] Mohri M, Koyanagi M, Egashira K, Tagawa H, Ichiki T, Shimokawa H, et al. Angina pectoris caused by coronary microvascular spasm. *Lancet* 1998;351:1165-9.

[17] Nugent L, Mehta PK, Bairey Merz CN. Gender and microvascular angina. *J. Thromb. Thrombolysis* 2011;31:37-46.

[18] Lanza GA, Crea F. Primary coronary microvascular dysfunction: clinical presentation, pathophysiology, and management. *Circulation* 2010;121:2317-25.

[19] Vaccarino V, Badimon L, Corti R, de Wit C, Dorobantu M, Hall A, et al. Ischaemic heart disease in women: are there sex differences in pathophysiology and risk factors?: Position Paper from the Working Group on Coronary Pathophysiology and Microcirculation of the European Society of Cardiology. *Cardiovasc. Res.* 2011.

[20] Vermeltfoort IA, Raijmakers PG, Riphagen, II, Odekerken DA, Kuijper AF, Zwijnenburg A, et al. Definitions and incidence of cardiac syndrome X: review and analysis of clinical data. *Clin. Res. Cardiol.* 2010;99:475-81.

[21] Zeiher AM, Krause T, Schachinger V, Minners J, Moser E. Impaired endothelium-dependent vasodilation of coronary resistance vessels is associated with exercise-induced myocardial ischemia. *Circulation* 1995;91:2345-52.

[22] Chauhan A, Mullins PA, Taylor G, Petch MC, Schofield PM. Both endothelium-dependent and endothelium-independent function is impaired in patients with angina pectoris and normal coronary angiograms. *Eur. Heart J.* 1997;18:60-8.

[23] Egashira K, Inou T, Hirooka Y, Yamada A, Urabe Y, Takeshita A. Evidence of impaired endothelium-dependent coronary vasodilatation in patients with angina pectoris and normal coronary angiograms. *N. Engl. J. Med.* 1993;328:1659-64.

[24] Rigo F, Pratali L, Palinkas A, Picano E, Cutaia V, Venneri L, et al. Coronary flow reserve and brachial artery reactivity in patients with chest pain and "false positive" exercise-induced ST-segment depression. *Am. J. Cardiol.* 2002;89:1141-4.

[25] Opherk D, Mall G, Zebe H, Schwarz F, Weihe E, Manthey J, et al. Reduction of coronary reserve: a mechanism for angina pectoris in patients with arterial hypertension and normal coronary arteries. *Circulation* 1984;69:1-7.

[26] Reis SE, Holubkov R, Conrad Smith AJ, Kelsey SF, Sharaf BL, Reichek N, et al. Coronary microvascular dysfunction is highly prevalent in women with chest pain in the absence of coronary artery disease: results from the NHLBI WISE study. *Am. Heart J.* 2001;141:735-41.

[27] Reis SE, Holubkov R, Lee JS, Sharaf B, Reichek N, Rogers WJ, et al. Coronary flow velocity response to adenosine characterizes coronary microvascular function in women with chest pain and no obstructive coronary disease. Results from the pilot phase of the Women's Ischemia Syndrome Evaluation (WISE) study. *J. Am. Coll. Cardiol.* 1999;33:1469-75.

[28] Camici PG, Marraccini P, Lorenzoni R, Buzzigoli G, Pecori N, Perissinotto A, et al. Coronary hemodynamics and myocardial metabolism in patients with syndrome X: response to pacing stress. *J. Am. Coll. Cardiol.* 1991;17:1461-70.

[29] Jadhav S, Ferrell W, Greer IA, Petrie JR, Cobbe SM, Sattar N. Effects of metformin on microvascular function and exercise tolerance in women with angina and normal coronary arteries: a randomized, double-blind, placebo-controlled study. *J. Am. Coll. Cardiol.* 2006;48:956-63.

[30] Buchthal SD, den Hollander JA, Merz CN, Rogers WJ, Pepine CJ, Reichek N, et al. Abnormal myocardial phosphorus-31 nuclear magnetic resonance spectroscopy in women with chest pain but normal coronary angiograms. *N. Engl. J. Med.* 2000;342:829-35.

[31] Johnson BD, Shaw LJ, Buchthal SD, Bairey Merz CN, Kim HW, Scott KN, et al. Prognosis in women with myocardial ischemia in the absence of obstructive coronary disease: results from the National Institutes of Health-National Heart, Lung, and Blood Institute-Sponsored Women's Ischemia Syndrome Evaluation (WISE). *Circulation* 2004;109:2993-9.

[32] Pries AR, Habazettl H, Ambrosio G, Hansen PR, Kaski JC, Schachinger V, et al. A review of methods for assessment of coronary microvascular disease in both clinical and experimental settings. *Cardiovasc. Res.* 2008;80:165-74.

[33] Daly C, Clemens F, Lopez Sendon JL, Tavazzi L, Boersma E, Danchin N, et al. Gender differences in the management and clinical outcome of stable angina. *Circulation* 2006;113:490-8.

[34] Pasternak RC, Abrams J, Greenland P, Smaha LA, Wilson PW, Houston-Miller N. 34th Bethesda Conference: Task force #1--Identification of coronary heart disease risk: is there a detection gap? *J. Am. Coll. Cardiol.* 2003;41:1863-74.

[35] Ridker PM, Buring JE, Rifai N, Cook NR. Development and validation of improved algorithms for the assessment of global cardiovascular risk in women: the Reynolds Risk Score. *JAMA* 2007;297:611-9.

[36] Angeli F, Angeli E, Ambrosio G, Mazzotta G, Reboldi G, Verdecchia P. Neutrophil count for the identification of postmenopausal hypertensive women at increased cardiovascular risk. *Obstet. Gynecol.* 2010;115:695-703.

[37] NHS-National Institute for health and Clinical Excellence. National Clinical Guideline Centre. Management of stable angina. *www.nice.org.uk/guidance/CG126* 2011.

[38] Zaman MJ, Junghans C, Sekhri N, Chen R, Feder GS, Timmis AD, et al. Presentation of stable angina pectoris among women and South Asian people. *CMAJ* 2008;179:659-67.

[39] Pepine CJ, Abrams J, Marks RG, Morris JJ, Scheidt SS, Handberg E. Characteristics of a contemporary population with angina pectoris. TIDES Investigators. *Am. J. Cardiol.* 1994;74:226-31.

[40] Kimble LP, McGuire DB, Dunbar SB, Fazio S, De A, Weintraub WS, et al. Gender differences in pain characteristics of chronic stable angina and perceived physical limitation in patients with coronary artery disease. *Pain* 2003;101:45-53.

[41] Sheps DS, Kaufmann PG, Sheffield D, Light KC, McMahon RP, Bonsall R, et al. Sex differences in chest pain in patients with documented coronary artery disease and exercise-induced ischemia: Results from the PIMI study. *Am. Heart J.* 2001;142:864-71.

[42] NHS-National Institute for health and Clinical Excellence. National Clinical Guideline Centre. Chest pain of recent onset. *www.nice.org.uk/guidance/CG95* 2010.

[43] Kwok Y, Kim C, Grady D, Segal M, Redberg R. Meta-analysis of exercise testing to detect coronary artery disease in women. *Am. J. Cardiol.* 1999;83:660-6.

[44] Morise AP, Dalal JN, Duval RD. Value of a simple measure of estrogen status for improving the diagnosis of coronary artery disease in women. *Am. J. Med.* 1993;94:491-6.

[45] Hlatky MA, Pryor DB, Harrell FE, Jr., Califf RM, Mark DB, Rosati RA. Factors affecting sensitivity and specificity of exercise electrocardiography. Multivariable analysis. *Am. J. Med.* 1984;77:64-71.

[46] Guiteras P, Chaitman BR, Waters DD, Bourassa MG, Scholl JM, Ferguson RJ, et al. Diagnostic accuracy of exercise ECG lead systems in clinical subsets of women. *Circulation* 1982;65:1465-74.

[47] Barolsky SM, Gilbert CA, Faruqui A, Nutter DO, Schlant RC. Differences in electrocardiographic response to exercise of women and men: a non-Bayesian factor. *Circulation* 1979;60:1021-7.

[48] Mieres JH, Shaw LJ, Arai A, Budoff MJ, Flamm SD, Hundley WG, et al. Role of noninvasive testing in the clinical evaluation of women with suspected coronary artery disease: Consensus statement from the Cardiac Imaging Committee, Council on Clinical Cardiology, and the Cardiovascular Imaging and Intervention Committee,

Council on Cardiovascular Radiology and Intervention, American Heart Association. *Circulation* 2005;111:682-96.

[49] Handberg E, Johnson BD, Arant CB, Wessel TR, Kerensky RA, von Mering G, et al. Impaired coronary vascular reactivity and functional capacity in women: results from the NHLBI Women's Ischemia Syndrome Evaluation (WISE) Study. *J. Am. Coll. Cardiol.* 2006;47:S44-9.

[50] Lichtlen PR, Bargheer K, Wenzlaff P. Long-term prognosis of patients with anginalike chest pain and normal coronary angiographic findings. *J. Am. Coll. Cardiol.* 1995;25:1013-8.

[51] Radice M, Giudici V, Marinelli G. Long-term follow-up in patients with positive exercise test and angiographically normal coronary arteries (syndrome X). *Am. J. Cardiol.* 1995;75:620-1.

[52] Johnson BD, Shaw LJ, Pepine CJ, Reis SE, Kelsey SF, Sopko G, et al. Persistent chest pain predicts cardiovascular events in women without obstructive coronary artery disease: results from the NIH-NHLBI-sponsored Women's Ischaemia Syndrome Evaluation (WISE) study. *Eur. Heart J.* 2006;27:1408-15.

[53] von Mering GO, Arant CB, Wessel TR, McGorray SP, Bairey Merz CN, Sharaf BL, et al. Abnormal coronary vasomotion as a prognostic indicator of cardiovascular events in women: results from the National Heart, Lung, and Blood Institute-Sponsored Women's Ischemia Syndrome Evaluation (WISE). *Circulation* 2004;109:722-5.

[54] Pepine CJ, Anderson RD, Sharaf BL, Reis SE, Smith KM, Handberg EM, et al. Coronary microvascular reactivity to adenosine predicts adverse outcome in women evaluated for suspected ischemia results from the National Heart, Lung and Blood Institute WISE (Women's Ischemia Syndrome Evaluation) study. *J. Am. Coll. Cardiol.* 2010;55:2825-32.

[55] Halcox JP, Schenke WH, Zalos G, Mincemoyer R, Prasad A, Waclawiw MA, et al. Prognostic value of coronary vascular endothelial dysfunction. *Circulation* 2002;106:653-8.

[56] Suwaidi JA, Hamasaki S, Higano ST, Nishimura RA, Holmes DR, Jr., Lerman A. Long-term follow-up of patients with mild coronary artery disease and endothelial dysfunction. *Circulation* 2000;101:948-54.

[57] Boden WE, O'Rourke RA, Teo KK, Hartigan PM, Maron DJ, Kostuk WJ, et al. Optimal medical therapy with or without PCI for stable coronary disease. *N. Engl. J. Med.* 2007;356:1503-16.

[58] Holubkov R, Laskey WK, Haviland A, Slater JC, Bourassa MG, Vlachos HA, et al. Angina 1 year after percutaneous coronary intervention: a report from the NHLBI Dynamic Registry. *Am. Heart J.* 2002;144:826-33.

[59] Curtis JP, Schreiner G, Wang Y, Chen J, Spertus JA, Rumsfeld JS, et al. All-cause readmission and repeat revascularization after percutaneous coronary intervention in a cohort of medicare patients. *J. Am. Coll. Cardiol.* 2009;54:903-7.

[60] Serruys PW, Morice MC, Kappetein AP, Colombo A, Holmes DR, Mack MJ, et al. Percutaneous coronary intervention versus coronary-artery bypass grafting for severe coronary artery disease. *N. Engl. J. Med.* 2009;360:961-72.

[61] Tritto I, Lanza GA, Rigo F, Favale S, Parodi O, Muiesan ML, et al. Long-Term Prognosis of Patients With Cardiac Syndrome X: Data From the Italian Registry of Syndrome X (RISX). *J. Am. Coll. Cardiol.* 2009;35:A343.

[62] Cocco G, Chu D. The anti-ischemic effect of metoprolol in patients with chronic angina pectoris is gender-specific. *Cardiology* 2006;106:147-53.

[63] Olson MB, Kelsey SF, Matthews K, Shaw LJ, Sharaf BL, Pohost GM, et al. Symptoms, myocardial ischaemia and quality of life in women: results from the NHLBI-sponsored WISE Study. *Eur. Heart J.* 2003;24:1506-14.

[64] Hemingway H, McCallum A, Shipley M, Manderbacka K, Martikainen P, Keskimaki I. Incidence and prognostic implications of stable angina pectoris among women and men. *JAMA* 2006;295:1404-11.

[65] Jochmann N, Stangl K, Garbe E, Baumann G, Stangl V. Female-specific aspects in the pharmacotherapy of chronic cardiovascular diseases. *Eur. Heart J.* 2005;26:1585-95.

[66] Luzier AB, Killian A, Wilton JH, Wilson MF, Forrest A, Kazierad DJ. Gender-related effects on metoprolol pharmacokinetics and pharmacodynamics in healthy volunteers. *Clin. Pharmacol. Ther.* 1999;66:594-601.

[67] Stramba-Badiale M. Women and research on cardiovascular diseases in Europe: a report from the European Heart Health Strategy (EuroHeart) project. *Eur. Heart J.* 2010;31:1677-81d.

[68] Heidenreich PA, McDonald KM, Hastie T, Fadel B, Hagan V, Lee BK, et al. Meta-analysis of trials comparing beta-blockers, calcium antagonists, and nitrates for stable angina. *JAMA* 1999;281:1927-36.

[69] Bugiardini R, Borghi A, Biagetti L, Puddu P. Comparison of verapamil versus propranolol therapy in syndrome X. *Am. J. Cardiol.* 1989;63:286-90.

[70] Lanza GA, Colonna G, Pasceri V, Maseri A. Atenolol versus amlodipine versus isosorbide-5-mononitrate on anginal symptoms in syndrome X. *Am. J. Cardiol.* 1999;84:854-6, A8.

[71] Fragasso G, Chierchia SL, Pizzetti G, Rossetti E, Carlino M, Gerosa S, et al. Impaired left ventricular filling dynamics in patients with angina and angiographically normal coronary arteries: effect of beta adrenergic blockade. *Heart* 1997;77:32-9.

[72] Sutsch G, Oechslin E, Mayer I, Hess OM. Effect of diltiazem on coronary flow reserve in patients with microvascular angina. *Int. J. Cardiol.* 1995;52:135-43.

[73] Masumoto A, Mohri M, Takeshita A. Three-year follow-up of the Japanese patients with microvascular angina attributable to coronary microvascular spasm. *Int. J. Cardiol.* 2001;81:151-6.

[74] Yoshio H, Shimizu M, Kita Y, Ino H, Kaku B, Taki J, et al. Effects of short-term aminophylline administration on cardiac functional reserve in patients with syndrome X. *J. Am. Coll. Cardiol.* 1995;25:1547-51.

[75] Elliott PM, Krzyzowska-Dickinson K, Calvino R, Hann C, Kaski JC. Effect of oral aminophylline in patients with angina and normal coronary arteriograms (cardiac syndrome X). *Heart* 1997;77:523-6.

[76] Pizzi C, Manfrini O, Fontana F, Bugiardini R. Angiotensin-converting enzyme inhibitors and 3-hydroxy-3-methylglutaryl coenzyme A reductase in cardiac Syndrome X: role of superoxide dismutase activity. *Circulation* 2004;109:53-8.

[77] Kaski JC, Rosano G, Gavrielides S, Chen L. Effects of angiotensin-converting enzyme inhibition on exercise-induced angina and ST segment depression in patients with microvascular angina. *J. Am. Coll. Cardiol.* 1994;23:652-7.

[78] Chen JW, Hsu NW, Wu TC, Lin SJ, Chang MS. Long-term angiotensin-converting enzyme inhibition reduces plasma asymmetric dimethylarginine and improves endothelial nitric oxide bioavailability and coronary microvascular function in patients with syndrome X. *Am. J. Cardiol.* 2002;90:974-82.

[79] Nalbantgil I, Onder R, Altintig A, Nalbantgil S, Kilicciogl u B, Boydak B, et al. Therapeutic benefits of cilazapril in patients with syndrome X. *Cardiology* 1998;89:130-3.

[80] Fabian E, Varga A, Picano E, Vajo Z, Ronaszeki A, Csanady M. Effect of simvastatin on endothelial function in cardiac syndrome X patients. *Am. J. Cardiol.* 2004;94:652-5.

[81] Kayikcioglu M, Payzin S, Yavuzgil O, Kultursay H, Can LH, Soydan I. Benefits of statin treatment in cardiac syndrome-X1. *Eur Heart J* 2003;24:1999-2005.

[82] Nash DT, Nash SD. Ranolazine for chronic stable angina. *Lancet* 2008;372:1335-41.

[83] Belardinelli L, Shryock JC, Fraser H. Inhibition of the late sodium current as a potential cardioprotective principle: effects of the late sodium current inhibitor ranolazine. *Heart* 2006;92 Suppl 4:iv6-iv14.

[84] Ju YK, Saint DA, Gage PW. Hypoxia increases persistent sodium current in rat ventricular myocytes. *J. Physiol.* 1996;497 (Pt 2):337-47.

[85] Undrovinas AI, Fleidervish IA, Makielski JC. Inward sodium current at resting potentials in single cardiac myocytes induced by the ischemic metabolite lysophosphatidylcholine. *Circ. Res.* 1992;71:1231-41.

[86] Murphy E, Perlman M, London RE, Steenbergen C. Amiloride delays the ischemia-induced rise in cytosolic free calcium. *Circ. Res.* 1991;68:1250-8.

[87] Bing OH, Keefe JF, Wolk MJ, Finkelstein LJ, Levine HJ. Tension prolongation during recovery from myocardial hypoxia. *J. Clin. Invest.* 1971;50:660-6.

[88] Hayashida W, van Eyll C, Rousseau MF, Pouleur H. Effects of ranolazine on left ventricular regional diastolic function in patients with ischemic heart disease. *Cardiovasc. Drugs Ther.* 1994;8:741-7.

[89] Belardinelli L, Shryock, J.C., Fraser, H. The mechanism of ranolazine action to reduce ischemia-induced distolic dysfunction. *Eur. Heart J.* 2006;8:A10-A3.

[90] Mehta PK, Goykhman P, Thomson LE, Shufelt C, Wei J, Yang Y, et al. Ranolazine Improves Angina in Women With Evidence of Myocardial Ischemia But No Obstructive Coronary Artery Disease. *J. Am. Coll. Cardiol. Img.* 2011;4:514-22.

[91] Chaitman BR, Skettino SL, Parker JO, Hanley P, Meluzin J, Kuch J, et al. Anti-ischemic effects and long-term survival during ranolazine monotherapy in patients with chronic severe angina. *J. Am. Coll. Cardiol.* 2004;43:1375-82.

[92] Chaitman BR, Pepine CJ, Parker JO, Skopal J, Chumakova G, Kuch J, et al. Effects of ranolazine with atenolol, amlodipine, or diltiazem on exercise tolerance and angina frequency in patients with severe chronic angina: a randomized controlled trial. *JAMA* 2004;291:309-16.

[93] Stone PH, Gratsiansky NA, Blokhin A, Huang IZ, Meng L. Antianginal efficacy of ranolazine when added to treatment with amlodipine: the ERICA (Efficacy of Ranolazine in Chronic Angina) trial. *J. Am. Coll. Cardiol.* 2006;48:566-75.

[94] Rousseau MF, Pouleur H, Cocco G, Wolff AA. Comparative efficacy of ranolazine versus atenolol for chronic angina pectoris. *Am. J. Cardiol.* 2005;95:311-6.

[95] Wenger NK, Chaitman B, Vetrovec GW. Gender comparison of efficacy and safety of ranolazine for chronic angina pectoris in four randomized clinical trials. *Am. J. Cardiol.* 2007;99:11-8.

[96] Koren MJ, Crager MR, Sweeney M. Long-term safety of a novel antianginal agent in patients with severe chronic stable angina: the Ranolazine Open Label Experience (ROLE). *J. Am. Coll. Cardiol.* 2007;49:1027-34.

[97] Morrow DA, Scirica BM, Karwatowska-Prokopczuk E, Murphy SA, Budaj A, Varshavsky S, et al. Effects of ranolazine on recurrent cardiovascular events in patients with non-ST-elevation acute coronary syndromes: the MERLIN-TIMI 36 randomized trial. *JAMA* 2007;297:1775-83.

[98] Mega JL, Hochman JS, Scirica BM, Murphy SA, Sloan S, McCabe CH, et al. Clinical features and outcomes of women with unstable ischemic heart disease: observations from metabolic efficiency with ranolazine for less ischemia in non-ST-elevation acute coronary syndromes-thrombolysis in myocardial infarction 36 (MERLIN-TIMI 36). *Circulation* 2010;121:1809-17.

[99] Manz M, Reuter M, Lauck G, Omran H, Jung W. A single intravenous dose of ivabradine, a novel I(f) inhibitor, lowers heart rate but does not depress left ventricular function in patients with left ventricular dysfunction. *Cardiology* 2003;100:149-55.

[100] Borer JS, Fox K, Jaillon P, Lerebours G. Antianginal and antiischemic effects of ivabradine, an I(f) inhibitor, in stable angina: a randomized, double-blind, multicentered, placebo-controlled trial. *Circulation* 2003;107:817-23.

[101] Tardif JC, Ponikowski P, Kahan T. Efficacy of the I(f) current inhibitor ivabradine in patients with chronic stable angina receiving beta-blocker therapy: a 4-month, randomized, placebo-controlled trial. *Eur. Heart J.* 2009;30:540-8.

[102] Tardif JC, Ford I, Tendera M, Bourassa MG, Fox K. Efficacy of ivabradine, a new selective I(f) inhibitor, compared with atenolol in patients with chronic stable angina. *Eur. Heart J.* 2005;26:2529-36.

[103] Ruzyllo W, Tendera M, Ford I, Fox KM. Antianginal efficacy and safety of ivabradine compared with amlodipine in patients with stable effort angina pectoris: a 3-month randomised, double-blind, multicentre, noninferiority trial. *Drugs* 2007;67:393-405.

[104] Koster R, Kaehler J, Meinertz T. Treatment of stable angina pectoris by ivabradine in every day practice: the REDUCTION study. *Am. Heart J.* 2009;158:e51-7.

[105] Fox K, Ford I, Steg PG, Tendera M, Ferrari R. Ivabradine for patients with stable coronary artery disease and left-ventricular systolic dysfunction (BEAUTIFUL): a randomised, double-blind, placebo-controlled trial. *Lancet* 2008;372:807-16.

[106] Fox K, Ford I, Steg PG, Tendera M, Robertson M, Ferrari R. Relationship between ivabradine treatment and cardiovascular outcomes in patients with stable coronary artery disease and left ventricular systolic dysfunction with limiting angina: a subgroup

analysis of the randomized, controlled BEAUTIFUL trial. *Eur. Heart J.* 2009;30:2337-45.

[107] Cannon RO, 3rd, Watson RM, Rosing DR, Epstein SE. Efficacy of calcium channel blocker therapy for angina pectoris resulting from small-vessel coronary artery disease and abnormal vasodilator reserve. *Am. J. Cardiol.* 1985;56:242-6.

[108] Montorsi P, Cozzi S, Loaldi A, Fabbiocchi F, Polese A, De Cesare N, et al. Acute coronary vasomotor effects of nifedipine and therapeutic correlates in syndrome X. *Am. J. Cardiol.* 1990;66:302-7.

[109] Cannon RO, 3rd, Brush JE, Jr., Schenke WH, Tracy CM, Epstein SE. Beneficial and detrimental effects of lidoflazine in microvascular angina. *Am. J. Cardiol.* 1990;66:37-41.

[110] Lanza GA, Manzoli A, Bia E, Crea F, Maseri A. Acute effects of nitrates on exercise testing in patients with syndrome X. Clinical and pathophysiological implications. *Circulation* 1994;90:2695-700.

[111] Radice M, Giudici V, Pusineri E, Breghi L, Nicoli T, Peci P, et al. Different effects of acute administration of aminophylline and nitroglycerin on exercise capacity in patients with syndrome X. *Am. J. Cardiol.* 1996;78:88-92.

[112] Russell SJ, Di Stefano EM, Naffati MT, Brown O, Saltissi S. The effects of the angiotensin II receptor (type I) antagonist irbesartan in patients with cardiac syndrome X. *Heart* 2007;93:253-4.

[113] Rosano GM, Peters NS, Lefroy D, Lindsay DC, Sarrel PM, Collins P, et al. 17-beta-Estradiol therapy lessens angina in postmenopausal women with syndrome X. *J. Am. Coll. Cardiol.* 1996;28:1500-5.

[114] Lerman A, Burnett JC, Jr., Higano ST, McKinley LJ, Holmes DR, Jr. Long-term L-arginine supplementation improves small-vessel coronary endothelial function in humans. *Circulation* 1998;97:2123-8.

[115] Botker HE, Sonne HS, Schmitz O, Nielsen TT. Effects of doxazosin on exercise-induced angina pectoris, ST-segment depression, and insulin sensitivity in patients with syndrome X. *Am. J. Cardiol.* 1998;82:1352-6.

In: Recent Advances in Cardiology
Editors: José Milei and Giuseppe Ambrosio
ISBN: 978-1-63117-282-3

Chapter 4

Major Clinical Aspects of Diabetic Cardiomyopathy

***Jelena P. Seferović Mitrović*[1], *Petar M. Seferović*[2,3], *Arsen D. Ristić*[2,3], *Katarina Lalić*[1,3], *Aleksandra Jotić*[1,3], *Ivan Milinković*[2], *Dejan Simeunović*[2] *and Nebojša M. Lalić*[1,3]**

[1]Department of Endocrinology, Diabetes and Metabolic Diseases, Clinical Center of Serbia, Belgrade, Serbia
[2]Department of Cardiology, Clinical Center of Serbia, Belgrade, Serbia
[3]Belgrade University, Faculty of Medicine, Belgrade, Serbia

Abstract

The cardiovascular complications of type 2 diabetes (T2DM) are contributing considerably to morbidity and mortality worldwide, heart failure (HF) being one of the most frequent. The adverse effect of T2DM on myocardium can develop early, and clinically present as left ventricular (LV) diastolic dysfunction in the absence of other heart disease. The pathophysiology of DC includes the major metabolic features of T2DM such as hyperglycemia, hyperinsulinemia, hyperlipidemia, and the formation of both reactive oxygen species and advanced glycation end-products. There are no pathognomonic diagnostic features of diabetic cardiomyopathy (DC) and no single imaging method exists for the accurate diagnosis. Clinical presentation is mostly mild, and majority of the patients are asymptomatic or with nonspecific complaints. The major hurdles in diagnosing DC are imprecise definition and dissimilar criteria for diagnosis of LV diastolic dysfunction. DC is best defined as myocardial disease in diabetic patients characterized by LV diastolic dysfunction in the absence of hypertension, coronary artery disease or any other cardiac disease. LV diastolic dysfunction is the most important element of diagnosis of DC, best assessed by tissue Doppler echocardiography (E/E' ratio). The prevalence of LV diastolic dysfunction in T2DM demonstrate the wide variations caused by diverse patient selection and heterogeneous criteria for its diagnosis. Patient selection varies in terms of age, duration, stage, and microvascular complications of T2DM. Several clinical correlates were reported as related to DC such as: age, duration of T2DM, parameters of glycoregulation, insulin resistance, and renal function.

The treatment of DC should be initiated as early as LV diastolic dysfunction is identified. Various therapeutic options include improving diabetic control with diet, daily physical activity, and reduction in body mass index. Both antiglycaemic (metformin and thiazolidinediones), and cardiovascular drugs (ACE inhibitors, beta blockers and calcium channel blockers) should be used to improve LV diastolic dysfunction.

Introduction

The cardiovascular complications of type 2 diabetes (T2DM) are contributing considerably to morbidity and mortality worldwide. At present, T2DM affects 246 million people [1] around the globe, and it is assessed that by the year 2025, this disease will have epidemic proportions [2], with 300 million diabetic patients. Among cardiovascular complications in T2DM, heart failure (HF) is one of the most frequent. In addition, T2DM is also listed as one of the most common comorbidities in patients with HF. The major etiological factors for development of HF in T2DM include arterial hypertension, coronary artery disease (CAD), the activation of neurohormonal systems, but also the direct detrimental effect of T2DM on the myocardium. HF with preserved left ventricular ejection fraction (LVEF) can be frequently diagnosed in T2DM. An analysis of 987 patients with HF and preserved LVEF, enrolled in the Digitalis Investigation Group ancillary study [3] revealed that T2DM was associated with significantly increased risk of developing adverse HF outcomes in this group.

In the general population 0.3-0.5% patients have both HF and T2DM [4], while among T2DM patients, almost 12% suffer from HF. The population studies revealed that in patients with HF the prevalence of T2DM varies from 12-30% [5]. In the clinical practice, T2DM is considered to be a major independent risk factor for the development of HF. In the Framingham study, the relative risk of HF in patients with T2DM (between 45–74 years), was doubled for men and five-fold higher in women [6]. The high incidence of HF in patients with T2DM was also confirmed in NHANES, which demonstrated T2DM as an independent risk factor for HF with HR of 1.85 (1.51–2.28) in T2DM, compared to non-DM [7].

The adverse effect of T2DM on myocardium can develop early, even before the other micro- and macro vascular complications arise. Rubler et al. [8] described more than 30 years ago, four cases with long standing T2DM, severe congestive HF, but normal coronary arteries. Later on, numerous reports confirmed the existence of specific heart muscle disease, mostly involving LV diastolic dysfunction in asymptomatic T2D patients [9–13]. The majority of the descriptions were referred to as LV diastolic dysfunction in the absence of coronary atherosclerosis and hypertension. In addition, in patients with idiopathic dilated cardiomyopathy T2DM was diagnosed much more frequently, in up to 75%, in comparison with controls of the same age [14]. This is confirmed in the study of Bertoni AG et al. [15], who analyzed the discharge data from 900 hospitals in USA. Among 45 254 patients with idiopathic dilated cardiomyopathy, the prevalence of T2DM in these patients vs. controls was 26.6% vs. 17.2%, respectively (OR 1.75, 95%CI 1.71-1.79).

This entity was also recognized in the Guidelines on diabetes, pre-diabetes, and cardiovascular diseases of the European Society of Cardiology (ESC) and of the European Association for the Study of Diabetes (EASD), in which diabetic cardiomyopathy (DC) was listed as a first among non-atherosclerotic cardiovascular disease [16]. However, despite solid epidemiological body of evidence for existence of DC, the causal relationship between metabolic abnormalities in T2DM and specific clinical presentation has been difficult to ascertain. Also, since the confirmation for DC are mostly experimental, further clinical and functional description of myocardial abnormalities is needed.

The Scope of the Chapter

Analyzing the clinical relevance of DC, the current literature was evaluated during the period 1995-2013., with the key word "diabetic cardiomyopathy" in title, English language, and using PubMed as a source. The total number of manuscripts regarding DC was small, with the approximately six-fold increase over 12 years period (from eight in 1995 to 36 in 2012), representing the growth in interest for the subject. The number of review articles, or articles covering experimental aspects of DC was much higher in comparison to the manuscripts describing the clinical features of DC (Figure 1.). This illustrates discrepancy between experimental data and basic, molecular hypotheses at one and the clinical knowledge about this condition on the other side.

The clinical features of DC discussed in these articles demonstrates wide variations, because the majority of this issues are not agreed upon. These dilemmas include basic clinical issues such as definition, incidence, diagnostic controversies, clinical correlates and accuracy of parameters of left ventricular diastolic dysfunction in DC. Therefore, the authors believe that elucidating this issues will help improve the knowledge in this field.

Cardiometabolic Continuum

Cardiometabolic (cardiodiabetic) continuum mostly refers to the development of the lesions in the structure and function of cardiovascular system, presumably myocardium, in patients with T2DM and metabolic syndrome. This spectrum of pathophysiological and morphological lesions, including HF, is rather wide, ranging from asymptomatic forms to the overt disease. From the clinical point of view, and by opinion of the most of the experts, T2DM and cardiovascular diseases can be considered as clinical equivalents.

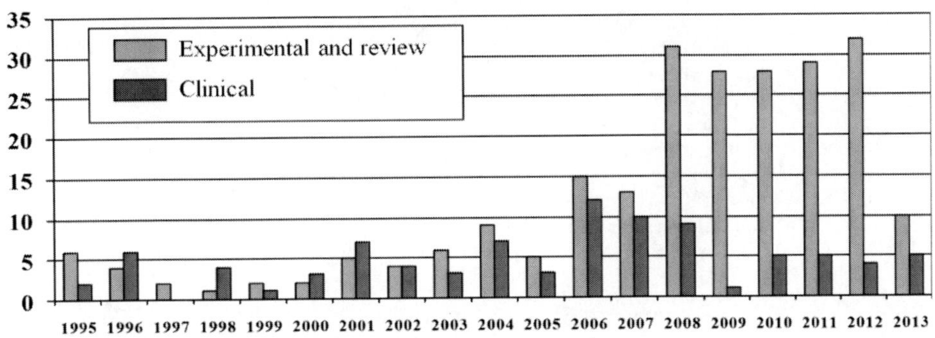

Figure 1. The total number of manuscripts regarding DC, using PubMed search in the period 1995-2013.

DC is placed at the very early stage of cardiometabolic continuum and its timely diagnosis may have a significant clinical implications.

In most of the patients, cardiometabolic continuum is initiated in the third and fourth decade, depending on the severity of T2DM and associated risk factors that promote cardiovascular diseases (arterial hypertension, dyslipidemia, sedentary lifestyle, diet rich in saturated fats and carbohydrates, high body mass index and smoking). Genetic predisposition for cardiovascular disease is often existing.

The majority of authors agree that the initial cardiovascular lesions appearing early in the cardiometabolic continuum is asymptomatic myocardial abnormality [5, 17]. The first clinical symptoms are the result of atherosclerosis, since T2DM causes 2-3 fold increase of risk for coronary artery disease (CAD) and 2-4 fold increase of risk for cerebrovascular insult [18-20]. Proteinuria, retinopathy and sympathetic neuropathy are often associated with coronary, cerebrovascular, and peripheral vascular disease [21, 22]. Also, T2DM is associated with 4-fold increase of risk for sudden death and complex ventricular arrhythmias.

There are several stages of progression of cardiometabolic continuum, in which various cardiac structures are affected (Figure 2.).

The early phase is characterized by the discrete myocardial lesions, featuring the physiological adaptation of myocardium on hyperglycemia, insulin resistance and low glucose transporter proteins 1 and 4 concentrations. Morphological and structural changes on myocites are minimal [23], with elevated level of plasma free fatty acids and carnitine concentrations. LV diastolic dysfunction can be detected, rarely associated with LV hypertrophy.

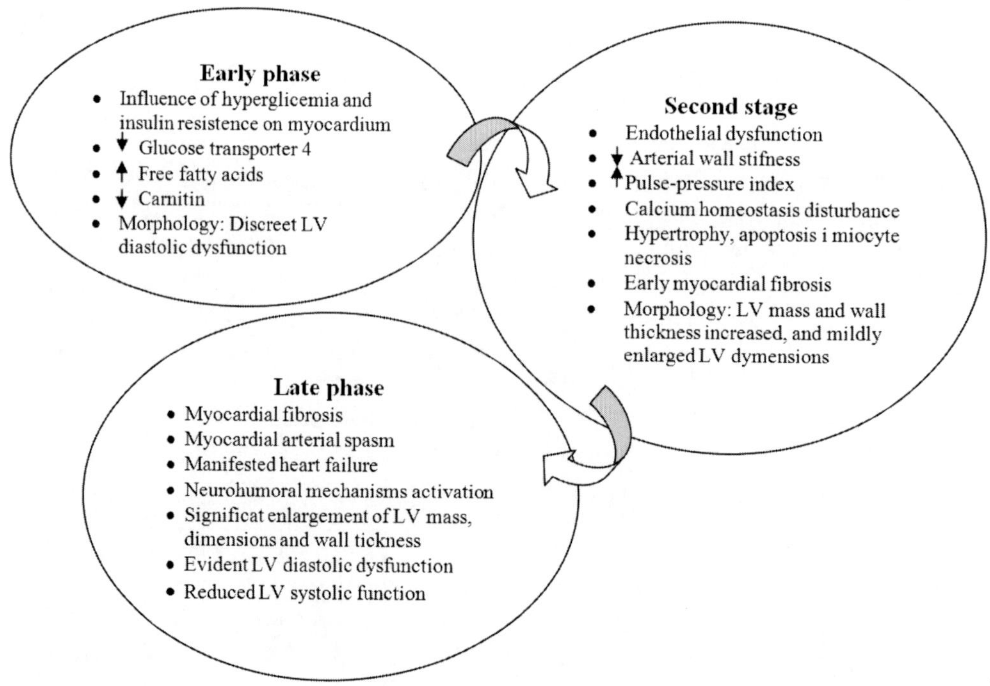

Figure 2. Stages of cardiometabolic continuum.

In the second stage, endothelial dysfunction progresses and worsens vascular function, increasing arterial stiffness and elevating pulse-pressure index. Vascular changes further promote not only myocardial damage, but also disturbances of calcium homeostasis, LV hypertrophy, myocyte apoptosis and necrosis with subsequent initial fibrosis [24]. Plasma angiotensin II and transforming growth factor 1 activity are increased, while insulin growth factor 1 concentration is reduced. On echocardiography, LV mass and wall thickness is mildly increased, LV diastolic dysfunction more evident, but systolic function is either normal or slightly reduced.

In third, late stage, metabolic disturbances are severe, myocardial fibrosis is progressive, and microvascular changes including arterial spasm are developing. Sympathetic neuropathy significantly affects vasodilatatory response of coronary arteries on sympathetic stimulation [25]. Manifested HF develops with the activation of neurohumoral mechanisms, increased afterload and reduced coronary blood flow. LV mass, dimensions and wall thickness are increased, diastolic dysfunction evident, and LV systolic function reduced.

Clinically Relevant Pathophysiological Mechanisms

The complexity of mechanisms underlining the pathophysiology of DC, causing structural and functional changes of the heart muscle, are still not completely elucidated. The major metabolic features of diabetic subjects which can lead to alteration of myocardial structure and function can be defined as hyperglycemia, hyperinsulinemia, hyperlipidemia, and the formation of both reactive oxygen species and advanced glycation end-products.

The Role of Hyperglycemia on Formation of Reactive Oxygen Species

Long-lasting hyperglycemia can cause glucose oxidation and mitochondrial generations of superoxide, which causes DNA damage and activation of poly-polymerase. This sequence of events diverts glucose from its glycolytic into alternative biochemical pathways. Hyperglycemia also act as an activator of the protein kinase C, which causes the phosphorylation of several proteins involved in contraction process, affecting Ca^{2+} handling in cardiomyocytes, [26] resulting in myocardial necrosis and fibrosis [27]. In addition, hyperglycemia stimulates the production of reactive oxygen species (ROS) in the myocardium, which impairs the endothelial function, reduces the nitric oxide concentration, and leads to an inflammatory reaction. Inflammation stimulates poly-(ADP-ribose) polymerase-1-enzyme (PARP) which inhibits glyceraldehydes 3-phosphate dehydrogenase, causing the accumulation of glycolytic intermediates and activation of protein kinase C. In addition, PARP activates nuclear factor kB and induces an over-expression of the vasoconstrictor endothelin 1 (ET-1) and its receptors [28]. ROS also accelerate the process of apoptosis triggered by glycosylation, phosphorylation of p53, and increased activity of angiotensin I [29].

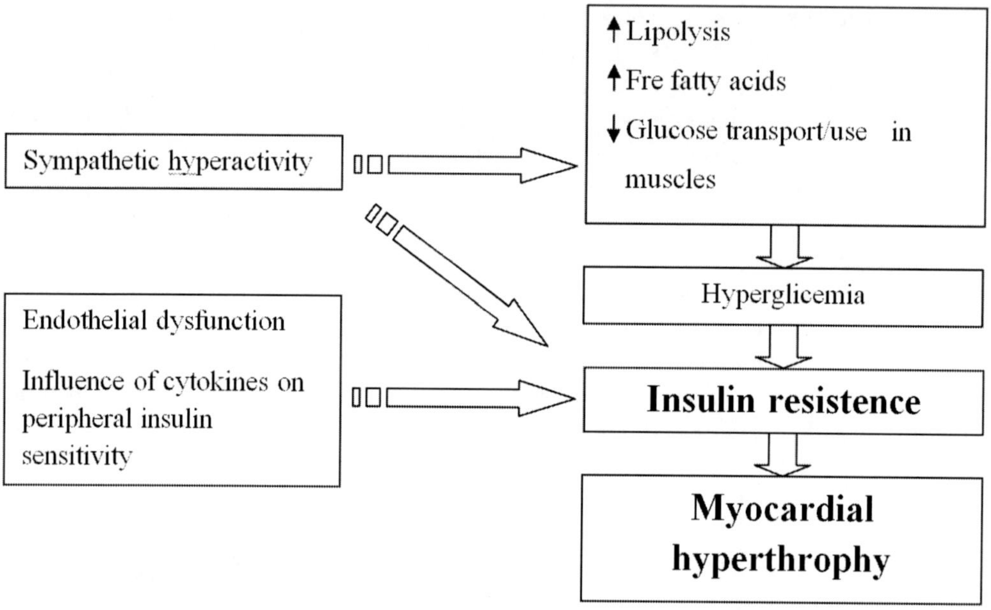

Figure 3. The role of insulin resistance in development of diabetic cardiomyopathy.

Hyperglycemia and Advanced Glycation End-Products

Hyperglycemia activates local myocardial renin-angiotensin and endothelin systems, contributing to myocyte necrosis and fibrosis (interstitial and perivascular) [30, 31]. The pathological lesions includes myocardial hypertrophy, interstitial fibrosis, capillary endothelial changes, and capillary basal laminae thickening [32]. Deposition of collagen type I and III predominates in the epicardial and perivascular regions, whereas type IV predominates in the endocardium [33]. Collagen interacts with glucose, forming Schiff bases, which reorganize over the following weeks into glycated collagen (Amadori products). The Amadori products transforms through chemical modification into advance glycation end-products (AGEs). AGEs are a stable form of collagen with the detrimental activity on blood vessels, finally resulting in arterial and myocardial stiffness, endothelial dysfunction, and atherosclerotic plaque formation. The further activity of AGEs affects cross-linking of collagen and circulating proteins (e.g., low-density lipoprotein), causing dysfunction in cellular nitric oxide signaling and exacerbate intracellular oxidative stress and cell damage [34].

The Importance of Increased Free Fatty Acid

As a result of depleted glucose transporter proteins (glucose transporter-1 and 4) in T2DM, myocardial glucose use is significantly reduced, with a shift in energy production from beta-oxidation of free fatty acids [35]. Prolonged hyperglycemia and high insulin resistance are associated with high free fatty acids concentration, which depresses myocardial function. Free fatty acids inhibit pyruvate dehydrogenase, which impairs myocardial energy production and leads to the accumulation of glycolytic intermediates and ceramide, enhancing apoptosis [36, 37]. Free fatty acids metabolism, also, requires large amounts of oxygen, producing toxic intermediates resulting in [35, 38] lipotoxicity that impair myocyte calcium handling and worsens myocardial mechanics [39-41]. The increased concentration of free fatty acids in diabetic myocardium is the result of high sympathetic activity, insulin resistance and lipolysis, caused by insulin deficiency [42, 43]. In the study of Di Bonito et al. [44], in patients with T2DM the negative correlation between LV diastolic dysfunction and index of insulin sensitivity was demonstrated. In addition, Goldstein et al. [45] revealed the association of insulin resistance and the high expression of the growth factor production and myocardial collagen deposition (Figure 3).

Insulin resistance and hyperinsulinemia are the major etiological factors in the development of LV hypertrophy [46]. In the Framingham Study women with diabetes had a 10% greater LV mass in comparison to females without diabetes [47, 48]. LV hypertrophy develops late in patients with DC, and correlates well with the degree of insulin resistance. Both insulin resistance and hyperinsulinemia are causing the elevation of free fatty acid concentrations and products of their degradation, resulting in myocardial dysfunction [49]. Diabetic state is characterized by low insulin-like growth factor-1 and elevated transforming growth factor-β1 levels. Resistance to insulin-like growth factor-1, leads to myocyte necrosis, LV hypertrophy, and myocardial dysfunction [50].

Beside these basic pathways in pathophysiology of DC there are several important additional mechanisms which contribute to its development such as: the disorders in copper metabolism, autonomic neuropathy, stem cell involvement, endothelial dysfunction, micro vascular disease, and carnitine deficiency.

Hyperglycemia can damage the copper binding properties of ceruloplasmin and albumin, resulting in increased copper levels in the extracellular matrix [51, 52]. Glycated proteins also might have an increased affinity toward copper [53, 54]. An abundance of copper in the extracellular matrix may activate the oxidation–reduction system, leading to an enhanced production of free radicals resulting in increased oxidative stress and fibrosis [55].

Diabetic autonomic neuropathy changes sympathetic innervations, adrenergic receptor expression and catecholamine levels in the myocardium. An increased expression of the β1-receptor results in enhanced apoptosis, fibrosis, hypertrophy, and impaired myocardial function [56]. In addition, elevated myocardial catecholamines [57] are increasing resting heart rate, resulting in loss of heart rate variability, the modification of chronotropic and inotropic myocardial response and impairment of myocardial perfusion.

Enhanced oxidative stress in T2DM can alter cardiac progenitor cell function, leading to defective cardiac progenitor cell growth and myocyte formation, leading to HF. In addition, cardiac progenitor cell apoptosis and HF are ameliorated by ablation of the p66 shc gene, possibly responsible for promoting the senescent phenotype [58].

T2DM is recognized by changes in microvasculature such as: abnormal capillary permeability, microaneurysm formation, subendothelial matrix deposition, and perivascular fibrosis. Coronary blood flow reserve in diabetic patients is reduced even in the absence of obstructive coronary artery disease and LV hypertrophy [59]. Hyperglycemia also can lead to an enhanced synthesis of vasoconstrictor prostanoids, and activation of protein kinase C, promoting myocardial hypertrophy, endothelial dysfunction, and ventricular hypertrophy [60, 61]. Protein kinase C activation cause endothelial dysfunction by reducing the bioavailability of nitric oxide while increasing oxygen-derived free radical production. It also can enhance leukocyte adhesion, increase albumin permeability, and impair fibrinolysis [62, 63]. Carnitine deficiency may have role in etiopathogenesis of DC, but more based on experimental and not on clinical evidence [64].

Diagnostic Approach

There are no pathognomonic diagnostic features of DC. Specific histological, clinical and/or diagnostic characteristics are lacking, and there is no single imaging or biochemical method for the accurate diagnosis, which implies that most cases are underdiagnosed.

Before establishing the diagnosis, two steps need to be taken: the exclusion of other causes of cardiomyopathy and the detection of LV diastolic dysfunction. It order to diagnose DC properly, it is important to exclude other forms/causes of LV diastolic dysfunction which may mimic DC. Both myocardial hypertrophy and fibrosis of various degrees may or may not be present, and are nonspecific, but could not porten the final diagnosis. Endomyocardial biopsy is rarely indicated, mostly in selected tertiary centers, but may be useful to exclude several causes of restrictive cardiomyopathy.

Clinical presentation of DC is mostly mild, majority of the patients are asymptomatic or with nonspecific complaints [24]. The most frequent symptoms include dyspnea, shortness of breath, fatigue, and tachycardia. Rarely, dizziness and nonspecific chest pain may occur.

From the didactic point of view, the major hurdles in diagnosing DC may be listed as follows: imprecise definition, technological inadequacies of imaging and the variability of parameters for diagnosis of LV diastolic dysfunction.

Definition

The lack of precise definition of DC is the result of several factors, which are related to the poor understanding of the nature of the disease, discrete and various clinical presentation, the non-convincing therapeutic or preventive strategies and absence of expert consensus of diagnostic criteria for DC.

The proper DC definition is critical, because it porten/allow to establish the precise diagnosis, stimulate the accurate selection of patients, homogenization of the study groups, and provides the characterization of various stages of DC.

In analyzing ten definitions of DC in most recent literature [65-72] five elements used as inclusion criteria of DC can be revealed: 1) T2DM (all ten); 2) stage of the disease (in one study-late, otherwise not reported); 3) LV systolic dysfunction (five); 4) LV diastolic dysfunction (four), and 5) absence of coronary artery disease, hypertension and other cardiac disorder (all ten).

Therefore, according to abovementioned criteria the following definition of DC seems to represent the current body of knowledge and experience:

> Diabetic cardiomyopathy is myocardial disease in diabetic patients characterized by LV diastolic dysfunction in the absence of hypertension, coronary artery disease or any other cardiac disease.

The Most Accurate Parameters of LV Diastolic Dysfunction

In clinical practice, LV diastolic dysfunction is often associated with diabetes, older age, female gender, obesity, arterial hypertension, coronary artery disease, and LV hypertrophy.

The accurate selection of parameters specifically representing LV diastolic function was in debate for a long time. After the publication of the Consensus statement of the ESC Heart Failure and Echocardiography Associations [73] most of the investigators are using tissue Doppler parameters as a standard. In the Consensus, it was stressed that LV diastolic dysfunction is an important part of diagnosis of diastolic heart failure, in association with signs and symptoms of congestive heart failure and near-normal LVEF.

LV diastolic dysfunction is the most important element in diagnosis of DC. With routine use of tissue Doppler echocardiography the diagnosis of LV diastolic dysfunction, presenting as abnormal LV relaxation and filling as well as impaired diastolic distensibility and stiffness became accurate and widely clinically available. According to the Consensus, when the ratio of early mitral valve flow velocity (E) divided by early diastolic lengthening velocity (E/E') is higher than 15, the diagnosis of LV diastolic dysfunction is established. If this ratio is lower than 8, this diagnosis is not likely, whereas the range of 8-15 is considered suggestive but not diagnostic. In these borderline cases additional Doppler echocardiographic measurements are necessary, including Doppler evaluation of mitral valve or pulmonary veins, LV mass index or left atrial volume index. In the study of Pritchett-a et al. [74] left atrial volume index correlated with severity of LV diastolic dysfunction, increasing from 23±6 in normals to 48±12 ml/m^2 in patients with LV diastolic dysfunction, The values less than 29 ml/m^2 could exclude this diagnosis.

Prevalence

One of the most important causes of confusion in the clinical understanding of DC is the lack of information about its prevalence. Due to the limited number of patients and nonconsistent patient selection in the studies, their statistical power and clinical implication were poor. Therefore, the prevalence of LV diastolic dysfunction in T2DM reported in the last decade clearly demonstrate the wide variation, from the early studies with high to the recent data with much lower prevalence [75]. By the most authors, the major causes of such variations are recognized as heterogeneous patient selection and diverse criteria for diagnosis of LV diastolic dysfunction. The precise parameters specifically representing LV diastolic function were previously discussed.

Patient Selection

Patient selection for DC should exclude those with arterial hypertension, CAD, and advanced age, because of the adverse effect of these diseases on myocardial morphology and function. In analyzing patient selection among studies, the significant heterogeneity in terms of age of the patients as well as duration and microvascular complications of T2DM can be recognized. In particular, essential are the variability of T2DM stages of patients included, which has different effect on myocardial structure and function.

The patient heterogeneity can be appreciated even from the initial report of Rubler at al [8] who investigated autopsy samples of 27 patients with T2DM, heart failure, and diabetic glomerulosclerosis. Four of these patients had congestive HF, but normal coronary arteries, and no other etiologies explaining HF. Based on the pathoanatomic and clinical findings it can be concluded that these patients were in the advanced stages of T2DM (glomerulosclerosis). This is in contrast to the contemporary understanding of the DC, which is defined as an early complication of T2DM in the absence of arterial hypertension and CAD. Recent studies which used criteria for LV diastolic dysfunction defined by the Consensus statement, revealed lower prevalence of DC.

From et al. [76] investigated 486 patients with T2DM, without hypertension and CAD, and detected E/E' ratio higher than 15 in 21% patients. Identical criteria were used in DADD study (Diabetes mellitus And Diastolic Dysfunction) [77] which studied the influence of strict glycaemic control on LV diastolic function. The study included 39 patients with T2DM, without CAD and HF, and detected LV diastolic function in 33% of patients. The investigation of Sharman et al. [78] included 155 patients with T2DM and no cardiovascular diseases, in whom LV diastolic dysfunction was detected in 51%, using E/E' ratio as diagnostic criteria, while 15% had pseudonormal diastolic filling.

In the study of Seferovic-Mitrovic et al. [79] which included 78 normotensive T2DM patients, tissue Doppler parameters to diagnose LV diastolic dysfunction were used and the prevalence of DC of 10.3 % (8 patients) was uncovered.

Cosson et al. [80] compared diastolic impairment in 48 patients with T2DM, without arterial hypertension, CAD and microangiopathic complications with controls, using tissue Doppler and transmitral flow parameters. The results demonstrated the absence of differences in LV diastolic function in compared groups.

In addition, Zabalgoitia et al. [81] investigated a group of 86 T2DM patients, without hypertension, CAD or HF, and revealed in 30% LV diastolic dysfunction (parameters of transmitral flow), while 17% had pseudonormal diastolic filling.

Di Bonito et al. [44] compared diastolic impairment in 40 patients with T2DM, who had normal blood pressure and body mass index, while control group included 20 healthy volunteers. Diastolic dysfunction was diagnosed using Doppler parameters, and the results implicated a significant impairment of LV diastolic function in patients with T2DM in comparison to controls.

The study of Schannwell et al. [82], which included 87 patients with type 1 diabetes and no cardiovascular disease, revealed significant early impairment of LV diastolic function (conventional Doppler echocardiography).

Using the similar methodology, Boyer et al. [83] showed that the prevalence of LV diastolic dysfunction was 75% in 61 normotensive, T2DM patients, with no CAD. However, when tissue Doppler methodology was used in this patient group, LV diastolic dysfunction prevalence was lower, 63%.

In the study of Poirier et al. [84] parameters of transmitral flow were used to assess LV diastolic dysfunction, in 46 patients with T2DM, in the absence of hypertension, CAD, thyroid or kidney dysfunction. The results detected LV diastolic dysfunction in 32% of patients, while 28% had pseudonormal diastolic filling.

In the work of Srivastava et al. [85] 229 T2DM patients were included. Microvascular complications were present in 64%, arterial hypertension in 78%, CAD in 12% and cerebrovascular disease in 33% of these patients. Myocardial dysfunction was revealed in 146 patients (64%), 37 patients (16%) had systolic and diastolic dysfunction, while 109 (48%) had only LV diastolic dysfunction.

Henry et al. [86] included 472 patients with different stages of glycoregulation impairment in the HOORN study. Systolic dysfunction was found in 14% of patients with impaired glucose tolerance and in 30% of patients with T2DM. Furthermore, 36% of patients with impaired glucose tolerance and 47% of patients with T2DM had LV diastolic dysfunction. These results indicated that systolic and diastolic impairment was more frequent in patients with glycoregulation disturbance.

Fang et al. [87] uncover global LV dysfunction (10%), systolic (16%), and LV diastolic dysfunction (21%) in 120 patients with T2DM.

Di Bonito et al. [44], detected LV diastolic dysfunction in all of 16 normotensive patients with T2DM, and no microvascular complications. On the contrary, Takenaka et al. [88] showed normal LV diastolic function in 60 normotensive patients with T2DM, without microvascular complications.

Investigation of Fonseca et al. [89] included 28 patients with T2DM with normal systolic and impaired LV diastolic function. Using magnetic resonance, LV diastolic dysfunction was diagnosed in 12–32% of patients, depending on the diagnostic parameter used.

Clinical Correlates

The most important clinical correlates of LV diastolic dysfunction identified in the literature are age, duration of diabetes, parameters of glycoregulation, insulin resistance and renal function.

Age

By the most investigators, age is considered to be an important risk factor for the development of diabetic LV diastolic dysfunction. Seferovic-Mitrovic et al. [79] studied 78 normotensive T2DM patients, and identified, by univariate regression analysis, age and value of apoprotein A1 as independent predictors for the development of DC. Also, significant correlation among E/E' ratio and patient age, HDL cholesterol and apolipoprotein A1 has been revealed. Furthermore, significant correlation between E/A and patient age, and the value of free fatty acids has been uncovered.

In the study of Yazici et al. [90], which investigated 72 patients with T2DM, without hypertension and CAD, a significant correlation of age, duration of T2DM, glycated hemoglobin (HbA1c) and LV diastolic function parameters was revealed. Similar results were confirmed by Masugata et al, who demonstrated the positive correlation of age with LV diastolic dysfunction in 77 normotensive patients with T2DM [91] and revealed that parameter of transmitral flow, E/A ratio, correlated with age and duration of disease.

Srivastava et al. [85] investigated 229 patients with T2DM and showed that age, obesity, antihypertensive drugs and impaired renal function were independent predictors of LV diastolic dysfunction, age being the most important. The risk for the development of LV diastolic dysfunction increased for 9% by year, over the age of 50.

The Duration of Diabetes

Duration of T2DM is one of the most important factors in the development of all diabetic complication, including myocardial lesions. Masugata et al. [91] studied 77 normotensive T2DM patients, and indicated the correlation of disease duration and LV diastolic dysfunction. Similar were the results of Yazici et al. [90] who uncovered the significant correlation of duration of T2DM and parameters of LV diastolic function.

From et al. [76] also confirmed, in 486 patients, the positive correlation between E/E' ratio and duration of T2DM, and increase of E/E' by 0, 23, yearly. Multivariate logistic analysis revealed that duration of T2DM for more than four years was linked with significant LV diastolic dysfunction, shown as the independent predictor of total mortality.

Liu et al. [92] analyzed Strong Heart Study and demonstrated the highest grade of LV diastolic dysfunction in patients with both T2DM and hypertension. The positive correlation between the duration of T2DM and LV diastolic dysfunction was also confirmed.

Glycoregulation

Study conducted by Markuszewski et al. [93] revealed the positive correlation between LV diastolic dysfunction and HbA1c in 57 patients with T2DM but without CAD. LV diastolic dysfunction was diagnosed in 43% of patients with HbA1c higher than 6.1%, but only in 4.5% with HbA1c lower than 6.1%.

Bajraktari et al. [94], revealed LV diastolic dysfunction in 27.6% of patients with normal glycoregulation, in 55% of those with impaired glucose tolerance and in 75.7% of patients with T2DM. Multiple regression analysis showed that postprandial glucose positively correlated with E/A ratio.

In analyzing Strong Heart Study, Liu et al. [92] demonstrated positive correlation of glycoregulation and LV diastolic dysfunction, while more severe forms of LV diastolic dysfunction were associated with higher HbA1c level, higher fasting glucose and increased arterial stiffness.

Guo et al. [95] revealed negative correlation of LV diastolic dysfunction and HbA1c level in patients with T2DM using pulse and tissue Doppler, and myocardial acoustic densitometry.

Insulin Resistance

Several studies demonstrated the strong correlation of insulin resistance with LV diastolic dysfunction and LV hypertrophy.

LV diastolic dysfunction negatively correlated with insulin resistance, using HOMA-IR [96] and positively using QUICKI (Quantitative Insulin Sensitivity Check Index, [97]) in 119 patients. Multiple linear regression analysis revealed insulin resistance as an independent predictor of LV diastolic dysfunction.

In the investigation of Di Bonito et al. [44] linear regression analysis demonstrated a significant negative correlation between LV diastolic dysfunction and HOMA-IR in 40 normotensive T2DM patients.

Ozasa et al. [98] confirmed that HbA1c and HOMA-IR had a positive correlation with LV mass index and LV diastolic dysfunction. Besides, HOMA-IR was an independent predictor of LV mass index and LV diastolic dysfunction in 40 patients with T2DM and without hypertension and CAD.

Renal Impairment

Srivastava et al. [85] concluded that renal dysfunction was an independent predictor of LV diastolic dysfunction in patients with T2DM. Also Poirier et al. [84] revealed a positive correlation of albuminuria and LV diastolic dysfunction in 46 patients with well controlled T2DM and without hypertension and CAD.

Similar results were found by Durman et al. [99] who included 140 patients with T2DM, without hypertension, renal dysfunction or CAD. The level of albuminuria positively correlated with LV diastolic dysfunction and increased arterial stiffness.

Treatment Strategies for Diabetic Cardiomyopathy

Glycemic Control

Chronic hyperglycemia is a basic pathophysiological disorder implicated in the development of DC in type 2 diabetic patients [100-102]. Thiazolidinediones activate peroxisome proliferator-activated receptor (PPAR-c) enabling increased peripheral insulin sensitivity and secondarily reduce hepatic glucose production. Despite thiazolidinediones are effective glycemic controllers, which improve adipocyte function and triglyceride levels, these drugs are contraindicated in advanced HF [103, 104]. Metformin decreases hepatic glucose production and has demonstrated improvements in survival of diabetic patients with HF. Studies do not offer direct information on the effects of metformin on DC, but the reduction in cardiovascular disease rates justifies its usage to treat DC [105, 106]. However, new incretin-based agents for glycemic control had beneficial effects and reduced heart failure in DC. Incretin mimics injectable glucagon-like peptide-1 (GLP-1) analogs that activate the GLP-1 receptors, therefore increasing glucose-dependent insulin secretion and decreasing glucagon secretion. Likewise, oral dipeptidyl peptidase inhibitors prolong the half-life of endogenous GLP-1, increasing its effect. Overall, these agents have a positive effect on myocardial function and LV ejection fraction in patients with HF and in animal models [107, 108]. Alpha-glucosidase inhibitors, like acarbose, prevent the absorption of glucose in the gastro-intestinal system, increasing the effect of insulin, decreasing stress on beta-cells, and reducing the cardiovascular risk due to postprandial hyperglycemia [109, 110]. Additionally, for type 1 DM, it has been shown that DC does not develop if the diabetes is well controlled with insulin therapy. Accordingly, hyperglycemia should be regarded as not only an exacerbating, but also a treatable cause of DC [111].

Beta-adrenergic Blockade

Multiple clinical trials have confirmed benefits of beta-blockade in HF patients with T2DM. It was also clearly demonstrated that beta-blockers with addition of angiotensin-converting enzyme inhibitors decrease mortality rates of diabetic congestive HF patients [112, 113].

Cholesterol Reduction

Statins reduce the synthesis of cholesterol and have a multitude of effects proven to reduce the not only the cardiovascular risk, but also the incidence of DC [114]. In the realm of DC, not enough studies have been performed to allow definitive indications for the preventive use of statins.

Fibrates

Since fibrates lower triglyceride/low-density lipoprotein (LDL) levels, raise high-density lipoprotein (HDL) levels, and increase insulin sensitivity they could be an attractive treatment option for hyperlipidemia and hyperinsulinemia that accompany T2DM [115, 116]. Importantly, clinical trials have shown that fibrate therapy may reduce cardiovascular risk factors associated with dyslipidemia and decrease occurrence of coronary events in the diabetic population [117]. Bezafibrate has been shown to prevent not only metabolic dysfunction in sucrose fed animals, but also prevent cardiomyocyte dysfunction seen in these T2DM models [118]. The clinical effects of fibrates and other classes of PPARa agonists should continue to be pursued to determine possible protective effects against type 2 DC.

Antioxidants

Antioxidants could be a promising strategy for the prevention of DC. Experimental data showed a significant increase in ROS production (pre-diabetic insulin-resistant mice), along with abnormal Ca^{2+} signaling and decreased Na^{+}/Ca^{2+} exchanger protein expression. Transgenic mice with an overexpression of catalase restored normal Ca^{2+} signaling and contractile properties despite the lack of effect on insulin sensitivity and post-insulin receptor signaling [119]. Metallothionein overexpression relieved cellular dysfunction in DC except for decreased SERCA2a function [120].

Zinc also acts as an antioxidant and as a part of other antioxidant-related proteins, such as metallothionein and zinc-copper superoxide dismutase. T2DM induced cardiac and renal oxidative damage, inflammation and fibrosis, can be reversed by zinc supplementation [121]. Several clinical observations also support the preventive effect of zinc in the development of DC and nephropathy providing protection against diabetes-induced oxidative damage, inflammation, and fibrosis.

Renin–Angiotensin Aldosterone System Modification

Hyperglycemia has been clearly confirmed as one of the triggers for the activation of the renin–angiotensin aldosterone system (RAAS). Angiotensin II depresses Ca^{2+} sparks and inhibits SERCA2a in heart failure. Candesartan has been shown to restore normal electrical activity in atrial tissue that are impaired by angiotensin II [122]. These results indicate that angiotensin II receptor blockers may show improvements in Ca^{2+} signaling parameters in DC. It is well known, that angiotensin-converting enzyme inhibitors (ACE) decrease cardiovascular risk and all-cause mortality in patients with diabetes, in particular diabetic hypertensive patients with HF. However, it is much less known that ACE inhibitors also increase insulin sensitivity of cells [123–125]. Furthermore, angiotensin II receptor blockers (ARBs) and ACE inhibitors can prevent coronary perivascular fibrosis and collagen deposition [126]. In addition, aldosterone antagonists have been shown to promote positive remodeling in patients with left-ventricular diastolic dysfunction, which may be applicable to T2DM [127]. These drugs modifying the RAAS system have significant positive effects for the treatment of DC.

Calcium Upregulation

Calcium channel blockers increase intracellular calcium to prevent diabetes-induced cardiomyocyte changes. Diltiazem showed possible suppression of muscle hypertrophy, degeneration, and fibrosis caused by hyperglycemia in animal type 1 DM models [128]. Early studies with verapamil demonstrated marked improvement of myosin/ myofibrillary ATPase and SERCA activity in ventricular tissue of STZ-induced type 1 DM animals. Additionally, decreases in diastolic ventricular pressure and increases in the rate of contraction and relaxation were all shown in STZ-treated mice [129, 130]. These data suggest the use of verapamil in treating type 1 DC. STZ-treated animals similarly saw a beneficial effect in insulin sensitivity and cardiac function, as well as reductions in hypertriglyceridemia from treatments with nifedipine [131, 132]. Accordingly, there is a potential for use of CCBs in DC, but additional studies are required to determine and verify the mechanisms of action of CCBs in DC.

Exercise Training

Exercise training has been proven to prevent and improve DC. Reviews of system studies show that exercise training reverses DM-induced free fatty acid metabolism, increases sensitivity to insulin, allows for increased glucose metabolism, increases cardiac output, and can even reverse contractile dysfunction observed in DC [100]. A study in T2DM mice found that interval training reverses myocyte Ca^{2+} handling dysfunction. Mice that underwent the training protocol exhibited a return to normal sarcoplasmic reticulum Ca^{2+} load and a decrease in spontaneous Ca^{2+} waves. The training did not lead to normal blood glucose or insulin levels, suggesting that it may have had a more direct effect on the heart [133]. In recent studies of vigorous long-lasting exercise in a T1DM model (STZ-induced), results demonstrated altered dynamics of cardiomyocyte contraction; however, they did not show a change in the amplitude of contraction or calcium transients, implicating a possible effect of exercise on other states of Ca^{2+} homeostasis [134]. These results illustrate positive overall effects of exercise training in combating DC.

Conclusion

Recent years have yielded new therapies for DC focusing on advanced glycation end products (AGEs) including AGE inhibitors and AGE cross-link breakers, which may provide future directions for DC intervention, treatment, and prevention [27]. The calcium signaling pathway lends itself to several potential DC treatment targets. The most obvious therapeutic strategy for impaired calcium signaling is improving SERCA2a function. Overexpression of SERCA2a in transgenic rats prevented drug-induced DM-induced contractile dysfunction by inhibiting changes in contractile function and calcium handling. A follow-up study showed that doxycycline- induced SERCA2a over expression following the induction of DC improved contractile and calcium signaling parameters [135]. This both confirms the importance of SERCA2a downregulation in diabetic cardiomyopathy and suggests a potential therapeutic target for patients. Overall, PKC inhibition in preventing DC via the calcium signaling pathway seems to be worth pursuing as PKC appears to prevent changes in the expression of calcium-handling proteins [136]. There are numerous options for the treatment of DC, but the best treatment option will depend on, among other things, the type of DM, the individual's response to prescribed therapies and complicating comorbidities.

References

[1] International Diabetes Federation. Diabetes Prevalence. (Available at: http://www.idf.org/home/index.cfm?node=264##.)

[2] Consentino F, Ryden L, Francia P. Diabetes mellitus and metabolic syndrome. In: Camm AJ, Luscher TF, Serruys PW (eds) The ESC Textbook of cardiovascular medicine, Blackwell, London, 2006;p 301–331.

[3] Aguilar D, Deswal A, Ramasubbu K, et al. Comparison of patients with heart failure and preserved left ventricular ejection fraction among those with versus without diabetes mellitus. *Am. J. Cardiol.* 2010;105(3):373-7.

[4] Thrainsdottir IS, Aspelund T, Thorgeirsson G, et al. The association between glucose abnormalities and heart failure in the population-based Reykjavik study. *Diabetes Care* 2005;28:612–616.

[5] Harris MI, Flegal KM, Cowie CC, et al. Prevalence of diabetes, impaired fasting glucose, and impaired glucose tolerance in U.S. adults. The Third National Health and Nutrition Examination Survey1988–1994. *Diabetes Care* 1998;21:518–524.

[6] Kengne AP, Turnbull F, MacMahon S. The Framingham Study, diabetes mellitus and cardiovascular disease: turning back the clock. *Prog. Cardiovasc. Dis.* 2010;53(1):45-51.

[7] He J, Ogden LG, Bazzano LA, et al. Risk factors for congestive heart failure in US men and women: NHANES-I epidemiologic follow-up study. *Arch. Intern. Med.* 2001; 161:996–1002.

[8] Rubler S, Dlugash J, Yuceoglu YZ, et al. New type of cardiomyopathy associated with diabetic glomerulosclerosis. *Am. J. Cardiol.* 1972;30:595–602.

[9] Tarquini R, Lazzeri C, Pala L, et al. The diabetic cardiomyopathy. *Acta Diabetol.* 2011;48(3):173–81.

[10] Boudina S, Abel ED. Diabetic cardiomyopathy revisited. *Circulation* 2007; 115(25):3213–23.
[11] Seferović PM, Lalić NM, Seferović JP, et al. Diabetic cardiomyopathy: old disease or new entity? *Srp. Arh. Celok. Lek.* 2007;135(9–10):576–82.
[12] Ernande L, Bergerot C, Rietzschel ER, et al. Diastolic dysfunction in patients with type 2 diabetes mellitus: is it really the first marker of diabetic cardiomyopathy? *J. Am. Soc. Echocardiogr.* 2011;24(11):1268–75.
[13] Bell DSH. Diabetic Cardiomyopathy. *Diabetes Care* 2003;26:2949–51.
[14] Poornima I, Parikh P, Shannon RP. Diabetic cardiomyopathy: The search for Unifying Hypothesis. *Circ. Res.* 2006;98;596-605.
[15] Bertoni AG, Hundley WG, Massing MW, et al. Heart failure prevalence, incidence, and mortality in the elderly with diabetes. *Diabetes Care* 2004; 27: 699-703.
[16] Rydén L, Standl E, Bartnik M. The Task Force on Diabetes and Cardiovascular Diseases of the European Society of Cardiology (ESC) and of the European Association for the Study of Diabetes (EASD). Guidelines on diabetes, pre-diabetes, and cardiovascular diseases: executive summary. *Eur. Heart J.* 2007;28(1):88–136.
[17] Rathmann W, Haastert B, Icks A, et al. High prevalence of undiagnosed diabetes mellitus in Southern Germany: target populations for efficient screening—The Kora survey 2000. *Diabetologia* 2003; 46: 182–89.
[18] Kannel WB, McGee DL. Diabetes and cardiovascular disease. The Framingham study. *JAMA* 1979; 241: 2035–38.
[19] Stegmayr B, Asplund K. Diabetes as a risk factor for stroke. A population perspective. *Diabetologia* 1995; 38: 1061–8.
[20] Mankovsky BN, Ziegler D. Stroke in patients with diabetes mellitus. *Diabetes Metab. Res. Rev.* 2004; 20: 268–87.
[21] Miettinen H, Haffner SM, Lehto S, et al. Proteinuria predicts stroke and other atherosclerotic vascular disease events in nondiabetic and non-insulin-dependent diabetic subjects. *Stroke* 1996; 27: 2033–9.
[22] Toyry JP, Niskanen LK, Lansimies EA, Partanen KP, Uusitupa MI. Autonomic neuropathy predicts the development of stroke in patients with non-insulin-dependent diabetes mellitus. *Stroke* 1996; 27: 1316–18.
[23] Russell RR 3rd, Yin R, Caplan MJ, et al. Additive effects of hyperinsulinemia and ischemia on myocardial GLUT 1 and GLUT 4 translocation in vivo. *Circulation* 1998; 98(20): 2180-6.
[24] Stevens MJ, Raffel DM, Allman KC et al, et al. Cardiac sympathetic dysinnervation in diabetes: implications for enhanced cardiovascular risk. *Circulation* 1998; 98(10): 961-8.
[25] Nakano S, Kitazawa M, Ito T, et al. Insulin resistant state in type 2 diabetes is related to advanced autonomic neuropathy. *Clin. Exp. Hypertens.* 2003; 25(3): 155-67.
[26] Braz JC, Gregory K, Pathak A, et al. PKC-alpha regulates cardiac contractility and propensity toward heart failure. *Nature Medicine* 2004;10(3):248–254.
[27] Aneja A, Tang WH, Bansilal S, et al. Diabetic cardiomyopathy: insights into pathogenesis, diagnostic challenges, and therapeutic options. *Am. J. Med.* 2008;121:748–757.
[28] Seddon M, Looi YH, Shah AM. Oxidative stress and redox signaling in cardiac hypertrophy and heart failure. *Heart* 2007;93(8):903–907.

[29] Chiu J, Farhangkhoee H, Xu BY, et al. PARP mediates structural alterations in diabetic cardiomyopathy. *J. Mol. Cell. Cardiol.* 2008;45(3):385–393.

[30] Frustaci A, Kajstura J, Chimenti C, et al. Myocardial cell death in human diabetes. *Circ. Res.* 2000;87:1123-1132.

[31] Chen S, Evans T, Mukherjee K, et al. Diabetes-induced myocardial structural changes: role of endothelin-1 and its receptors. *J. Mol. Cell Cardiol.* 2000;32:1621-1629.

[32] Fischer VW, Barner HB, Larose LS. Pathomorphologic aspects of muscular tissue in diabetes mellitus. *Hum. Pathol.* 1984;15:1127-1136.

[33] Shimizu M, Umeda K, Sugihara N, et al. Collagen remodeling in myocardia of diabetic patients. *J. Clin. Pathol.* 1993;46:32-36.

[34] Zieman SJ, Kass DA. Advanced glycation endproduct crosslinking in the cardiovascular system: potential therapeutic target for cardiovascular disease. *Drugs.* 2004;64:459-470.

[35] Rodrigues B, Cam MC, McNeill JH. Metabolic disturbances in diabetic cardiomyopathy. *Mol. Cell Biochem.* 1998;180:53-57.

[36] Eckel J, Reinauer H. Insulin action on glucose transport in isolated cardiac myocytes: signaling pathways and diabetes-induced alterations. *Biochem. Soc. Trans.* 1990; 18:1125-1127.

[37] Liedtke AJ, DeMaison L, Eggleston AM, et al. Changes in substrate metabolism and effects of excess fatty acids in reperfused myocardium. *Circ. Res.* 1988;62:535-542.

[38] Yazaki Y, Isobe M, Takahashi W, et al. Assessment of myocardial fatty acid abnormalities in patients with idiopathic dilated cardiomyopathy using I123 BMIPP SPECT: correlation with clinicopathological findings and clinical course. *Heart.* 1999;81:153-159.

[39] Malhotra A, Sanghi V. Regulation of contractile proteins in diabetic heart. *Cardiovasc. Res.* 1997;34:34-40.

[40] Takeda N, Nakamura I, Hatanaka T, et al. Myocardial mechanical and myosin isoenzyme alterations in streptozotocin-diabetic rats. *Jpn. Heart J.* 1988;29:455-463.

[41] Abe T, Ohga Y, Tabayashi N, et al. Left ventricular diastolic dysfunction in type 2 diabetes mellitus model rats. *Am. J. Physiol. Heart Circ. Physiol.* 2002;282:H138-H148.

[42] Murray AG, Anderson RE, Watson GC, et al. Uncoupling proteins in human heart. *Lancet* 2004; 364: 1786–8.

[43] Swan GW, Anker SD, Walton C, et al. Insulin resistance in chronic failure: relation to severity and etiology of heart failure. *J. Am. Coll. Cardiol.* 1997; 30: 527–32.

[44] Di Bonito P, Moio N, Cavuto L, et al. Early detection of diabetic cardiomyopathy: usefulness of tissue Doppler imaging. *Diabet Med.* 2005; 22(12): 1720-5.

[45] Goldstein RH, Poliks CF, Pilch PF, et al. Stimulation of collagen formation by insulin and insulin-like growth factor I in cultures of human lung fibroblasts. *Endocrinology* 1989; 124: 964–70.

[46] Rutter MK, Parise H, Benjamin EJ, et al. Impact of glucose intolerance and insulin resistance on cardiac structure and function: sex-related differences in the Framingham Heart Study. *Circulation* 2003;107:448–454.

[47] Voulgari C, Moyssakis I, Papazafiropoulou A, et al. The impact of metabolic syndrome on left ventricular myocardial performance. *Diabetes Metab. Res. Rev.* 2010; 26:121–127.

[48] Paternostro G, Pagano D, Gnecchi-Ruscone T, et al. Insulin resistance in patients with cardiac hypertrophy. *Cardiovasc. Res.* 1999;42:246–253.

[49] Malone JI, Schocken DD, Morrison AD, et al. Diabetic cardiomyopathy and carnitine deficiency. *J. Diabetes Complications* 1999;13:86–90.

[50] Kajstura J, Fiordaliso F, Andreoli AM, et al. IGF-1 overexpression inhibits the development of diabetic cardiomyopathy and angiotensin II-mediated oxidative stress. *Diabetes.* 2001;50:1414-1424.

[51] Islam KN, Takahashi M, Higashiyama S, et al. Fragmentation of ceruloplasmin following nonenzymatic glycation reaction. *J. Biochem.* 1995;118:1054-1060.

[52] Argirova MD, Ortwerth BJ. Activation of protein-bound copper ions during early glycation: study on two proteins. *Arch. Biochem. Biophys.* 2003;420:176-184.

[53] Eaton JW, Qian M. Interactions of copper with glycated proteins: possible involvement in the etiology of diabetic neuropathy. *Mol. Cell Biochem.* 2002;234-235:135-142.

[54] Qian M, Eaton JW. Glycochelates and the etiology of diabetic peripheral neuropathy. *Free Radic. Biol. Med.* 2000;28:652-656.

[55] Yim MB, Yim HS, Lee C, et al. Protein glycation: creation of catalytic sites for free radical generation. *Ann. N. Y. Acad. Sci.* 2001;928:48-53.

[56] Bisognano JD, Weinberger HD, Bohlmeyer TJ, et al. Myocardial directed overexpression of the human _(1)-adrenergic receptor in transgenic mice. *J. Mol. Cell Cardiol.* 2000;32:817-830.

[57] Kurata C, Okayama K, Wakabayashi Y, et al. (1997) Cardiac sympathetic neuropathy and effects of aldose reductase inhibitor in streptozocin-induced diabetic rats. *J. Nucl. Med.* 38:1677–1680.

[58] Rota M, LeCapitaine N, Hosoda T, et al. Diabetes promotes cardiac stem cell aging and heart failure, which are prevented by deletion of the p66shc gene. *Circ. Res.* 2006;99:44-52.

[59] Park JY, Takahara N, Gabriele A, et al. Induction of endothelin-1 expression by glucose: an effect of protein kinase C activation. *Diabetes.* 2000;49:1239-1248.

[60] Hattori Y, Kawasaki H, Abe K, et al. Superoxide dismutase recovers altered endothelium-dependent relaxation in diabetic rat aorta. *Am. J. Physiol.* 1991;261: H1086-H1094.

[61] Bucala R, Tracey KJ, Cerami A. Advanced glycosylation products quench nitric oxide and mediate defective endothelium dependent vasodilatation in experimental diabetes. *J. Clin. Invest.* 1991;87:432- 438.

[62] Tesfamariam B, Jakubowski JA, Cohen RA. Contraction of diabetic rabbit aorta caused by endothelium-derived PGH2-TxA2. *Am. J. Physiol.* 1989;257:H1327-H1333.

[63] Tesfamariam B, Brown ML, Cohen RA. Elevated glucose impairs endothelium-dependent relaxation by activating protein kinase C. *J. Clin. Invest.* 1991;87:1643-1648.

[64] Sunni S, Bishop SP, Kent SP, et al. Diabetic cardiomyopathy. A morphological study of intramyocardial arteries. *Arch. Pathol. Lab. Med.* 1986; 110:375–381.

[65] King H, Aubert RE, Herman WH. Global burden of diabetes, 1995–2025: prevalence, numerical estimates, and projections. *Diabetes Care* 1998; 21: 1414–31.

[66] Wild S, Roglic G, Green A, et al. Global prevalence of diabetes: estimates for the year 2000 and projections for 2030. *Diabetes Care* 2004; 27: 1047–53.

[67] Qiao Q. Epidemiology and geography of type 2 diabetes mellitus. In DeFronzo QA, et al., ed. International textbook of diabetes mellitus. Milan: John Wiley & Sons, 2004. p. 33–56.

[68] The DECODE Study Group. Age- and sex-specific prevalences of diabetes and impaired glucose regulation in 13 European cohorts. *Diabetes Care* 2003; 26: 61–9.

[69] Garcia MJ, McNamara PM, Gordon T, et al. Morbidity and mortality in diabetics in the Framingham population. Sixteen year follow-up study. *Diabetes* 1974; 232: 105-11.

[70] Kannel WB, McGee DL. Diabetes and cardiovascular disease. The Framingham study. *JAMA* 1979; 241: 2035–38.

[71] Laakso M. Hyperglycaemia and cardiovascular disease in type 2 diabetes. *Diabetes* 1999; 48: 937–42.

[72] Morrish NJ, Wang SL, Stevens LK, et al. Mortality and causes of death in the WHO multinational study of vascular disease in diabetes. *Diabetologia* 2001; 44 (20): S14–S21.

[73] Paulus WJ, Tschöpe C, Sanderson JE, et al. How to diagnose diastolic heart failure: a consensus statement on the diagnosis of heart failure with normal left ventricular ejection fraction by the Heart Failure and Echocardiography Associations of the European Society of Cardiology. *Eur. Heart J.* 2007; 28: 2539–50.

[74] Pritchett AM, Mahoney DW, Jacobsen SJ, et al. Diastolic dysfunction and left atrial volume: a population based study. *J. Am. Coll. Cardiol.* 2005; 45: 87–92.

[75] Kiencke S, Handschin R, von Dahlen R, et al. Pre-clinical diabetic cardiomyopathy: prevalence, screening, and outcome. *Eur. J. Heart Fail.* 2010 Sep;12(9):951-7.

[76] From AM, Scott CG, Chen HH. Changes in diastolic dysfunction in diabetes mellitus over time. *Am. J. Cardiol.* 2009; 103(10): 1463-6.

[77] Jarnert C, Landstedt-Hallin L, Malmberg K, et al. A randomized trial of the impact of strict glycaemic control on myocardial diastolic function and perfusion reserve: a report from the DADD (Diabetes mellitus And Diastolic Dysfunction) study. *Eur. J. Heart Fail.* 2009; 11(1): 39-47.

[78] Sharman JE, Haluska BA, Fang ZY, et al. Association of arterial wave properties and diastolic dysfunction in patients with type 2 diabetes mellitus. *Am. J. Cardiol.* 2007; 99(6): 844-8.

[79] Seferović Mitrović JP, Seferović PM, Vujisić Tešić B, et al. Predictors of diabetic cardiomyopathy in asymptomatic patients with type 2 diabetes. *Int. J. Cardiol.* 2012 Apr 19;156(2):219-21.

[80] Cosson S, Kevorkian JP, Virally ML, et al. No evidence for left ventricular diastolic dysfunction in asymptomatic normotensive type 2 diabetic patients: a case-control study with new echocardiographic techniques. *Diabetes Metab.* 2007; 33(1): 61-7.

[81] Zabalgoitia M, Ismaeil MF, Anderson L, et al. Prevalence of diastolic dysfunction in normotensive, asymptomatic patients with well-controlled type 2 diabetes mellitus. *Am. J. Cardiol.* 2001; 87(3): 320-3.

[82] Schannwell CM, Schneppenheim M, Perings S, et al. Left ventricular diastolic dysfunction as an early manifestation of diabetic cardiomyopathy. *Cardiology* 2002; 98(1-2): 33-9.

[83] Boyer JK, Thanigaraj S, Schechtman KB, et al. Prevalence of ventricular diastolic dysfunction in asymptomatic, normotensive patients with diabetes mellitus. *Am. J. Cardiol.* 2004; 93(7): 870-5.

[84] Poirier P, Bogaty P, Garneau C, et al. Diastolic dysfunction in normotensive men with well-controlled type 2 diabetes: importance of maneuvers in echocardiographic screening for preclinical diabetic cardiomyopathy. *Diabetes Care* 2001; 24: 5–10.

[85] Srivastava PM, Thomas MC, Calafiore P, et al. Diastolic dysfunction is associated with anaemia in patients with Type II diabetes. *Clin. Sci.* (Lond) 2006; 110(1): 109-16.

[86] Henry RM, Paulus WJ, Kamp O, et al. Deteriorating glucose tolerance status is associated with left ventricular dysfunction-the Hoorn Study. *Neth. J. Med.* 2008; 66(3): 110-7.

[87] Fang ZY, Schull-Meade R, Downey M, et al. Determinants of subclinical diabetic heart disease. *Diabetologia* 2005; 48(2): 394-402.

[88] Takenaka K, Sakamoto T, Amano K, et al. Left ventricular filling determined by Doppler echocardiography in diabetes mellitus. *Am. J. Cardiol.* 1988; 61: 1140–3.

[89] Fonseca CG, Dissanayake AM, Doughty RN, et al. Three-dimensional assessment of left ventricular systolic strain in patients with type 2 diabetes mellitus, diastolic dysfunction, and normal ejection fraction. *Am. J. Cardiol.* 2004; 94(11): 1391-5.

[90] Yazici M, Ozdemir K, Gonen MS, et al. Is there any relationship between metabolic parameters and left ventricular functions in type 2 diabetic patients without evident heart disease? *Echocardiography* 2008; 25(7): 675-82.

[91] Masugata H, Senda S, Goda F, et al. Left ventricular diastolic dysfunction in normotensive diabetic patients in various age strata. *Diabetes Res. Clin. Prac.* 2008; 79(1): 91-6.

[92] Liu JE, Palmieri V, Roman MJ, et al. The impact of diabetes on left ventricular filling pattern in normotensive and hypertensive adults: the Strong Heart Study. *J. Am. Coll. Cardiol.* 2001; 37(7): 1943-9.

[93] Markuszewski L, Grycewicz T, Pietruszyński R, et al. Glycosylated hemoglobin and left ventricular diastolic dysfunction in patients with type 2 diabetes mellitus. *Pol. Merkur Lekarski* 2006; 21(121): 8-11.

[94] Bajraktari G, Koltai MS, Ademaj F, et al. Relationship between insulin resistance and left ventricular diastolic dysfunction in patients with impaired glucose tolerance and type 2 diabetes. *Int. J. Cardiol.* 2006; 110(2): 206-11.

[95] Guo CY, Shen LH, Li HW, et al. Relation of Hemoglobin A1c to myocardial acoustic densitometry and left ventricular diastolic function in patients with type 2 diabetes mellitus and without evident heart disease. *Diabetes Res. Clin. Pract.* 2009; 83(3): 365-70.

[96] Matthews DR, Hosker JP, Rudenski AS, et al: Homeostasis model assessment: insulin resistance and beta-cell function from fasting plasma glucose and insulin concentrations in man. *Diabetologia* 1985; 28: 412-9.

[97] Katz A, Nambi SS, Mather K, et al. Quantitative insulin sensitivity check index: a simple, accurate method for assessing insulin sensitivity in humans. *J. Clin. Endocrinol. Metab.* 2000; 85: 2402–10.

[98] Ozasa N, Furukawa Y, Morimoto T, et al. Relation among left ventricular mass, insulin resistance, and hemodynamic parameters in type 2 diabetes. *Hypertens. Res.* 2008; 31(3): 425-32.

[99] Duman D, Demirtunç R, Karadağ B, Karataş M. Association of albuminuria with impaired aortic elasticity and left ventricular diastolic dysfunction in type 2 diabetes. *Anadolu Kardiyol. Derg.* 2008; 8(1): 10-5.

[100] Isfort M, Stevens SC, Schaffer S, Jong CJ, Wold LE. Metabolic dysfunction in diabetic cardiomyopathy. *Heart Fail Rev*. 2013 Feb 27. [Epub ahead of print].

[101] von Bibra H, Hansen A, Dounis V, et al. Augmented metabolic control improves myocardial diastolic function and perfusion in patients with non-insulin dependent diabetes. *Heart* 224;90:1483–1484.

[102] von Bibra H, Siegmund T, Hansen A, et al. Augmentation of myocardial function by improved glycemic control in patients with type 2 diabetes mellitus. *Dtsch. Med. Wochenschr.* 2007;132:729–734.

[103] McGuire DK, Inzucchi SE. New drugs for the treatment of diabetes mellitus: part I: thiazolidinediones and their evolving cardiovascular implications. *Circulation* 2008;117:440–449.

[104] Sharma AM, Staels B. Review: peroxisome proliferator-activated receptor gamma and adipose tissue–understanding obesity-related changes in regulation of lipid and glucose metabolism. *J. Clin. Endocrinol. Metab.* 2007;92:386–395.

[105] Masoudi FA, Inzucchi SE. Diabetes mellitus and heart failure: epidemiology, mechanisms, and pharmacotherapy. *Am. J. Cardiol.* 2007;99:113B–132B.

[106] Masoudi FA, Inzucchi SE, Wang Y, et al. Thiazolidinediones, metformin, and outcomes in older patients with diabetes and heart failure: an observational study. *Circulation* 2005;111:583–590.

[107] Nikolaidis LA, Elahi D, Hentosz T, et al. Recombinant glucagon- like peptide-1 increases myocardial glucose uptake and improves left ventricular performance in conscious dogs with pacing-induced dilated cardiomyopathy. *Circulation* 2004;110:955–961.

[108] Sokos GG, Nikolaidis LA, Mankad S, et al. Glucagon-like peptide-1 infusion improves left ventricular ejection fraction and functional status in patients with chronic heart failure. *J. Card. Fail.* 2006;12:694–699.

[109] Chiasson JL, Josse RG, Gomis R, et al. Acarbose for prevention of type 2 diabetes mellitus: the STOP-NIDDM randomised trial. *Lancet* 2002;359:2072–2077.

[110] Hanefeld M, Josse RG, Chiasson JL. Alpha-glucosidase inhibitors for patients with type 2 diabetes: response to van de Laar, et al. *Diabet Care* 2005;28:1840 (author reply 1).

[111] Konduracka E, Gackowski A, Rostoff P, et al. Diabetes-specific cardiomyopathy in type 1 diabetes mellitus: no evidence for its occurrence in the era of intensive insulin therapy. *Eur. Heart J.* 2007;28:2465–2471.

[112] Haas SJ, Vos T, Gilbert RE, et al. Are beta-blockers as efficacious in patients with diabetes mellitus as in patients without diabetes mellitus who have chronic heart failure? A meta-analysis of large-scale clinical trials. *Am. Heart J.* 2003;146:848–853.

[113] Fonseca V, Bakris GL, Bell DS, et al. Differential effect of beta-blocker therapy on insulin resistance as a function of insulin sensitizer use: results from GEMINI. *Diabet. Med.* 2007;24: 759–763.

[114] Ramasubbu K, Estep J, White DL, et al. Experimental and clinical basis for the use of statins in patients with ischemic and nonischemic cardiomyopathy. *J. Am. Coll. Cardiol.* 2008;51:415–426.

[115] Rubenstrunk A, Hanf R, Hum DW, et al. Safety issues and prospects for future generations of PPAR modulators. *Biochim. Biophys. Acta* 2007;1771:1065–1081.

[116] Goa KL, Barradell LB, Plosker GL. Bezafibrate. An update of its pharmacology and use in the management of dyslipidaemia. *Drugs* 1996;52:725–753.

[117] Gross B, Staels B. PPAR agonists: multimodal drugs for the treatment of type-2 diabetes. *Best Pract. Res. Clin. Endocrinol. Metab.* 2007;21:687–710.

[118] Davidoff AJ, Mason MM, Davidson MB, et al. Sucroseinduced cardiomyocyte dysfunction is both preventable and reversible with clinically relevant treatments. *Am. J. Physiol. Endocrinol. Metab.* 2004;286:E718–E724.

[119] Dong F, Fang CX, Yang X, et al. Cardiac overexpression of catalase rescues cardiac contractile dysfunction induced by insulin resistance: role of oxidative stress, protein carbonyl formation and insulin sensitivity. *Diabetologia* 2006;49:1421–1433.

[120] Wold LE, Ceylan-Isik AF, Fang CX, et al. Metallothionein alleviates cardiac dysfunction in streptozotocin-induced diabetes: role of Ca^{2+} cycling proteins, NADPH oxidase, poly(ADPRibose) polymerase and myosin heavy chain isozyme. *Free Radic. Biol. Med.* 2006; 40:1419–1429.

[121] Li B, Tan Y, Sun W, Fu Y, Miao L, Cai L. The role of zinc in the prevention of diabetic cardiomyopathy and nephropathy. *Toxicol. Mech. Methods*. 2013;23(1):27-33.

[122] Yaras N, Bilginoglu A, Vassort G, et al. Restoration of diabetes-induced abnormal local Ca^{2+} release in cardiomyocytes by angiotensin II receptor blockade. *Am. J. Physiol. Heart Circ. Physiol*. 2007;292:H912–H920.

[123] Shekelle PG, Rich MW, Morton SC, et al. Efficacy of angiotensin-converting enzyme inhibitors and beta-blockers in the management of left ventricular systolic dysfunction according to race, gender, and diabetic status: a meta-analysis of major clinical trials. *J. Am. Coll. Cardiol.* 2003;41:1529–1538.

[124] Sowers JR, Epstein M, Frohlich ED. Diabetes, hypertension, and cardiovascular disease: an update. *Hypertension* 2001;37:1053–1059.

[125] Murarka S, Movahed MR. Diabetic cardiomyopathy. *J. Card. Fail.* 2010;16:971–979.

[126] Zaman AK, Fujii S, Goto D, et al. Salutary effects of attenuation of angiotensin II on coronary perivascular fibrosis associated with insulin resistance and obesity. *J. Mol. Cell Cardiol.* 2004;37:525–535.

[127] Orea-Tejeda A, Colin-Ramirez E, Castillo-Martinez L, et al. Aldosterone receptor antagonists induce favorable cardiac remodeling in diastolic heart failure patients. *Rev. Invest. Clin.* 2007;59:103–107.

[128] Shimada T. Correlation between metabolic and histopathological changes in the myocardium of the KK mouse. Effect of diltiazem on the diabetic heart. *Jpn. Heart J.* 1993;34:617–626.

[129] Afzal N, Ganguly PK, Dhalla KS, et al. Beneficial effects of verapamil in diabetic cardiomyopathy. *Diabetes* 1988;37:936–942.

[130] Afzal N, Pierce GN, Elimban V, et al. Influence of verapamil on some subcellular defects in diabetic cardiomyopathy. *Am. J. Physiol*. 1989;256:E453–E458.

[131] Shah TS, Satia MC, Gandhi TP, et al. Effects of chronic nifedipine treatment on streptozotocin-induced diabetic rats. *J. Cardiovasc. Pharmacol*. 1995;26:6–12.

[132] Higa S, Shimabukuro M, Shinzato T, et al. Long-term nifedipine treatment reduces calcium overload in isolated reperfused hearts of diabetic rats. *Gen. Pharmacol*. 1995; 26:1679–1686.

[133] Stolen TO, Hoydal MA, Kemi OJ, et al. Interval training normalizes cardiomyocyte function, diastolic Ca^{2+} control, and SR Ca^{2+} release synchronicity in a mouse model of diabetic cardiomyopathy. *Circ. Res*. 1999;105:527–536.

[134] Howarth FC, Almugaddum FA, Qureshi MA, et al. The effects of heavy long-term exercise on ventricular myocyte shortening and intracellularCa^{2+}in streptozotocin-induced diabetic rat. *J. Diabet Complicat.* 2010; 24:278–285.

[135] Suarez J, Scott B, Dillmann WH. Conditional increase in SERCA2a protein is able to reverse contractile dysfunction and abnormal calcium flux in established diabetic cardiomyopathy. *Am. J. Physiol. Regul. Integr. Comp. Physiol.* 2008;295:R1439–R1445.

[136] Wang M, Zhang WB, Zhu JH, et al. Breviscapine ameliorates cardiac dysfunction and regulates the myocardial Ca(2+)-cycling proteins in streptozotocin-induced diabetic rats. *Acta Diabetol.* 2010;47:209–218.

In: Recent Advances in Cardiology
Editors: José Milei and Giuseppe Ambrosio

ISBN: 978-1-63117-282-3

Chapter 5

Chronic Chagasic Cardiomyopathy

G. Risso, F. Azzato and J. Milei[*]
Instituto de Investigaciones Cardiológicas
"Prof. Dr. Alberto C. Taquini," Buenos Aires, Argentina

Abstract

Chronic chagasic cardiomyopathy (ChrChC) is the most serious and most common type of chronic myocarditis in the world. Our experience, both clinical and experimental for more than 30 years, is summarized in the present chapter.

The disease is caused by the flagellate parasite Trypanosoma cruzi (*T cruzi*). The insect vectors are present throughout most of South and Central America, and their zone of distribution extends across the southern United States. Other forms of transmission include blood transfusion, intravenous drug abuse, digestive, transplacentary, breast feeding, and organ transplant. Considering these varied forms of transmission and the increasing immigration rates this disease gains importance in the United States and Europe as well.

The infection is characterized by an acute symptomatic phase with high parasitemia, and is followed by a lifelong indeterminate phase in which low numbers of parasites are sequestered in tissues; however, the acute phase often is clinically silent. Chronic progressive Chagas' disease develops in 10% to 20% of previously asymptomatic patients, 15 to 30 years after the infection. It is manifested by a chronic, diffuse, progressive fibrosing myocarditis that involves not only the working myocardium but also the atrioventricular conduction system. This leads to cardiomegaly, cardiac failure, arrhythmias, thromboembolic phenomena, and death. Megacolon and megaesophagus may also occur, considering that Chagas disease is not restricted to the cardiovascular region.

Given the fact that in the chronic phase there is low parasitemia, the diagnosis relies on serologic studies. Nevertheless direct studies can be used in reactivations of the disease in patients with HIV or immunosuppression states. Patients with higher mortality risk showed clinical manifestations such as third tone, right bundle branch block with left anterior hemiblock and left ventricle dilation. Chronic recurrent ventricular tachycardia

[*] E-mail: ininca@fmed.uba.ar.

often occurs in patients with chagasic aneurysms, and ventricular mapping indicates that these arrhythmias originate in regions adjacent to those aneurysms. ChrChC is characterized by the presence of multifocal inflammatory infiltrates, composed mainly by mononuclear cells, adhered to myocytes and leading to myocytolysis, and by interstitial fibrosis with or without apical ventricular aneurysms. These lesions seems to be mediated by immune phenomena rather than by continuing parasitic invasion of the heart. The treatment is limited to the acute phase using benznidazole or nifurtimox; although some authors support this treatment also in the undetermined phase. Heart transplantation might be a useful therapy for end-stage ChrChC; however, disease reactivation remains a mayor complication.

Introduction

Chronic chagasic cardiomyopathy is the most serious and most common type of chronic myocarditis in the world [1]. It has been extensively reviewed in the last years by our team and our experience, both clinical and experimental for more than 30 years, will be summarized in the present chapter [2-21].

Chagas disease, a chronic illness caused by the flagellate parasite Trypanosoma cruzi (*T cruzi*), was first described in 1909 by the Brazilian physician Carlos Chagas [4]. The insect vectors of the disease are present throughout most of South and Central America, and their zone of distribution extends across the southern United States. Several animal species in this zone are affected by the disease in their natural habitats. [6].

In the endemic areas, approximately 90 million people are estimated to be at risk of infection, being 16-18 million already infected. Due to the parasite distribution throughout Central and South America, it is commonly known as the 'American trypanosomiasis'. In non-endemic countries, the disease is transmitted through blood transfusions, organ donations, and from mother to child at birth. As such, it is considered to be an exotic' disease in Europe and USA, where it is virtually undiagnosed. However, thanks to free circulation of individuals and employment opportunities Europe and USA are a magnet for millions of immigrants, many of whom are from South America. However, besides possible occurrence of new cases of infection, substantial concern exists regarding the progressive development of cardiomyopathy in many individuals who had already become infected in their native country, and then move to Europe and USA [2, 9, 10].

The infection is characterized by an acute symptomatic phase with high parasitemia, and is followed by a lifelong indeterminate phase in which low numbers of parasites are sequestered in tissues [11]; however, the acute phase often is clinically silent. Chronic progressive Chagas' disease develops in 10% to 20% of previously asymptomatic patients, 15 to 30 years after the infection. It is manifested by a chronic, diffuse, progressive fibrosing myocarditis that involves not only the working myocardium but also the atrioventricular conduction system [7, 12, 13, 15]. This leads to cardiomegaly, cardiac failure, arrhythmias, thromboembolic phenomena, and death [1, 5, 14]. Megacolon and megaesophagus may also occur, considering that Chagas disease is not restricted to the cardiovascular region.

Pathology

In a series of pathological, immunohistochemical, ultrastructural and morphological studies completed by Milei et al. [5-7, 11-17] that involved endomyocardial biopsies and autopsies of patients suffering from chronic chagasic cardiomyopathy (ChrChC), the pathogenic mechanism underlying this disease was explained.

All the autopsied hearts presented severe dilatation (Figure 1A), flattening of the papillary muscles and a marked subendocardial sclerosis related to an increased end diastolic pressure.

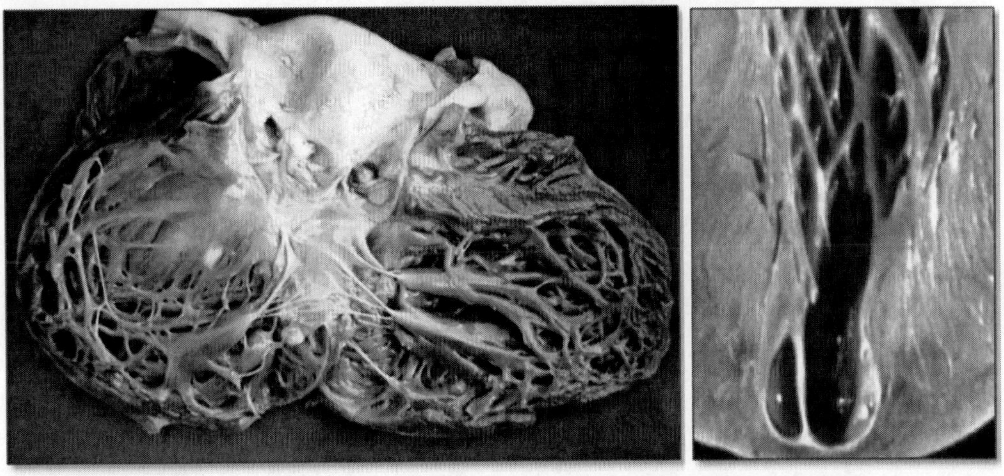

A B

Reproduced from Milei et al. [5] with permission.

Figure 1. A. High grade heart dilatation. Thinning of the apical wall of the left ventricle and cavitary thrombus. B. Characteristic apical aneurysm..

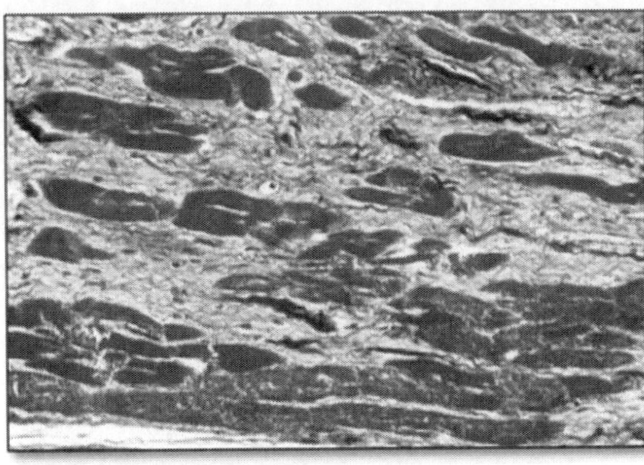

Figure 2. Endomyocardial biopsy showing atrophy of myocytes, myocitolysis and extensive replacement of myocardium by fibrosis. Masson Trichome. X100.

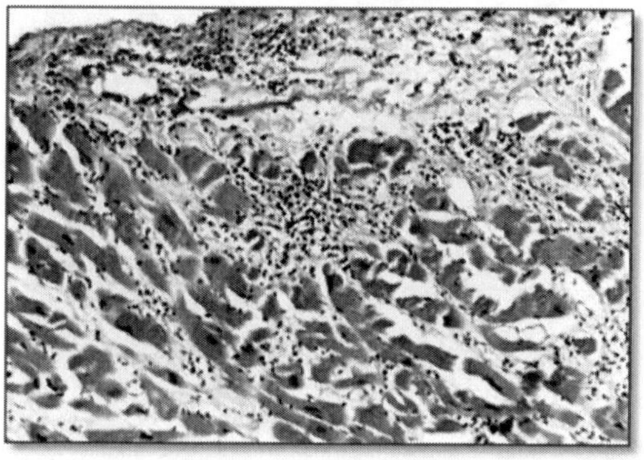

Reproduced from Milei et al. [5] with permission.

Figure 3. Severe myocarditis. Extensive mononuclear infiltrates, myocyte loss, and subendocardial fibrosis. Hematoxylin and eosin stain, X25.

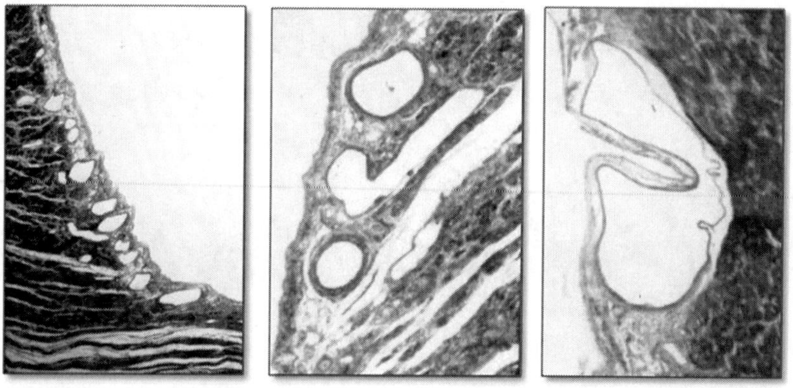

Reproduced from Milei et al. [5] with permission.

Figure 4. Severe dilation of lymphatic vessels belonging to subepicardium (A) and apex of the left ventricle (B, C).

A remarkable thinning of the left ventricular wall was characteristic at the apical areas. Intracavitary thrombi were also found. Microscopically, myocardial lesions consisted of a chronic inflammatory process with fibrotic scars (Figure 2) and extensive mononuclear infiltrates (Figure 3). No amastigote nests were found. Extensive myocytolysis and spotty contraction band necrosis were observed. Cell hypertrophy in the apparently preserved myocytes was revealed by hyperthrophic bizarre nuclei. Dilated lymphatic channels widespread in the ventricular septum and in the AV node, His bundle, and in the root of the right and left bundles branch were observed. In the case of apical aneurysm of the left ventricle, dilated lymphatic were distributed in the subepicardium (Figure 4)

The serial sectioning of the conducting system showed mild to moderate diffuse fibrosis of the AV node (Figure 5) and of the penetrating and branching portions of the His bundle, complete destruction of the proximal segments of the right and left bundles branch by varying degrees of replacement by dense collagen tissue (Figure 6). The remaining specialized fibers presented atrophy and mild fatty infiltration and were surrounded in most cases by infiltrates consisting mainly of lymphocytes and macrophages. The subendocardial Purkinje fibers were usually damaged by chronic inflammation and fibrosis. A statistical significant difference ($p<0.05$) was obtained when the percentage of fibrosis was compared in the specialized vs. contracting myocardiums (51.6% vs. 43.4%). Eosinophils were scarce in infiltrates reaching 5%, and they were associated with necrotic myocardium. Mast cells also were scarce or absent in specialized and in contracting myocardium. Almost all the lymphocytic population was T lymphocytes. Such infiltrates were more prominent in the working myocardium (39%) and in the specialized cells of the left branch of the His bundle than in the atrioventricular node and in the right Hisian branch (34.4%). The 31% of mononuclear cells were CD68 positive, thus corresponding to macrophages.

A set of endomyocardial biopsy studies were performed [7, 15-17].

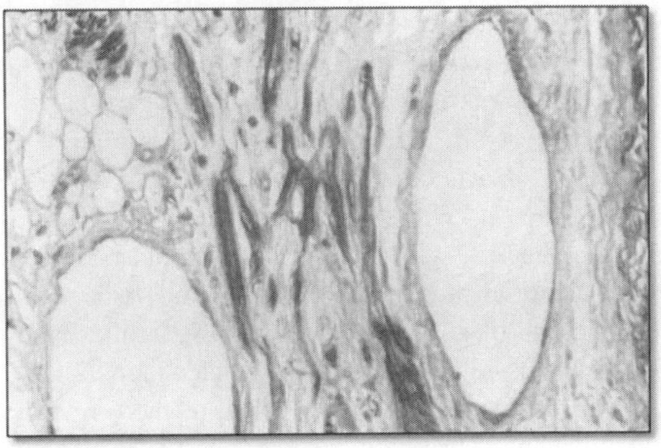

Reproduced from Milei et al. [5] with permission.

Figure 5. Serial sectioning of the conducting system showing mild to moderate diffuse fibrosis of the AV node.

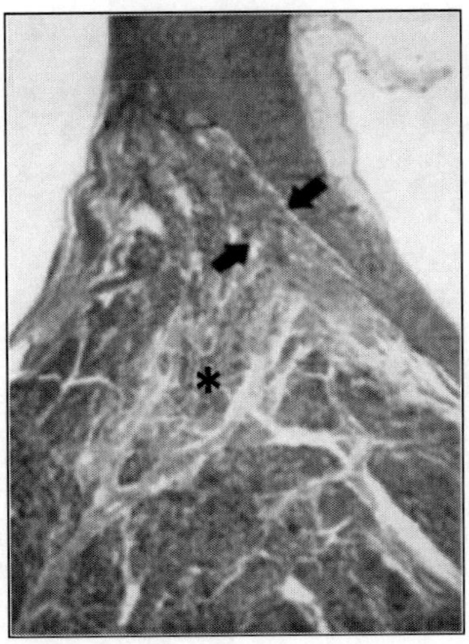

Reproduced from Milei et al. [5] with permission.

Figure 6. Bifurcating His bundle showing severe fibrosis at the left branch (between arrows). The right branch (asterisk) is intramyocardial and surrounded by connective tissue. Mallory trichome, X25.

Endomyocardial biopsies specimens showed mild to moderate hypertrophy of the myocytes and variable degrees of interstitial fibrosis. Lesions consisted of a chronic inflammatory process with fibrotic areas and mononuclear cellular infiltrates. The lesions showed a microfocal disposition. Coagulative necrosis and myocytolysis were frequently observed. A marked subendocardial sclerosis, presumably due to an increased end diastolic pressure was also observed (Figure 7). Tissue forms of trypanosomes were not found. Mononuclear cell infiltrates were found in 83% of the samples (Figure 8). The percentage of fibrous tissue was 24.1%. Eosinophils were scarce, but associated with necrotic areas of the myocardium. Mast cells were scarce or absent. They were always situated in fibrotic areas. The most remarkable finding was the presence of infiltrates consisting of macrophages and common leucocyte antigen (CLA) positive mononuclear cells. Twenty-six and one-half percent of them were T lymphocytes and 10.5% were B lymphocytes. Lymphocytic infiltration was particularly associated with necrotic and degenerative myocardial lesions. Thirty percent of the infiltrate was composed of macrophages (positive CD68 cells). The remaining infiltrate was composed of mononuclear cells resembling macrophages and CLA-negative mononuclear cells. Contacts between CD68 positive cells and T lymphocytes were frequently found (Figure 9 and 10). CD31 antibodies clearly pointed out normal endothelial cells, in either normal or damaged vessels (Figure 11). Rare platelet thrombi were observed in capillaries. Other striking alteration was the thickening of the basement membranes of cardiac myocytes, endothelium and vascular smooth muscle up to 20 times their normal thickness of 500 Å (Figure 12 A-C) [13]. Light (peroxidase-labeled antibodies) and electron (gold conjugated antibody) microscopic immunohistochemical methods revealed a positive reaction for laminin in these thickened basement membranes [13]. The thickened basement membranes appeared structurally homogeneous, without being multilayered or subdivided into a lamina rara and a lamina densa. They were of relatively low electron density, had a finely fibrillar appearance at high magnification and measured up to 1 um in thickness. These were confirmed by later studies using ultrastructural immunohistochemistry [15-17].

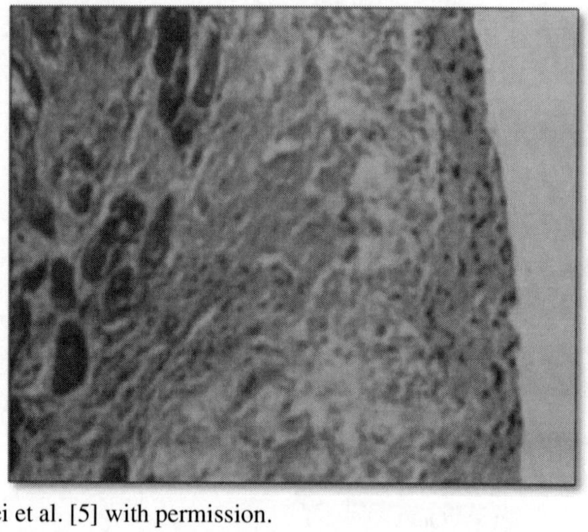

Reproduced from Milei et al. [5] with permission.

Figure 7. A marked subendocardial sclerosis is observed. Masson Trichome. X100.

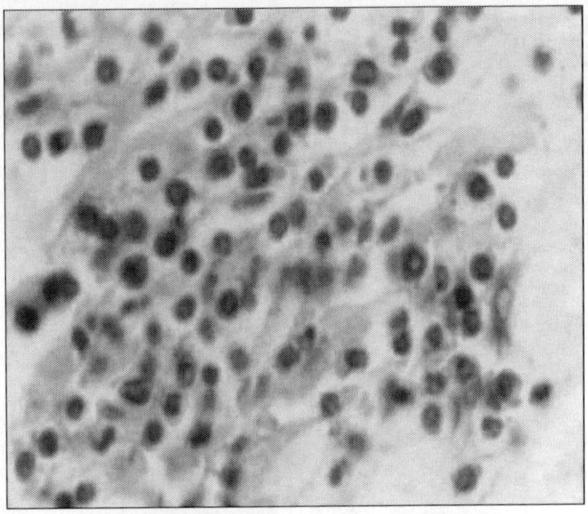

Reproduced from Milei et al. [5] with permission.

Figure 8. Serial section as in Figure 6. A detail of the left bundle of His is shown. Immunostaining for T lymphocyte. Positive cells express CD45R0 antigen (brown); specialized myocardial cells have almost disappeared. Extensive mononuclear infiltrate, the majority of them being T lymphocytes. X20.

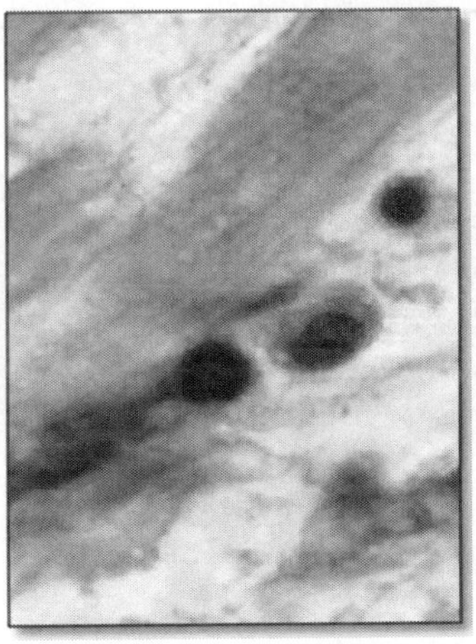

Reproduced from Milei et al. [5] with permission.

Figure 9. Double immunostaining for the simultaneous demonstration of T lymphocytes (CD45RO) and macrophages (CD68). Two close mononuclear cells in the neighbourhood of damaged myocytes. The T lymphocyte (brown) has a close contact with the sarcolemma. The macrophage, negative for CD68 antibody (large nucleus and pinky cytoplasm) is also very close to a round cell, presumably a B lymphocyte. X1000.

This thickening of basement membranes may develop as a consequence of: (1) an immunologic reaction that is triggered by the presence of a laminin-like molecule on the surfaces of *T cruzi* amastigotes and trypomastigotes; (2) an immunologic response to direct injury of basement membranes causing some of their components to become antigenic; (3) myocardial fibrosis, with synthesis of new connective tissue components; and (4) a combination of the preceding factors [4, 18]. The relationship of these changes to antilaminin antibodies requires clarification.

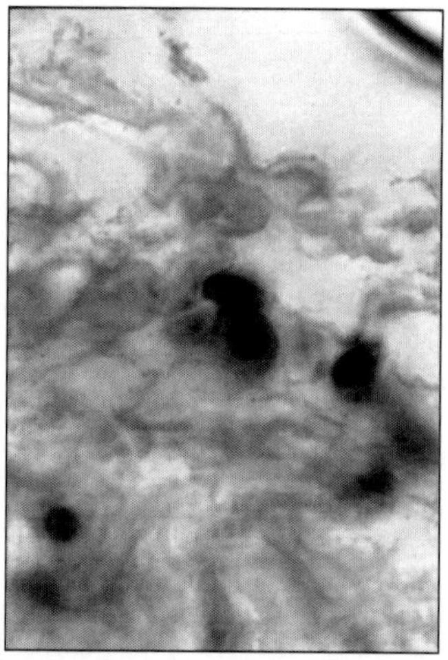

Reproduced from Milei et al. [5] with permission.

Figure 10. Double immunostaining for the simultaneous demonstration of T lymphocytes (CD45RO) and macrophages (CD68). T lymphocytes (brown) in close contact with a macrophage (pinky cytoplasm). X1000.

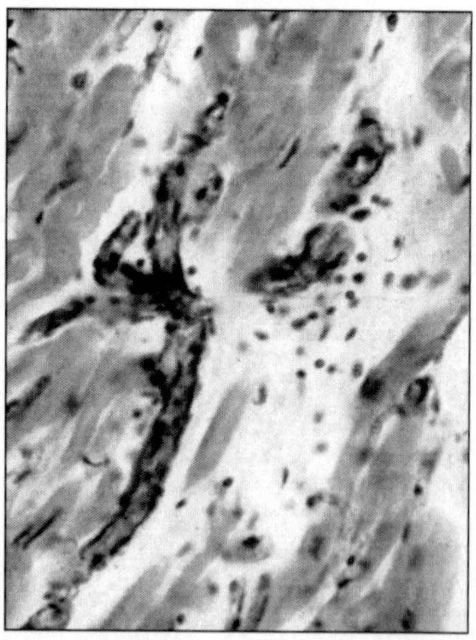

Reproduced from Milei et al. [5] with permission.

Figure 11. Immunostaining for endothelial cells. Capillaries and small vessels are clearly showed by the expression of CD31. Vessels are mildly or moderately distorted because of the surrounding fibrosis. X100.

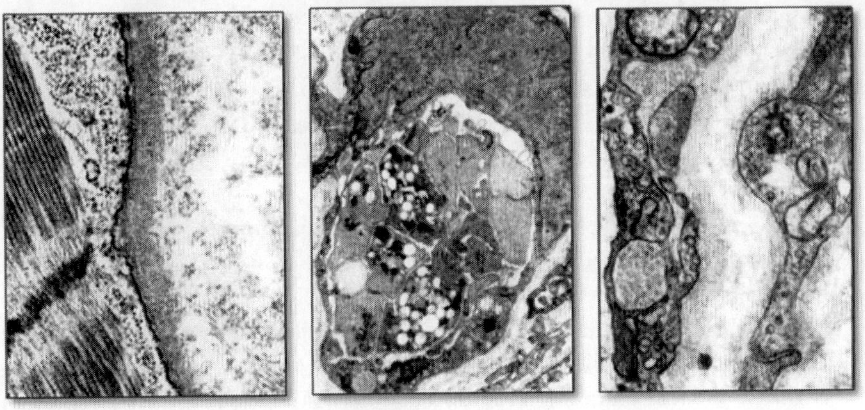

Reproduced from Milei et al. [5] with permission.

Figure 12. A. Myocardial fibre with thickened basement membrane. B. Platelet thrombus within a capillary. C. Thickened basement membranes in a myocardial fibre and a capillary.

Pathogenesis

Milei et al. [4, 7] proposed a combined theory that could explain the pathogenic mechanism in chronic ChrChC. This theory is based on three ingredients: the parasite, macrophages and lymphocytes and the fibrosis (Figure 13).

First ingredient: The parasite. The role of *T cruzi* in the chronic phase has been previously underestimated due to the fact that its presence was believed to be scarce and unrelated to the inflammatory infiltrate present at this stage [6]. Nowadays, the involvement of the parasite in the chronic phase has been well documented. Using dissimilar methods, different authors demonstrated either the persistence of *T cruzi* or parasite antigens in mice [22], the parasite DNA sequence amplified by the polymerase chain reaction (PCR) [23], *T cruzi* antigens from inflammatory lesions in human chagasic cardiomyopathy [24] or the immunohistochemical finding of the parasite in endomyocardial biopsies with PCR confirmation [25]. This would suggest a direct role for the parasite in the perpetuation of myocardial inflammation. In other words, the antigen stimulation would persist throughout the chronic stage, even though the parasites are not morphologically detectable by light microscopy. A delayed type of hypersensitivity reaction might also play an important role in this pathology [26]. Teixeirá et al. [27] have postulated the insertion of *T cruzi* DNA sequences into the host cell genome. Regardless the form of lesional parasite DNA, the ChrChC may be a consequence of the continued persistence of *T cruzi* or its parts at the site of the lesion [23]. Studies like the one performed by Garcia et al. [28], which demonstrate that treatment with benznidazole in the chronic phase of Chagas disease prevents the development of severe chronic cardiomyopathy are also able to highlight the role of the parasite persistence in this stage of the disease. In addition, several studies showed a correlation in between parasite infection and the clinical manifestation. Jones et al. [23] showed that *T cruzi* DNA was consistently amplified in 18 of 21 hearts of patients with severe ChrChC but it was never amplified in hearts of seropositive patients with no cardiac involvement.

Second ingredient: Macrophages and lymphocytes. Is chronic ChrChC an autoimmune mediated disease? As described earlier, mononuclear cells persist in the chronic stage of the disease, contributing to the inflammation through its products of secretion or through its own cytotoxicity (suppressor T cells) and cytolytic action (macrophages) [22]. Apparently only autoimmunity may explain that all the process is restricted to the myocardium [29]. Autoimmunity may be explained by the presence of cross-reactivity antigens between myocardium and T. *cruzi* or because the polyclonal activation might liberate antiautoclones during the acute phase that may persist a long time in the host [30]. Various reports support the hypothesis that circulating antibodies in Chagasic patients interact with myocardial ß adrenergic and muscarinic cholinergic receptors. Borda and Borda et al. [31, 32] have shown that the interaction of antibodies with cardiac neurotransmitter receptors behaving as an agonist, triggers intracellular signal transductions in the cells that could produce physiological, biochemical and pharmacological alteration of the heart. These antibodies could induce desensitization or down regulation of the receptors producing sympathetic or parasympathetic alterations seen in Chagas disease [31].

Third ingredient: The fibrosis. Fibrosis causes the progressive loss of the contracting capacity of the heart [33]. Patients with ChrChC exhibit heart failure in the late stage of the disease [2, 22]. Ultrastructural studies have described degeneration of organelles, hyperthrophy of myocytes with thickening of the basement membranes of these cells, endothelium and vascular smooth muscle cells and increased fibrosis [13, 34]. Schaper et al. [35] in chronic dilated cardiomyopathy showed impairment of the myocardial ultrastructure and changes of the cytoskeleton. They concluded that the increase of fibrosis, the degeneration of hypertrophied myocytes, and the alterations of the cytoskeleton (increase of desmin, tubulin and vinculin) are the morphologic correlates of reduced myocardial function in chronic heart disease. A similar pattern may be suspected in ChrChC.

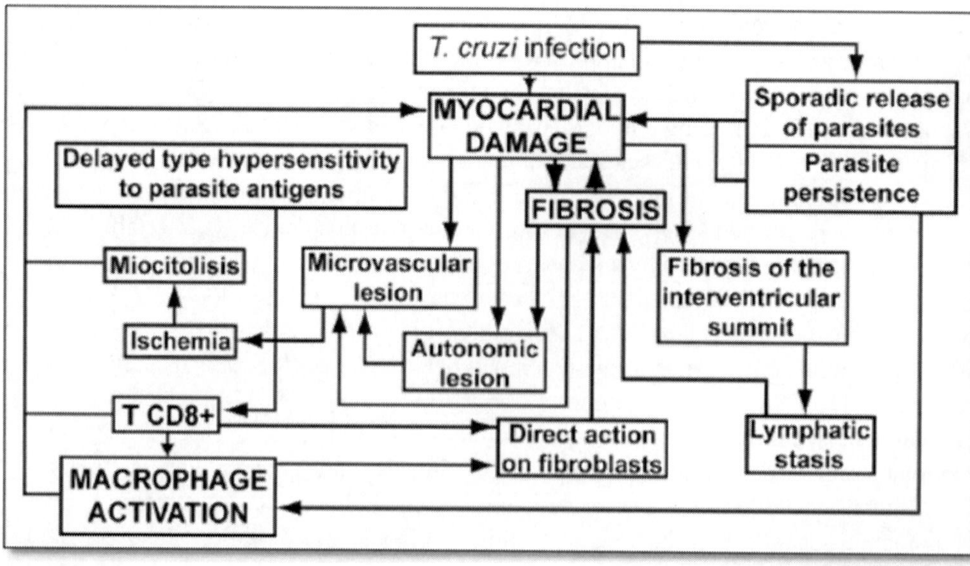

Reproduced from Milei et al. [4] with permission.

Figure 13. Combined theory. Factors involved in the production of myocardial damage in chronic Chagas' cardiomyopathy.

Ventricular Aneurysm

An apical aneurysm (Figure 1B) is generally accepted as the cardinal sign of cardiac involvement in ChrChC. The lesion varies from a fibrotic, localized thinning of the wall to a saccular aneurysm; frequently the involvement reaches an extent that only a layer of tissue remains. According to different authors, the incidence of this lesion varied from 30 to 60%. Oliveira et al. [36] reported an overall incidence of 52% of aneurysms in 1078 autopsies from patients suffering from chronic Chagasic cardiomyopathy. The site of the aneurysm was found as being at the left ventricular apex in 82%, the right ventricular apex in 9% and in both apices in 9%. Acquatella [37], in an echocardiographic study reported that 47-64% of the symptomatic patients and 1.6-8.6% of the asymptomatic patients with ChrChC had ventricular aneurysms. Concordantly, Carod-Artal et al. [38] reported that out of 94 patients diagnosed with ischemic stroke who were seropositive for Chagas disease, 35 of them (37%) presented ventricular aneurysms. These findings appeared in 19 patients with cardiac symptoms of chagasic cardiomyopathy and in 16 patients with chronic indetermined form of Chagas' disease.

Chronic recurrent ventricular tachycardia often occurs in patients with Chagasic aneurysms. Ventricular mapping indicates that these arrhythmias originate in regions adjacent to those aneurysms [14]. In a study performed by Milei et al. [14] attention was paid to the morphology of chronic Chagasic aneurysms in terms of their role as a source of malignant arrhythmias. The study was performed in surgically removed apical aneurysms from patients with ChrChC. All the patients had been resuscitated from an episode of near-miss sudden death occurring out of hospital before surgery. The endocardium of all surgically excised aneurysms was thickened. The thickness of myocardial bundles varied from 42 (very few atrophic myocytes) to 457.8 μm (approximately 12 cells across its diameter). These bundles were separated completely by the matrix of collagenous tissue. Thick and thin bundles were randomly distributed throughout the width of the excised aneurysms. The diameter of myocytes ranged from 4.5 to 56.6 μm. The myocardium showed a chronic inflammatory reaction and scattered polynuclear cells. There was myocytolysis and extensive fibrosis, more often seen in the subendocardial layers. The presence of "islets" was common. They consisted of normal, damaged or necrotic myocytes surrounded by fibrous tissue. These islets predominated in the areas previously identified as arrhythmogenic. It was assumed that these fibers had abnormal morphologic characteristics related to the myocardial damage produced by Chagas' disease [13]. Both thick and thin bundles consisted of small foci of established necrosis and layers of myocardium showing early damage separated by thick strands of apparently normal myocytes. The histological picture, therefore, is one of heterogeneous layers of interwoven myocardial cells. When serial sections were reconstituteda clear continuity of the different layers was demonstrated. The electron microscopic studies showed hypertrophy of myocytes, manifested by an increased transverse diameter and a variety of alterations, such as partial or complete loss of myofibrils; large thickenings of the Z band to almost complete loss of the myofibrils and swelling of mitochondria and disruption of mitochondrial cristae, accumulation of lipofuscin granules, focal accumulations of glycogen particles, and areas of intracellular edema. Most of the cells had intact sarcolemmas and normal nuclei, with well dispersed chromatin strongly suggesting that some were still viable. Purkinje fibers were rarely seen and, when found, appeared to be structurally normal.

Ventricular tachycardia is usually prevented by surgical resection of subendocardial regions of aneurysms. This suggests that those cardiac fibers causing the arrhythmia are removed by the procedure. These fibers have abnormal morphologic and electrophysiological characteristics and may be the origin of tachycardia. Degenerative changes are probably caused by autoimmune phenomena in the chronic stage of the disease. It is not possible to determine more precisely how the structure of the subendocardium is related to the origin of ventricular tachycardia. As previously suggested, it might be caused by abnormal transmembrane potentials due to alterations in ultrastructural changes, by abnormal arrangement of muscle bundles trapped in fibrous tissue, or both.

Electrophysiological studies in patients with sustained ventricular tachycardia and Chagasic aneurysm suggest that the arrhythmia is caused by reentry. Myocardial fibers surviving on the endocardial surface of Chagasic aneurysms probably receive blood supply from retrograde perfusion through subendocardial sinusoidal channels. The prominent thickening of the endocardium may impair the possibility of perfusion from the ventricular cavity. Muscles bundles with surviving myocytes in the subendocardium are trapped in the scar and, together with Purkinje fibers, remain embedded in dense connective tissue.

If there are interconnections between the bundles, they might form discrete reentrant circuits around an anatomic obstacle. These subendocardial circuits are probably connected to the normal ventricular subendocardium only at the lateral borders of aneurysms. The interlaced fronts and myocytes showing early damage (slow conducting) as demonstrated the study performed by Milei et al. [14], produce the ideal configuration for reentry.

It is not yet clear if the reentrant circuits are made up of Purkinje fibers, ventricular muscle fibers, or both. Experimental studies demonstrated that Purkinje fibers surviving on the endocardial surface of extensive canine infarcts reduced resting potentials and prolonged potential actions duration, facilitating reentry "in vitro" [39].

Investigations of spontaneous depolarization and delayed after potentials is not suited for a histological approach [40]. In contrast, reentry depends upon localized dromotropic impairment within a precise geometric setting, which can be strongly suspected on the basis of morphological investigations. Different properties of conduction in the opposite limbs of reentry loops may appear, by light microscopy, as heterogeneous layers of interwoven myocardial cells. Likewise, tracts of macroreentrant circuits can either appear as partially jeopardized myocardial bundles, or recognized as accessory or dual atrioventricular pathways, or both. Blocks in intracardiac conduction, however, are usually related to destruction and disruption of the specialized tissues. In contrast, the viability of decrementally conducting myocardial cells is a prerequisite for the occurrence of reentry. Some of these damaged but viable cells might even have fired or after depolarized (or both) and are presumed to underlie the phenomenon of reentry [40, 41].

The exact size and anatomic course of the reentrant circuits, nonetheless, has yet to be defined. It was calculated to be between 2 and 3 [42, 43] and 10 and 12 cm [44]. Direct demonstration of anatomic circuits would require demonstration of differences in structure between the site of earliest activation during the arrhythmia and other areas in the resection.

The final proof that the arrhythmias originate in these endocardial regions is their abolition by aneurysm resection that Milei et al. [14] showed in their research, where no recurrences could be shown during the 19 to 51 month period of follow-up.

The clinical importance of ventricular aneurysms and the genesis of cardiac arrhythmias are not limited to the cardiomyopathy. Carod-Artal et al. [38] suggested that apical aneurysm, cardiac insufficiency and arrhythmias are important risk factors in the genesis of ischemic stroke related to Chagas disease, whereas hipercoagulable states are unlikely to be major contributors to the excess in stroke risk seen in chagasic patients.

Diagnosis

Acute phase: In the acute phase, the level of parasitemia is high; motile trypomastigotes can be detected by microscopy examination of a fresh drop of anticoagulated blood allowing the observation of *T cruzi*. Alternative methods include microhematocrit and Strout methods [45]. The level of parasitemia decreases within 90 days of infection, even without treatment, and is undetectable by microscopy in the chronic phase [46]. PCR is a sensitive diagnostic tool in the acute phase of Chagas disease, generally demonstrates positive results days to weeks before circulating trypomastigotes are detectable on peripheral blood smears [47]. It may also be used to monitor for acute infection in the recipient of an infected organ or after accidental exposure [48, 49].

Direct demonstration of parasite by hemoculture or xenodiagnosis in a reliable laboratory indicates true infection, although the sensitivity of these techniques in chronic *T cruzi* infection is generally less than 50 percent [50, 51]. Hemoculture consists of inoculation of a small volume (e.g., 0.2 cc) of whole blood or buffy coat in a standard parasitic medium such as Novy-MacNeal-Nicolle (NNN), followed by incubation at 28°C. Microscopic examination for motile epimastigotes is performed at 14 days and then weekly until at least 35 days post-inoculation.

Xenodiagnosis requires the availability of a laboratory-reared colony of uninfected triatomine bugs (usually Triatoma infestans or Dipetalogaster maxima) [52]. Bugs should be starved for at least 14 days before use. Direct xenodiagnosis consists of placing 5 to 10 fifth nymphs in a mesh box, which is then attached to the patient's arm or leg, and allowed to feed for 30 minutes. The process is not usually painful but often causes local irritation. Indirect xenodiagnosis consists of allowing the nymphs to feed on anticoagulated patient blood through a membrane feeding device. Direct xenodiagnosis generally has higher sensitivity, but indirect xenodiagnosis is more acceptable to patients. In either case, the triatomine nymphs are then kept for at least 28 days to allow them to pass to the adult stage. Their fecal contents are then examined for motile trypomastigotes and/or epimastigotes. If negative, the insects can be maintained for an additional period of time and examined at intervals for parasites.

Chronic phase: Serological methods to detect IgG antibodies to *T cruzi* like indirect hemaglutination, immunofluorescence (IFI) and enzyme-linked immunosorbent assay (ELISA) are the three test routinely used for detecting a *T cruzi* infection in the chronic phase of the disease where parasitemia is low. At least two positive results with two serologic techniques that use different antigens or a positive result in parasitology are necessary for the diagnosis [4, 53].The sensitivity of serological assays varies by geographical location, possibly due to strain *T cruzi* differences and resulting antibody responses [54-55].

In general, PCR is not a useful diagnostic test for chronic infection. The sensitivity is highly variable and depends on patient characteristics as well as PCR primers and methods [56-61].

Congenital Chagas disease: The technique traditionally used to diagnose congenital *T cruzi* infection is micromethod (or microhematocrit method) [61-62].This technique consists of centrifugation of fresh cord or neonatal blood sealed in four to six heparinized microhematocrit tubes (12, 000 rpm for 7 minutes), followed by light microscopic examination of the buffy coat layer [61]. However, the sensitivity of examination of a single infant specimen by this technique is less than 50 percent; repeated sampling may increase the sensitivity [63].

Molecular techniques have substantially higher sensitivity and detect congenital infections earlier in life compared with the micromethod [63-65]. Although not yet widely implemented in congenital Chagas disease screening programs, PCR is increasingly used for the early diagnosis of congenital Chagas disease in Latin America and is the method of choice in industrialized countries [66].For infants not diagnosed at birth, conventional IgG serology is recommended after nine months of age, when transferred maternal antibody has disappeared [67].

Clinical Findings

Signs and Symptoms

Figure 14 shows the most common signs and symptoms of ChrChC according to studies performed by Storino and Milei [4] in 132 patients, Pondé et al. [68] in 161 patients, and Amorin et al. [69] in 108 patients.

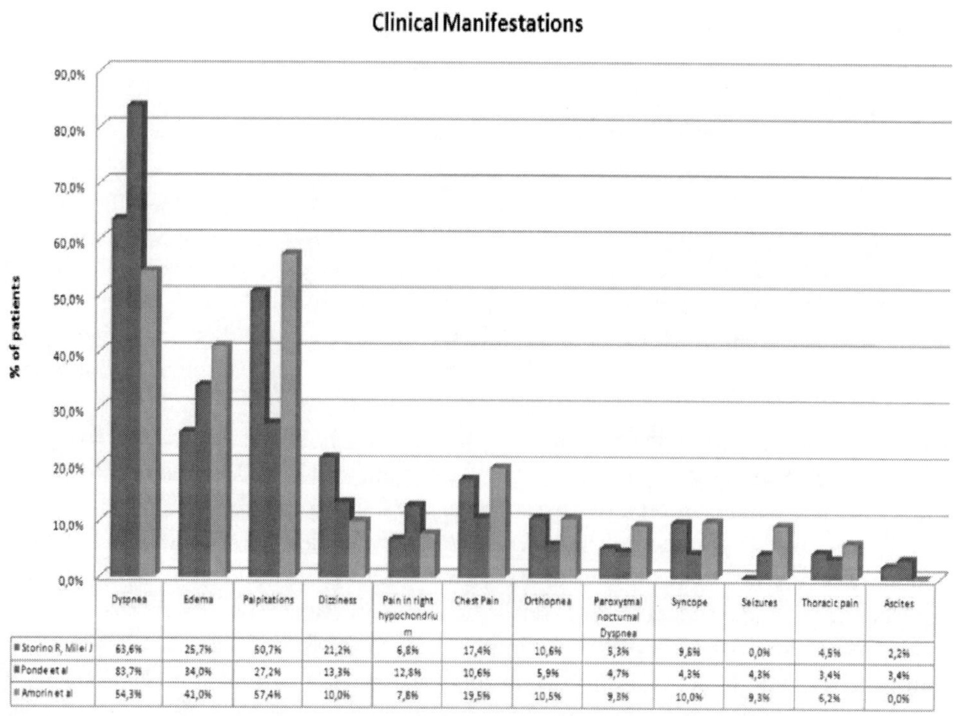

Figure 14. Clinical Manifestations of Chagas disease according to Storino and Milei [4], Ponde et al. [68] and Amorin et al. [69].

Physical Examination

Physical examination should not be restricted to the cardiovascular system, considering that Chagas disease can present digestive manifestations or less frequently neurological symptoms. However, given that this chapter deals with ChrChC only cardiac examination will be described.

The inspection of the patient is important as it can reveal if he is in acute distress, how is his breathing, if accessory muscles are being used, if there are signs of congestion or peripheral hypoperfusion and if there are signs of cardiac cachexia. The Romaña's sign, can also be easily found while inspecting the patient and reveals an acute infection of Chagas disease. The sign consists of a non-painful palpebral edema, erythema, adenopathy (of the same side of the ocular inflammation), conjunctivitis and dacryocystitis. This sign occurs whenever the parasite is inoculated in the orbital region. Another less frequent sign may also occur when the parasite is inoculated in exposed regions of the skin. This sign, known as "inoculation chagoma", is produced by a local inflammatory reaction and a lymphoreticular response triggered by the parasite and is clinically identified as an indurate erythematous area.

The percussion of the heart (actually rarely used) was performed at the third, fourth and fifth intercostals spaces from the left anterior axillary line to the right anterior axillary line. Percussion dullness of more than 10.5cm in the fifth intercostals space had a sensitivity of 94.4% and a specificity of 67.2% in detecting cardiomegaly [70].

Palpation is also essential. The point of maximum impulse could be laterally displaced or felt in two interspaces during the same phase of respiration suggesting cardiomegaly. Thrills may also be present indicating a loud murmur.

Auscultation may reveal a high pitched holosystolic murmur in 43% of the patients and an S3 in 31% of them. In contrast with the ChrChC, dilated cardiomyopathy (DCM) has an S3 present 75% of the cases [4].

Electrocardiographic Findings

Carlos Chagas in 1909 was the first to study the electrocardiographic changes in Chagasic patients. Since then, many authors have contributed with their studies. These reports agree in the electrocardiographic changes but do not coincide in the frequency in which they are found, most probably due to the fact that different diagnostic criteria, patients with different evolution of their disease, and from different regions (endemic and non-endemic) were considered. In this section a brief comment on the more frequent ECG alterations will be made. In Figure 15 the results of the study performed by Storino et al. [4, 19, 20] can be observed.

Incomplete right bundle branch block (IRBBB): This conduction abnormality is most frequently found in asymptomatic patients without cardiomegaly. Generally it appears in the latent or indetermined phase of the disease as a consequence of the acute myocarditis, and represents a good prognosis for the patient.

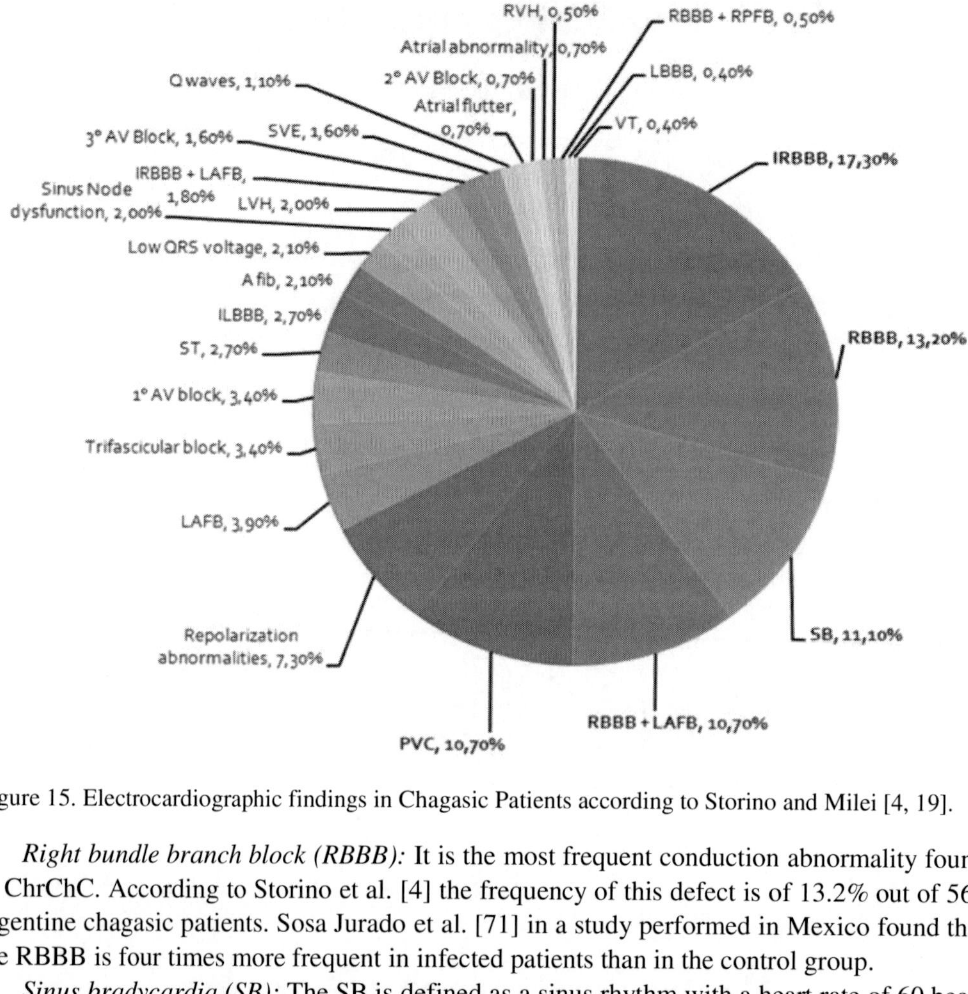

Figure 15. Electrocardiographic findings in Chagasic Patients according to Storino and Milei [4, 19].

Right bundle branch block (RBBB): It is the most frequent conduction abnormality found in ChrChC. According to Storino et al. [4] the frequency of this defect is of 13.2% out of 560 argentine chagasic patients. Sosa Jurado et al. [71] in a study performed in Mexico found that the RBBB is four times more frequent in infected patients than in the control group.

Sinus bradycardia (SB): The SB is defined as a sinus rhythm with a heart rate of 60 beats per minute or less and it is present in 11.1% of the Chagasic patients [4].

Bifascicular block (RBBB + LAFB): This electrocardiographic finding is the most frequent conduction abnormality after the isolated RBBB [4]. In a patient with the proper background this finding is suggestive of ChrChC. Patients who are candidates for pacemakers present a higher incidence of this conduction abnormality [4].

Premature ventricular contraction (PVC): The PVC is one of the most frequent electrocardiographic findings in ChrChC. Unifocal PVCs generally appear in stable patients and are 3 times more frequent than multifocal PVCs. This last group has a worse prognosis and is more frequently found in hospitalized patients rather than in seropositive patients detected by screening of endemic areas [4].

Chest X-Ray

This type of radiological imaging is used to assess the heart size, the pulmonary circulation and the presence of pericardial effusion.

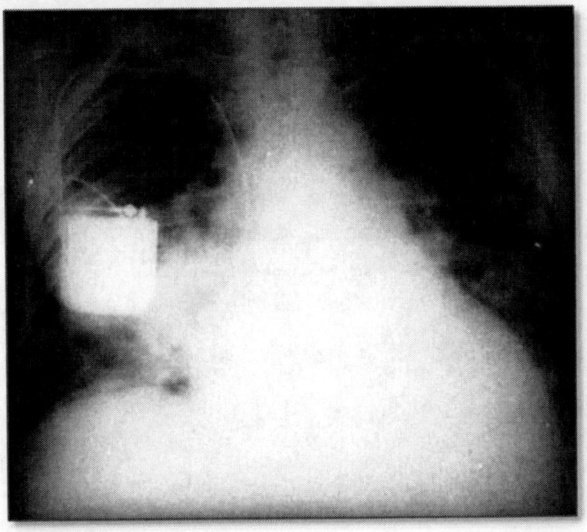

Reproduced from Milei et al. [5] with permission.

Figure 16. Chext x-ray of a Chagasic patient showing a cardiomegaly. Note the presence of a pacemaker.

Its findings should be correlated with the medical history and the electrocardiographic studies considering that the ChrChC is characterized for damaging the conduction system and/or the contracting myocardium. Hence, the damage of the conduction system will provoke electrocardiographic abnormalities with normal heart size while the damage of the myocardial fibers would result in cardiomegaly (Figure 16) without changes in the ECG. Generally the cardiomegaly observed in the ChrChC is purely caused by a left ventricular enlargement.

Álvarez and Rosenbaum [72], found that electrocardiographic changes always preceded radiological changes in chagasic patients. They also found in concordance with Schapachnik [72, 73] that the age of the patients is directly proportional to the cardiomegaly. On the other hand, Storino and Milei in a study performed in 560 patients found that 30.4% presented cardiomegaly and 16% of these cases an advanced enlargement of the heart. Thirty-three percent of the patients presented electrocardiographic abnormalities without evident radiologic changes. Once again, it was found that the age of the patient was associated with the magnitude of the disease [4, 19].

These findings would suggest that Chagas disease produces a selective damage over the conduction system of the heart in the first stages of the disease, or that the involvement of the contracting myocardium does not express ECG changes. Because of these reasons, ECG alterations precede the radiologic cardiomegaly. Hence, electrocardiographic studies could be used to rule out advance stages of cardiomegaly in chronic patients [4, 73].

Echocardiography

This widely available non invasive technique that uses ultrasound to generate cardiac images is useful in the assessment of Chagasic patients due to the following reasons [4]:

Detection of abnormalities in the asymptomatic phase of the disease where other cardiologic studies such as electrocardiograms and chest x-rays are negative. It is to note that in a study [35], more than half of the symptomatic patients with ChrChC presented a left ventricular apical aneurysm and other segmental contractile abnormalities similar to those seen in coronary heart disease.

The study permits the assessment of systolic and diastolic functions in the chronic and indeterminated phase by means of a non invasive technique. Left and right ventricular systolic function ranges from normal to severely impaired. Abnormalities of the ventricular function may be detected even in patients with NYHA functional classes of I/II and it is highly accurate in detecting ventricular aneurysms.

It is accepted that the echocardiography should be used to follow the indeterminated phase and to control therapeutic responses of patients in the chronic phase.

Acquatella [37] found that ventricular involvement in symptomatic individuals may range from an isolated small left ventricular apical aneurysm to a globally dilated heart without segmental scars. The author suggests that chagasic origin should be considered in the differential diagnosis in patients with a positive epidemiological history and serology, suggestive ECG abnormalities and the presence of an apical aneurysm [36].

Myocardial Biopsy

At present, this invasive technique is not used to diagnose ChrChC given its risks and the fact that focal myocarditis may be missed by the biopsy. Nevertheless, in patients with AIDS where a reactivation of Chagas disease is suspected, given the high mortality of this group and the immediate need of treatment, the benefits of performing a myocardial biopsy may outweigh its risks. It is important to note that in a non endemic country like USA, to diagnose the fourth and fifth cases of Chagas disease transmitted through organ donations, an endomyocardial biopsy was performed resulting positive in the first case and negative in the second [74].

HIV/AIDS, Organ Transplantation and Chagasic Cardiomyopathy

The immunosuppressed state of these patients usually reactivates Chagas' disease. Ferreira et al. [75] reported that reactivation of Chagas' disease affects mainly the central nervous system (75%) followed by the heart (44%). In their review, not all patients were systematically examined for cardiac involvement. Nevertheless, Sartori et al. [76] found that as a manifestation of the re-activation, myocarditis was as common as the meningo-encephalitis.

The problem lays on the fact that acute myocarditis as the major manifestation of the re-activation of T *cruzi* may be misdiagnosed as a progression state of the ChrChC. As the treatment and management of these conditions are dissimilar a differential diagnosis is mandatory. Parasitemia levels may help, considering that in a re-activation of the disease the T *cruzi* is elevated in blood. Unfortunately, this is not always the case [75, 76]. An endomyocardial biopsy may also support the diagnosis, since numerous nests of T *cruzi* amastigotes amidst areas of intense tissue inflammation are not usually observed in the chronic disease [76]. However, in some cases the myocarditis may be focal and hence, missed by the endomyocardial biopsy.

The mean survival rate of patients with AIDS and reactivation of Chagas' disease among 16 reported cases was of 10 days and only three patients survived as long as or longer than 3 months [75].

Reactivation of Chagas disease can also occur in transplanted patients. Benvenutti et al. [77] reported reactivation of Chagas disease after heart transplantation in 20% of the patients usually during the first year after surgery and it accounts for 4.2% of the causes of mortality amongst this group.

Differential Diagnosis

Mauricio Rosenbaum, an argentine cardiologist who revolutionized the knowledge of the heart conduction system by first describing the hemiblocks, made a comparative analysis in between the ChrChC and the DCM (table 1) [78].

On the other hand, various studies performed by Milei and Storino et al. [4, 13, 20] revealed other clinical differences in between these two pathologies (table 2).

Table 1. Comparison in between Chronic Chagasic Cardiomyopathy and Primary Idiopathic Dilated Cardiomyopathy according to Mauricio Rosenbaum [78]

Findings	Chronic Chagasic cardiomyopathy	Primary Idiopathic Dilated Cardiomyopathy
Dilatation	+	+
Systolic Function	↓	↓
Cardiac insufficiency	+	+
Ventricular Aneurysm	+	±
Autonomous nervous system involvement	+	-
Other organs involved	+	-
Sinus node disfunction	+	-
Conduction system alterations	RBBB+LAFB	LBBB
Q wave abnormalities	+	±
Ventricular arrhythmias	+	±
Inflamatory cells, infiltrate	+	±

Key: +:present. ±: sporadic finding. –: absent.↓:reduced. RBBB+ LAFB : Right bundle branch block associated with a left anterior fascicular block. LBBB: Left Bundle Branch Block.

Table 2. Comparison in between ChrChC and DCM according to Milei and Storino [4]

Clinical Studies	Chronic Chagasic Cardiomyopathy	Primary Idiopathic Dilated Cardiomyopathy
Serology for *T cruzi*	Positive	Negative
Mean age	48	40
Clinical Findings		
NYHA Class II	26%	60%
Symptom that predominates	Palpitations 89%	Dyspnea 100%
ECG findings	RBBB + LAFB	LBBB or incomplete LBBB
A-fib or Aflutter	2%	26%
Chest x-ray with cardiomegaly	Extreme 10%	Extreme: 53%
Holter monitoring	PVC: 48% SB: 28%	PVC: 50% Afib: 33%
Heart Sounds	High pitched holosystolic murmur: 46% S3: 31%	High pitched holosystolic murmur: 58% S3: 75%
Echocardiogram		
Left ventricular dilatation	87%	100%
Left ventricular diastolic diameter	63 mm	67 mm
Ventricular Aneurysm	30%	0%
Gamma Camera	Regional hypokinesia 38%	Global Hypokinesia 54%
Need of Pacemaker	13% for trifascicular block	13% for 3° AV block
Annual Mortality	5.2% (17% for 5 year mortality)	13%

Electrocardiogram [4]: The electrocardiographic differences in between the ChChC and the DCM rely on the fact that this last entity presents more damage in the myocardium fibers than on the conduction system. This is why left ventricular hypertrophy, biventricular hypertrhophy and anomalous P waves will prevail in the DCM while conduction alterations will predominate in the ChChC. The left bundle branch block (LBBB) is more frequent in the DCM than the right bundle branch block (RBBB). Complete AV blocks have a very low prevalence in the DCM. The most frequent arrhythmias present in the DCM are PVCs, Atrial Flutter (A-flutter) and atrial fibrillation (A-fib).

Chest X-ray [4]: Even though a differential diagnosis of cardiomyopathies cannot be made with a chest x-ray, the DCM has some radiologic characteristics which are not frequently seen in the ChChC. Firstly, the DCM usually presents an enlargement of the four heart chambers while the ChChC only presents LVH and only in very severe cases presents enlargement of further chambers. Secondly, biventricular hypertrophy is seen in 90% of the DCM and only in 40% of the ChChC. Thirdly, radiological signs present in the lungs that suggest congestive heart failure (CHF) are more frequent and appear earlier in the DCM than in the ChChC. Finally, the mean age in which radiologic alterations are found is lower in the DCM than in the ChChC.

Prognosis

A study made by Storino et al. [19] evaluated the course of Chagas disease in 350 Chagasic patients where 120 of them had been followed for 12 years and 270 had been followed for at least 5 years. The patients were grouped according to the Argentine Society of Cardiology former classification (table 1). A total of 103 infected patients with no cardiomyopathy were classified in Group I. Group II was formed by 115 infected patients with mild cardiomyopathy with no dilatation. Finally, Group III had 132 infected patients with dilated Chagasic cardiomyopathy. Only 8.6% of the patients knew about the triatoma *infestans*, commonly referred to as "vinchuca". In addition, 5.1% of the patients had never visited an endemic region but had eventually received blood transfusions.

Five Year Prognosis of Infected Patients without Cardiomyopathy (Group I)

The mean age of the patients from this group was 29.4. Fifteen percent of the patients in this group evolved to Group II for presenting electrocardiographic findings that suggested mild non-dilated cardiomyopathy. Five percent of Group I evolved to Group III for presenting not only electrocardiographic changes but for having radiological changes suggesting dilated Chagasic cardiomyopathy. The other studies performed (stress test, Holter monitoring, echocardiogram, gamma camera) also confirmed the myocardial damage. It is worthwhile mentioning that the patients who evolved to group III were of significantly older age ($p < 0.001$) than those who remained in group I. This finding remarks the importance of age in the prognosis of cardiac lesions.

Five Year Prognosis of Infected Patients with Mild Cardiomyopathy but No Dilatation (Group II)

The mean age of the patients from this group was 36 years. Ten percent of this group presented further alterations in their conducting system clinically represented by the worsening of their electrocardiographic alterations. Twenty percent of this group evolved to Group III given that they presented a dilated cardiomyopathy.

Prognosis of Infected Patients with Dilated Cardiomyopathy (Group III)

The mean age of the patients from this group was 48.9. Seventeen percent of this group died.

According to a study performed in mice it was demonstrated that the parasite strain and number of reinfections clearly determine a differential clinical course and either of these factors or both are involved in the severity of the clinical picture and the prognosis of the disease [79]. In other words, it was hypothesized that the 30% of the chagasic patients who develop cardiac lesions could be the ones who had been reinfected multiple times and the severity could be related to the parasitic strain as well [79]. If these results are applicable to humans, identifying the strain of the *T cruzi* could be helpful to determine the prognosis of the disease. At the same time, as it was discussed in the Epidemiology section, identifying if the patient comes from an endemic area where they could have multiple reinfections would also be helpful in order to assess the course of the disease.

By showing that infected patients with normal ECG and without evidence of myocardial damage have the same life expectancy than the general population these results support the WHO's suggestion published in 1971 of not preserving these patients from a normal lifestyle and regular jobs [80]. In other words, there is no reason for discriminating infected patients and preventing them from being active workers. Regarding the most deteriorated group, it should be taken into account the prolonged tolerance to the disease that they present and find appropriate jobs for them to do according to their physical condition.

Mortality

A recent study revealed that the lack of ß-blocking agent use, serum sodium levels, left ventricular ejection fraction, digoxin treatment and New York Heart Association (NYHA) Functional Class IV are independent predictors of all cause mortality for patients with moderate-to-severe chronic heart failure secondary to ChrChC [81].

Meanwhile, Cardinally-Neto et al. [82] showed that the number of shocks per patient per 30 days predicts outcome in Chagas disease patients treated with implantable cardioverter defibrilator (ICD) therapy.

In a systematic review of 12 observational studies recently performed by Rassi et al. [1] it was shown that risk stratification for Chagasic patients can be refined by combining prognostic factors related to three major clinical-pathophysiological characteristics of the disease: symptoms of heart failure (expressed by NYHA functional class III/IV), measures of ventricular dysfunction (cardiomegaly on chest x-ray, decreased LV contractility or increased LV diameter on echocardiography), and a measure of ventricular electrical instability (presence of non-sustained ventricular tachycardia on 24-hour Holter monitoring). These authors consider that patients who present a NYHA class III/IV or measures of ventricular dysfunction combined with non-sustained ventricular tachycardia on Holter monitoring are at the highest risk of death and should be candidates for aggressive therapy management. On the other hand, patients with normal or abnormal ECG with a NYHA functional class of I/II with neither LV dysfunction on the echocardiography nor non-sustained ventricular tachycardia on the 24 hour Holter monitoring are at low risk of death [1]. According to this author the score for assessment of risk is the following :

- NYHA class III/IV (5 points)
- Cardiomegaly on chest X-ray (5 points)
- Left ventricular systolic dysfunction on echocardiogram (3 points)
- Nonsustained ventricular tachycardia (NSVT) on Holter monitoring (3 points)
- Low QRS voltage (2 points)
- Male gender (2 points)

Ten-year mortality in patients with 12 to 20 points was 84 to 85 percent; for patients with 7 to 11 points it was 37 to 44 percent and for patients with 0 to 6 points it was 9 to 10 percent. The combination of left ventricular systolic dysfunction and NSVT was associated with particularly high risk (15.1 fold increased risk of death).The presence of NSVT alone was associated with a 2.15-fold increased risk of death [1, 83]

In a study made in Argentina the causes of mortality within Chagasic patients were, in order of prevalence: 1) cardiac insufficiency 2) sudden death 3) acute encephalitis in patients with Chagas disease and AIDS and 4) pulmonary embolism [84]. Likewise, a study performed in Brazil showed that sudden death was the first cause of mortality in chagasic patients followed by cardiac insufficiency, acute encephalitis in patients with AIDS and pulmonary embolism [85].

Bruno Linetzky et al. [86] performed a systematic review of the risk of cardiovascular events associated with positive serology for Chagas. They analysed 14 studies including patients with heart failure; 6 with severe symptoms and 9 with mild symptoms or asymptomatic patients with low ejection fraction. In 4 studies of patients in functional class III or IV and in 3 studies of patients with mild symptoms, a higher risk of death was reported among those with positive serology for Chagas. Of the 11 studies of patients without symptoms or low ejection fraction, 3 showed a higher risk of mortality related to Chagas exposure. Two of these were based on the same cohort of people aged >60 years. In 8 out of the 14 heart failure studies and 2 out of the 11heart damage studies adjusted for confounding factors. They concluded that positive serology for Chagas is associated with a higher risk of death for patients with heart failure, but there is little evidence to associate positive serology for Chagas with cardiovascular events in asymptomatic subjects.

Regarding the broad group of most patients that present the indeterminate form of the disease and remain without symptoms for decades, Milei et al. [87] have answered to some groups who believe that patients these patients are at high risk for developing sudden death although no studies have been designed to investigate this issue. A systematic review of follow-up studies in patients with asymptomatic Chagas disease, normal ECG and known cause of death was conducted and fifteen articles including 9382 patients were selected [87]. Mortality rate in asymptomatic patients with normal ECG was very low (0.92%) and similar to that of controls without Chagas disease (p=0.38).Therefore, sudden death is uncommon in the indeterminate form of the disease and the risk of death is similar to that of the general population [87].Thus, these patients should be allowed to lead a normal working life and to practice physical activity, without alarming them unnecessarily about their condition or indicating sophisticated and expensive studies. Anyhow, regular follow-up is necessary when the disease progresses to the cardiac form.

Emergencies

Storino's team [84] made a study to evaluate the most frequent causes of emergency in patients with Chagas disease in the city of Buenos Aires. Out of 1680 emergency admissions, 6% presented positive serology for Chagas disease. This number is alarming considering that in this non-endemic city 2.3% of its habitants are seropositive for *T cruzi*. The clinical events that resulted in the admission of these patients to the emergency room were syncope (32%), cardiac insufficiency (29%), coronary events (19%), stroke (5%), acute edema of hypertensive lung (3%) and acute encephalitis associated with AIDS (2%) [84].

Treatment

Symptomatic Treatment

The symptomatic treatment of the ChrChC involves the management of ventricular dysfunction and heart failure, management and prevention of thromboembolism, of bradyarrhythmias, ventricular arrhythmias and management of angina pain. This section is beyond the objectives of the chapter.

Etiologic Treatment of Chronic Chagas' Disease

Nifurtimox (Nx, Bayer®) a nitrofuran and Benznidazole (Bz, Roche®) a nitroimidazole derivative are the currently available chemotherapy against *T cruzi.* Nifurtimox acts producing highly toxic reduced oxygen metabolites [88]. *T cruzi* is deficient in detoxification mechanisms for oxygen metabolites, and is thus more sensitive to oxidative stress than are vertebrate cells [89]. Benznidazole acts via covalent modification of macromolecules by nitroreduction intermediates [89]. In the United States, these drugs are not FDA approved and are available only from Centers for Disease Control and Prevention (CDC) under investigational new drug protocols.

They are highly effective in treating the acute stage of the disease; nevertheless their use in the chronic stage is controversial. The reason why chemotherapy agents started to be tested for the chronic stage of the disease is related to the fact that, as stated in the Pathology section of this chapter, the parasite is one of the three main ingredients that explain the pathogenesis of ChrChC. The parasite persistence in the chronic stage was detected in endomyocardial biopsies [12, 15, 27], and some authors suggest that although the number of parasites is low in patients with ChrChC, their potential for heart damage may be comparable with those present during the acute phase [27, 28, 90-92], while others believe that there is not enough evidence to support their use [93-95]. Table 3 summarizes the studies that evaluated the treatment of ChrChC.

Cançado [90] performed a study in 21 patients with acute Chagas disease that were treated with benznidazole for at least 32 days and were post examined for a period of at least 13 years, and in 113 patients with chronic Chagas disease treated for at least 40 consecutive days and followed for a period of 6 to 18 years. As a result 76% of the acute cases were considered cured of infection after the treatment. On the other hand, for only 8% of the chronic cases did serological test became completely and consistently negative, indicating cure. Fifteen percent of the chronic cases were doubtful (results oscillated between negative and positive) and 77% had no serologic response to Bz. The author concluded that until a better drug is available Bz should be used also in the treatment of chronic patients, due to its high efficacy against both the acute and recent disease, its proved activity in at least 8% of the chronic cases, its suppressive effect of the parasitemia in chronic patients, its possible favourable effect on the clinical evolution of the disease and the fact that its side effects are well known and can be controlled [90].

Three years later, Garcia et al. [28], in a mouse model of *T cruzi* infection, demonstrated that although parasite eradication could not be achieved with Bz treatment in the chronic phase, a decrease in cardiac dysfunction (ECG alterations) and myocarditis was achieved with this drug. The authors concluded that Bz treatment is important to decrease or retard the development of experimental ChrChC [28].

In 2007, Fabbro et al. [91] performed a retrospective and prospective cohort study to evaluate the efficacy of treatment with Nx and/or Bz among 111 adults from northern Argentina over a mean follow-up of 21 years. Fifty-seven untreated patients remained with a positive serology with constant titers. From the 54 treated patients 37% had a negative seroconversion, 27.8% had a final serology with decreased titers and only 35.2% presented a positive final serology with constant titers. There were no significant differences as regards the cure percentage in patients treated with Bz and Nx. This study not only showed a very high seroconversion rate but it also showed a statistically significant difference in the clinical evolution of the treated patients and the controls [92].

Viotti et al. [96] performed a non randomized trial with 566 adult patients, half of them treated with Bz for 30 days. As a result, the treated group presented a 15% negative seroconversion rate and significantly less progression to the disease ($p<0.002$) and ECG alterations ($p<0.001$) than the untreated group.

Sgambatti de Andrade et al. [97] performed a randomized placebo controlled trial in 129 positive children (120 indeterminate and 9 early Chagas heart disease), 7 to 12 years old from 1990 children Presumably the patients were in their first year of infection. Sixty-four patients were treated with Bz for 60 days and the rest with placebo. A negative seroconversion was obtained for 55.8% of the treated patients. The remaining 44.2% of the Bz group presented a significant reduction in antibodies concentrations.

Likewise, Sosa Estani et al. [54] performed a study in 106 children from 6 to 12 years old in the indeterminate phase of the disease who most likely contracted the infection more than six years before beginning treatment with Bz. After 6 and 48 months, 37.5 and 62% of the treated group were seronegative, respectively. No untreated children had a negative seroconversion at the end of the study [54].

Therapeutic effectiveness as assessed by serological cure seems to depend on the delay between infection and the start of treatment [98].

Previous studies show that parasite persistence plays an important role in the pathogenesis of ChrChC [28]. The fact that reinfections aggravate heart dysfunction [81] also corroborates this idea.

On the other hand, Lauria Pires et al. [95] after performing a study in 91 patients and 41 uninfected controls concluded that treatment of chronic Chagas patients with nitroderivates was unsatisfactory. Every treated and 93.7% of the untreated patients yielded a specific PCR amplification product with primers that annealed to *T cruzi* nDNA, indicating active infection. One year after treatment ECG alterations were present in 79% of treated and 67.4% of untreated chagasic patients. Ten years thereafter, ECG alterations where found in 80.5% of treated and 75% of untreated patients ($p<0.05$). In addition, the differences between mean parasitemia of treated and untreated Chagasic patients were not significant [95].

Table 3. Studies evaluating the efficacy of treating chronic Chagas disease with benznidazole

Author (year) Country	Material and Method	Outcome of treated group	Conclusion
de Andrade et al. [97] (1996) Brazil	129 seropositive children from 7 to 12 years old (resulted from screening of 1990), 64 treated with benznidazole. 65 untreated	Negative seroconversion in 55.8%	Authors recommend the treatment of seropositive children.
Sosa Estani et al. [51] (1998) Argentina	106 children from 6 to 12 years old 55 treated with Bz for 60 days, 51 untreated	Negative seroconversion in 62% 4.7% of the treated group had a positive xenodiagnosis versus a 51.2% in the placebo group.	Infected children may successfully be treated with Bz.
Lauria Pires et al[95] (2000) Brazil	91 Chagasic patients 41 uninfected patients	100% of treated patients showed presence of the parasite by PCR. Not significant difference in between treated and untreated patients concerning ECG alterations and parasitemia levels.	Treatment of chronic Chagas with nitroderivatives is unsatisfactory and cannot be recommended
Cançado [90] (2002) Brazil	21 acute chagasic patients 113 chronic chagasic patients	Cure in 8% of chronic chagasic patients and 76% of acute cases.	Authors consider that Bz should be used in the treatment of chronic patients.
Reyes et al. [93] (2005) Mexico	Review of the literature	Considered a single double blind randomized clinical trial and 5 case control or case series.	Treatment of chronic Chagas with these drugs is not sufficiently well supported.
García et al. [28] (2005)	8 infected mice 8 infected mice treated with Bz 18 healthy mice	Decrease in the parasite load Decrease in ECG alterations Decrease in myocarditis	Authors emphasize the importance of Bz in chronic chagasic patients in order to decrease or retard the development of ChrChC.
Viotti et al. [96] (2006) Argentina	566 patients from 30 to 50 283 untreated	15% negative seroconversion Significantly less progression to the disease ($p<0.002$) and ECG alterations ($p<0.001$) than the untreated group.	Bz treatment is associated with a reduced risk for progression of ChrChC.
Fabbro et al. [92] (2007) Argentina	Total 111 patients. 57 untreated. 54 treated. Santa Fe (Argentina)	37% seroconversion (cured) 27.8% decreased titers 35.2% remained positive with constant titers Favorable clinical evolution in the treated group	This study favors the treatment of chronic Chagas disease.
Bern et al[102] (2007) United States	Review of the literature	Refer to text	

The existence of strains naturally resistant to Nx and Bz could help to explain the different responses to treatment [92]. Additional studies show that the efficacy of therapeutic treatment is related to the indemnity of the host immune system [98-101].

After a review of the literature Reyes et al. [93] considered that there is insufficient evidence to support the use of Nx drugs as trypanocidal agents as a recommended treatment for infection in the chronic stage of Chagas disease, especially when an overt heart disease is present.

Nevertheless, a recent systematic review performed by Bern et al. [102], concluded that despite gaps in the evidence base, current knowledge is sufficient to make recommendations to guide appropriate evaluation, management, and etiologic treatment of Chagas disease.

Treatment should always be offered (strength of recommendation graded A) in acute *T cruzi* infection in early congenital *T cruzi* infection, children up to 18 years old with chronic *T cruzi* infection and in reactivated *T cruzi* infection in patients with HIV/AIDS or other immunosupression [102].

Treatment should generally be offered (strength of recommendation graded B) in reproductive-age women, adults aged 19-50 years old with indeterminate form, or mild to moderate cardiomyopathy and in patients with impending immunosuppressant [102].

Evidence for efficacy is insufficient to support a recommendation for or against treating adults above 50 years of age without advanced cardiomyopathy, and for patients with Chagas gastrointestinal tract disease but without advanced cardiomyopathy [102].

Moderate evidence for lack of efficacy or for adverse outcome supports a recommendation against treating advance chagasic cardiomyopathy with congestive heart failure, and megaesophagus with significant impairment of swallowing [102].

Good evidence for lack of efficacy or for adverse outcome is available to recommend never treating a pregnant woman or patients with severe renal or hepatic insufficiency [102].

Of note from 2004, in order to clarify the role of trypanocidal therapy in preventing cardiac disease progression and death, The BENznidazole Evaluation For Interrupting Trypanosomiasis (BENEFIT), is being conducted. The design of this multicenter, randomized, double-blind, placebo-controlled clinical trial includes 3, 000 patients with Chagas' cardiomyopathy in Latin America. Patients were randomized to receive benznidazole (5 mg/kg per day) or matched placebo, for 60 days. The primary outcome is the composite of death; resuscitated cardiac arrest; sustained ventricular tachycardia; insertion of pacemaker or cardiac defibrillator; cardiac transplantation; and development of new heart failure, stroke, or systemic or pulmonary thromboembolic events. The average follow-up time was 5 years, and the trial has a 90% power to detect a 25% relative risk reduction. The BENEFIT program also comprises a substudy evaluating the effects of benznidazole on parasite clearance and an echo substudy exploring the impact of etiologic treatment on left ventricular function. More than one thousand patients have been enrolled in 35 centers from Argentina, Brazil, and Colombia [103] and results will appear in 2014.

Non-Pharmacological Treatment

Given that trypanocidal agents as Nx or Bz are not recommended to treat patients with advance cardiomyopathy and further drugs are still under clinical investigation, the need to find new therapeutic possibilities for these patients is of outmost importance. Cardiac transplantation has been the sole therapeutic possibility for these patients so far. Promising experimental studies show that bone marrow cell therapy produces beneficial effects in the treatment of ChrChC.

Limited data are available on the efficacy of heart failure therapies in Chagas disease. In a trial of 42 patients randomized to receive either carvedilol or placebo in addition to ACE inhibitor (or ARB) and spironolactone treatment, carvedilol plus ACE inhibitor was generally tolerated with associated improvements in Framingham heart failure score and quality of life [103]. However, because all therapies employed are empirically extrapolated from trials performed in patients with heart failure of other etiologies, the real benefit associated to each class of drugs remains to be demonstrated, both in terms of morbidity and mortality. This is especially relevant in the case of beta-blockers, since ChrChCpatients often have bradycardia that may limit their use, particularly with concomitant amiodarone therapy [105].

Bradyarrhythmias and Heart Block

Patients with second- or third-degree atrioventricular block or symptomatic sinus node dysfunction require permanent cardiac pacing.

Ventricular Arrhythmia and Sudden Cardiac Arrest

The first step in treating patients with ChrChC at risk for arrhythmia is optimization of medical therapy for heart failure (including beta blockers) since this may improve survival and reduce ventricular arrhythmias. The optimal approach for management of arrhythmia due to Chagas heart disease is uncertain. Potentially beneficial treatment tools include heart failure therapy, antiarrhythmic drugs, radiofrequency catheter ablation, implantable cardioverter-defibrillator device (ICD) placement, and surgical intervention.

The 2011 Latin American guidelines for Chagas' heart disease do not recommend ICD therapy for primary prevention of sudden cardiac arrest (SCA) [106]. For secondary prevention, the guidelines note that pharmacologic therapy should be an adjunct to ICD in patients with sustained ventricular tachycardia and LVEF <35 percent. For patients with well-tolerated sustained ventricular tachycardia with preserved LVEF, the guidelines suggest ICD implantation as the safest option, with amiodarone and ablation as other options.

The 2008 American College of Cardiology/American Heart Association/Heart Rhythm Society (ACC/AHA/HRS) guidelines for device-based therapy of cardiac rhythm abnormalities recommend an ICD for secondary prevention in patients who are survivors of SCA due to ventricular fibrillation or who have spontaneous sustained VT [107]. These guidelines also recommend an ICD for primary prevention in patients with nonischemic DCM with an LVEF ≤35 percent and NYHA functional class II or III.

Antiarrhythmic Drugs

Use of amiodarone in patients with Chagas' heart disease is based upon evidence that it improves survival free of cardiac arrest or ICD shocks in patients with other types of heart disease. Observations from in vitro and animal studies and a case report suggest that amiodarone might have an antitrypanosomal effect, although its efficacy as an antiparasitic agent has not been established [108].

Indications [109]: Amiodarone plus beta blocker therapy for patients with CCC with an LVEF ≤35 percent and a Rassi score of >10 or nonsustained VT on Holter (Grade 2C).

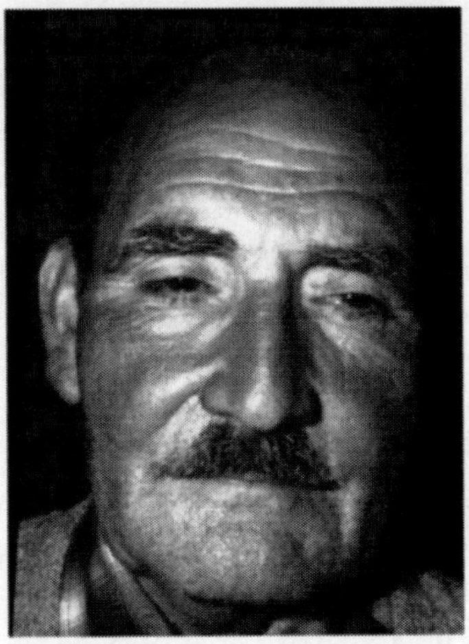

Reproduced from Milei et al. [5] with permission.

Figure 17. Blue-Gray skin discoloration as a side effect of long term treatment with Amiodarone.

Amiodarone for patients who survive an episode of SCA or have sustained ventricular tachycardia not treated with ICDs (due to physician or patient preference or because they are not candidates for an ICD) (Grade 2C).

Amiodarone plus beta blocker therapy to reduce shocks in patients treated with ICDs (Grade 2C).

Apart from the its well known side effects the blue-gray skin discoloration must be taken into in ChrChC patients treated with amiodarone (Figure 17).

Implantable Cardioverter Defibrillator

Treatment of patients with Chagas disease at risk for sudden cardiac death is controversial. Although ICD therapy has been empirically used for primary and secondary prevention of sudden cardiac arrest (SCA), there may be potential adverse effects of pacing and/or ICD therapy on pump function. Thus, deciding whether to implant an ICD would seem to represent a very important aspect of clinical management of these patients. However, thus far ICDs have been used only sporadically in this condition, even for secondary prevention of patients with previous episode of VT or VF); the largest single describes less than 100 patients. Furthermore, randomized clinical trials of ICD implantation have not included patients with ChrChC. Therefore, there is a need for getting better insights into the role of ICD in this condition [110]

Muratore et al. [111] presented data from a multi-centre South American registry of 89 chagasic patients who received an ICD, mostly (91%) for secondary prevention.

Over a mean follow-up of 12+7 months, 42% of patients received appropriate ICD therapy. Only six patients died (6.7%). Three due to congestive heart failure, one due to sudden death, and two due to non-cardiac cause. Importantly, 15.7% of patients experienced one or more episodes of electrical storm.

In a study of 116 patients with CD undergoing ICD implantation for secondary prevention were followed for a mean of 45 months [112]. The baseline mean LVEF was 42%.

Fifty % of patients had appropriate shocks and 11 percent had inappropriate ICD therapy. The annual mortality rate was 7 percent, with 45 percent of deaths caused by heart failure with no sudden deaths. Survival was worse in patients with more severe heart failure symptoms (NYHA class III), lower left ventricular ejection fraction, and more frequent right ventricular pacing.

Milei et al. [21] concluded that in patients with ChrChC, ICD therapy for secondary prevention is safe and effective, and it provides protection by effectively terminating life-threatening arrhythmias.

Given the potential implications of these results, these data need to be carefully considered.

One obvious comparison is with the already mentioned report by Cardinalli-Neto et al. [82] of 90 patients with ChrChC receiving ICD therapy for secondary prevention. Over an average follow-up of 756+581 days 64% of patients received appropriate shock. Thirty-four per cent died, suddenly in 7%, whereas heart failure was the prevailing cause of death (93%).

Finally, current evidence does not seem to be solid enough to dictate mandatory indications for ICD therapy in chagasic patients, nor can recommendations be immediately extrapolated from the results from patients with conditions other than Chagas' disease. In fact, although this condition shares many clinical features of classical DCM, it must be kept in mind that it is profoundly different in terms of mechanisms of disease, pathophysiology, and progression [21].

In this respect, in addition to obvious economical and logistic considerations, one must bear in mind the disturbing fact of a very high frequency of electrical storms in these patients, and that this may be a mechanism of cardiac injury and disease progression [21].

Indications [112]: patients with ChrChC who survive an episode of SCA or have sustained VT, particularly if the patient has already been treated with amiodarone and/or beta blocker therapy (Grade 2B). For patients with an LVEF $\leq$ 35 percent, and a Rassi score of >10 and NSVT on Holter, and a reasonable likelihood of survival of at least one year, ICD implantation is suggested (Grade 2C).

Conclusion

The etiologic agent of Chagas disease is present in South America, Central America, Mexico and south of United States of America. Due to immigration this disease can be found everywhere, especially in Europe. Although it is the most frequent type of chronic myocarditis in the world, there is a low awareness of the disease among physicians.

Two statements are clear: As long as there is poverty in the Latin American countries there will be Chagas disease and as long as this disease is neglected by other countries, or considered a problem restricted to South Americans, many patients will remain undiagnosed.

Despite recent advances in the understanding of the pathogenesis of ChrChC, which indicate that all seropositive patients in the acute form should receive specific treatment to reduce their parasite loads, treatment coverage of Chagas disease patients remains extremely low (currently estimated at <1 %), as the guidelines inmost endemic countries (with the exception of Brazil and Chile) still exclude chronic patients in endemic areas (reinfected), who are by far the large majority. Although observational studies have shown that treatment of chronic patients with currently available drugs, although hindered by frequent side effects and variable efficacy, can slow the clinical deterioration of the patients and reduce the occurrence of electrocardiographic alterations, there is not a scientific definition. A rigorous, randomized study to evaluate this issue (BENEFIT trial) is about to be completed in next year 2014.

In acute form the access to specific treatment of Chagas disease, with currently available or safer and more potent drugs is a medical priority in both endemic and non-endemic countries. Regarding the indeterminate phase, sudden death is uncommon and the risk of death is similar to that of the general population Thus, these patients should be allowed to lead a normal working life and to practice physical activity, without alarming them unnecessarily about their condition or indicating sophisticated and expensive studies.

Treatment of patients with Chagas cardiomyopathy at risk for cardiac death with ICD can be safe and effective. Given the potential implications of this therapy, these data need to be carefully considered.

References

[1] Rassi, AJ, Rassi A., and Rassi SG. Predictors of Mortality in Chronic Chagas Disease: A systematic review of observational studies. *Circulation.* 2007;115:1101-1108.

[2] Milei J, Mautner B, Storino RA, et al. Does Chagas' disease exist as an undiagnosed form of cardiomyopathy in the United States? *Am. Heart J.* 1992;123:1732-1735.

[3] Storino RA, Barragan H, and Milei J. Aspectos epidemiológicos de la enfermedad de Chagas en la Argentina y America Latina. Revista Federación Argentina de Cardiología. 1992; 21: 239-246.

[4] Storino RA, Milei J. Enfermedad de Chagas. Mosby-Doyma: Buenos Aires.1994.

[5] Milei J, Guerri-Guttenberg RA, Azzato F, et al. Chagasic cardiomyopathy: new trends for an old burden. Cardiomyopathies: Causes, Effects and Treatment.Editors: Bruno PH, Giordano MT. Hauppauge, New York: Nova Science Publishers. 2009.

[6] González J, Azzato F, Milei J.Pathogenesis and Pathology of Chagas' Chronic Myocarditis.In Myocarditis. Editor: Cihakova D. 2011; chapter 6, 119-150.

[7] Milei J, Alonso GF, Vanzulli S, et al. Myocardial inflammatory infiltrate in human chronic chagasic cardiomyopathy: immunohistochemical findings. *Cardiovasc. Pathol.* 1996; 5: 209-219.

[8] González J, Azzato F, Ambrosio G and Milei J. Pathogenesis of Chronic Chagasic Myocarditis. In Diagnosis and Treatment of Myocarditis. Editors: Milei J & Ambrosio G. Intech Europe. Rijeka, Croatia. 2013.

[9] Guerri-Guttenberg R, Milei J, Ambrosio G, et al. Chagas cardiomyopathy: Europe is not spared! *European Heart J.* 2008; 29: 2587–2591.

[10] Milei J, Grana DR, Storino R, et al. Prognostic impact of Chagas disease in the United States. *Am. Heart J.* 2009; 157:22-9.

[11] Milei J, Storino RA, Beigelman R, et al. Histopathology of specialized and ordinary myocardium and nerves in chronic Chagas disease, with a morphometric study of inflammation and fibrosis. *Cardiologia.* 1991;36:107-115.

[12] Ferrans VJ, Milei J, Tomita Y, et al. Basement membrane thickening in cardiac myocytes and capillaries in chronic Chagas' disease. *Am. J. Cardiol.* 1988;61:1137–1140.

[13] Sanchez JA, Milei J, Yu Z, et al. Immunohistochemical localization of laminin in the hearts of patients with chronic chagasic cardiomyopathy: relationship to thickening of basement membranes. *American Heart Journal.* 1993;126:1392 – 1401.

[14] Milei J, Pesce R, Valero E, et al. Electrophysiologic-structural correlations in chagasic aneurysms causing malignant arrhythmias. *International Journal of Cardiology.* 1991; 32: 65-74.

[15] Milei, J, Storino RA, Beigelman R, et al. Endomyocardial biopsies in chronic chagasic cardiomyopathy. Immunohistochemical and ultrastructural findings. *Cardiology.* 1992; 80: 424-37.

[16] Molina H, Milei J, and Storino R. Chronic Chagas' myocardiopathy. Demonstration of in vivo bound immunoglobulins in heart structures by the immunoperoxidase technique. *Cardiology.* 1984; 71: 297-306.

[17] Milei J, Sánchez J, Storino R, et al. Antibodies to laminin and immunohistochemical localization of laminin in chronic chagasic cardiomyopathy: a review. *Mol. Cell. Biochem.* 1993; 129: 161-70.

[18] Milei J. and Storino R. A. Laminin in chagasic autoimmunity? *Parasitol. Today.* 1987; 3: 119.

[19] Storino R, Milei J, Beigelman R, et al. Enfermedad de Chagas: doce años de seguimiento en área urbana. Revista Argentina de Cardiología. 1992; 60:205-216.

[20] Storino R.A. and Milei J. Mortalidad en la enfermedad de Chagas. Estudio longitudinal con 10 años de seguimiento. *Medicina.*1989; 49: 467.

[21] Milei J, Ambrosio G. Chagas cardiomyopathy and implantable cardioverter defibrillator implantation: similarities and differences with dilated cardiomyopathy. *Europace.* 2009 ;11:140-1.

[22] Younées-Chennoufi AB, Hontebeyre-Joskowicz M, Tricottet V, et al. Persistence of Trypanosoma cruzi antigens in the inflammatory lesions of chronically infected mice. *Trans. Roy Soc. Trop. Med. Hyg.* 1988; 82: 77.

[23] Jones EM, Colley DG, Tostes S, et al. Amplification of Trypanosoma cruzi DNA sequence from inflammatory lesions in human chagasic cardiomyopathy. *Am. J. Trop. Med. Hyg.* 1993; 48: 348-357.

[24] Higuchi ML, Brito T, and Martins Reis M. Correlation between trypanosoma cruzi parasitism and myocardial inflammatory infiltrate in human chronic chagasic myocarditis: in light microscopy and immunohistochemical findings. *Cardiovasc. Pathol.* 1993; 2: 101-106.

[25] Añez N, Carrasco H, Parada H. et al. Myocardial parasite persistence in chronic chagasic patients. *Amer. J. Trop. Med. Hyg.* 1999; 60: 726-732.

[26] Andrade Z. Novos aspectos sobre a patogenia da doenca de Chagas. *Rev. Soc. Bras. Med. Trop.* 1992; 25: 8.

[27] Teixeira ARL, Lacava ZL, Santana JM, et al. Insercao de DNA de trypanooma cruzi no genoma de celula hospedeira de mamifero por meio de infeccao. *Rev. Soc. Bras. Med. Trop.* 1991; 24: 55-61.

[28] Garcia S, Ramos C, Senra J, et al. Treatment with benznidazole during the chronic phase of experimental chagas disease decreases cardiac alterations. *Antimicrobial agents and chemotherapy*. 2005; 9:1521-1528.
[29] Andrade ZA. Pathogenesis of Chagas'disease. *Immunol.* 1991; 142: 126.
[30] Minoprio PM, Eisen H, Forni L, et al. Polyclonal lymphocyte responses to murine Trypaosoma cruzi infectio. Quantification of both T- and B-cell responses. *Scand. J. Immunol.* 1986; 24:661-666.
[31] Borda ES. and Sterin-Borda L. Antiadrenergic and mucarinic receptor antibodies in Chagas' cardiomyopathy. *Int. J. Cardiol.* 1996; 54:149-156.
[32] Sterin-Borda L, Gorelik G, and Borda ES. Chagasic IgG binding with cardiac muscarinic cholinergic receptors modifies cholinergic-mediated cellular transmembrane signals. *Clin. Immnol. Immunopathol.* 1991; 61: 387-397.
[33] Tafuri, WL. Patogenese. VIII Reunao Anual de Pesquisa Aplicada em Doenca de Chagas. *Rev. Soc. Bras. Med. Trop.* 1992; 25: 19.
[34] Carrasco Guerra HA, et al. Clinical, histochemical, and ultrastructural correlation in septal endomycardial biopsies from chronic cagasic patients: detection of early myocardial damage. *Am. Heart J.* 1987; 113:716-724.
[35] Schaper J, Froede R, and Hein S.T. Impairment of the myocardial ultrastructure and changes of the cytoskeleton in dilated cardiomyopathy. 1991; 83: 504.
[36] Oliveira JS, Mello De Oliveira JA, Frederigue U Jr, et al.. Apical aneurysm of Chagas' heart disease. *Br. Heart J.* 1981; 46:432-7.
[37] Acquatella H. Echocardiography in Chagas Heart Disease. *Circulation.* 2007; 115: 1124-1131.
[38] Carod-Artal FJ, Vargas AP, Horan TA, et al. Chagasic Cardiomyopathy is independently associated with ischemic stroke in Chagas disease. *Stroke.* 2005; 36: 965-970.
[39] Friedman PL, Fenoglio JJ Jr, Wit AL. Time course for reversal of electrophysiological and ultrastructural abnormalities in subendocardial punkinje fiber surviving extensive myocardial infarction in dogs. *Circ. Res.* 1975; 63:127-144.
[40] Rossi, L. The pathologic basis of cardiac arrhythmias. *Cardiol. Clin.* 1983; 1: 13-37.
[41] Reimer K. A. and Ideker R. E. Myocardial ischemia and infarction: anatomic and biochemical substrates for ischemic cell death and venticular arrhythmias. *Human Pathol.* 1987; 18: 462-475.
[42] Josephson ME, Horowitz LN, and Farchidi A. Sustained ventricular tachycardia: evidence for protected localized reentry. *Am. J. Cardiol.* 1978; 42:416-424.
[43] Josephson ME, Horowitz LN, and Farchidi A. Continuous local electrical activity: a mechanism of recurrent ventricular tachycardia. *Circulation*. 1978; 57: 659-665.
[44] Horowitz LN, Josephson ME, and Harken AH. Epicardial and endocardial activation during sustained ventricular tachycardia in man. *Circulation*. 1980; 61: 1227-1233.
[45] WHO Expert Committee. Control of Chagas Disease. World Health Organization, Brasilia, Brazil 2002. p. 1.
[46] Wegner DH, Rohwedder RW. The effect of nifurtimox in acute Chagas' infection. *Arzneimittelforschung* 1972; 22:1624.
[47] Schijman AG, Vigliano C, Burgos J, et al. Early diagnosis of recurrence of Trypanosoma cruzi infection by polymerase chain reaction after heart transplantation of a chronic Chagas' heart disease patient. *J. Heart Lung Transplant.* 2000; 19:1114.

[48] Kun H, Moore A, Mascola L, et al. Transmission of Trypanosoma cruzi by heart transplantation. *Clin. Infect. Dis.* 2009; 48:1534.

[49] Herwaldt BL. Laboratory-acquired parasitic infections from accidental exposures. *Clin. Microbiol. Rev.* 2001; 14:659.

[50] Hoff R, Mott KE, Silva JF, et al. Prevalence of parasitemia and seroreactivity to Trypanosoma cruzi in a rural population of Northeast Brazil. *Am. J. Trop. Med. Hyg.* 1979; 28:461.

[51] Sosa Estani S, Segura EL, Ruiz AM, et al. Efficacy of chemotherapy with benznidazole in children in the indeterminate phase of Chagas' disease. *Am. J. Trop. Med. Hyg.* 1998; 59:526.

[52] Williams JE. Leishmania and Trypanosoma. In: Medical Parasitology: A Practical Approach, Gillespie SH, Hawkey PM (Eds), Oxford University Press, Oxford, UK 2009. p.151.

[53] Gascón J, Albajar P, Canas E, et al. Diagnosis, Management, and Treatment of Chronic Chagas' Heart Disease in Areas Where Trypanosoma cruzi Infection is Not Endemic. *Rev. Esp. Cardiol.* 2007; 60: 285-93.

[54] Sosa-Estani S, Gamboa-León MR, Del Cid-Lemus J, et al. Use of a rapid test on umbilical cord blood to screen for Trypanosoma cruzi infection in pregnant women in Argentina, Bolivia, Honduras, and Mexico. *Am. J. Trop. Med. Hyg.* 2008; 79:755.

[55] Verani JR, Seitz A, Gilman RH, et al. Geographic variation in the sensitivity of recombinant antigen-based rapid tests for chronic Trypanosoma cruzi infection. *Am. J. Trop. Med. Hyg.* 2009; 80:410.

[56] Umezawa ES, Bastos SF, Camargo ME, et al. Evaluation of recombinant antigens for serodiagnosis of Chagas' disease in South and Central America. *J. Clin. Microbiol.* 1999; 37:1554.

[57] Junqueira AC, Chiari E, Wincker P. Comparison of the polymerase chain reaction with two classical parasitological methods for the diagnosis of Chagas disease in an endemic region of north-eastern Brazil. *Trans. R. Soc. Trop. Med. Hyg.* 1996; 90:129.

[58] Basquiera AL, Sembaj A, Aguerri AM, et al. Risk progression to chronic Chagas cardiomyopathy: influence of male sex and of parasitaemia detected by polymerase chain reaction. *Heart.* 2003; 89:1186.

[59] Wincker P, Telleria J, Bosseno MF, et al. PCR-based diagnosis for Chagas' disease in Bolivian children living in an active transmission area: comparison with conventional serological and parasitological diagnosis. *Parasitology.* 1997; 114: 367.

[60] Sosa-Estani S. Congenital transmission of Trypanosoma cruzi infection in Argentina. *Rev. Soc. Bras. Med. Trop.* 2005; 38 Suppl 2:29.

[61] Feilij H, Muller L, Gonzalez Cappa SM. Direct micromethod for diagnosis of acute and congenital Chagas' disease. *J. Clin. Microbiol.* 1983; 18:327.

[62] Luquetti AO, Dias JC, Prata A. Diagnosis and treatment of congenital infection caused by Trypanosoma cruzi in Brazil. *Rev. Soc. Bras. Med. Trop.* 2005; 38 Suppl 2:27.

[63] Bern C, Verastegui M, Gilman RH, et al. Congenital Trypanosoma cruzi transmission in Santa Cruz, Bolivia. *Clin. Infect. Dis.* 2009; 49:1667.

[64] Duffy T, Bisio M, Altcheh J, et al. Accurate real-time PCR strategy for monitoring bloodstream parasitic loads in chagas disease patients. *PLoS Negl. Trop. Dis.* 2009; 3:419.

[65] Russomando G, de Tomassone MM, de Guillen I, et al. Treatment of congenital Chagas' disease diagnosed and followed up by the polymerase chain reaction. *Am. J. Trop. Med. Hyg*. 1998; 59:487.

[66] Schijman A.G. Congenital Chagas Disease. In: Congenital and Other Related Infectious Diseases of the Newborn, Mushahwar IK (Ed), Elsevier, Amsterdam, Netherlands 2006;13:223.

[67] Carlier, Y. Torrico F. Congenital infection with Trypanosoma cruzi: from mechanisms of transmission to strategies for diagnosis and control. *Rev. Soc. Bras. Med. Trop*. 2003; 36:767.

[68] Pondé, A. A cardiopatía crónica na molesstias de Chagas. Hospital (Rio de Janeiro), 1960; 6: 58.

[69] Amorin DS, Manco JC, Gallo L, et al. Clínica: Forma crónica cardiaca. En: Braner Z, Andrade ZA. Trypanosoma cruzi e Doença de Chagas. Río de Janeiro, Brasil: Guanabara-Koogan, 1979: 265-311.

[70] Heckerling, PS, Stanley L, Vijai K. et al., Accuracy of precordial percussion in detecting cardiomegaly. *Am. J. Med.* 1991. 91:328-334.

[71] Sosa-Jurado F, Mazariego-aranda M, Hernández-BecerrilN., et. al. Electrocardiographic findings in Mexican chagasic subjects living in high and low endemic regions of Trypanosoma cruzi infection. *Mem. Inst. Oswaldo Cruz.* 2003; 98: 605-610.

[72] Álvarez J. and Rosenbaum M. Radiología cardiovascular en la miocarditis crónica chagásica. *Rev. Arg. Cardiol.* 1953; 20: 146.

[73] Schapachnik E. Enfermedad de Chagas crónica. correlación radiológica y electrocardiográfica. *Rev. Arg. Cardiol.* 1980; 48: 256.

[74] Centers-for-Disease-Control-and-Prevention-(CDC). Blood donor screening for Chagas disease - United States, 2006-2007. MMWR Morb. *Mortal. Wkly. Rep*. 2007; 56: 141-3.

[75] Ferreira M, Nishioka S, Silvestre MT, et al. Reactivation of Chagas' disease in patients with AIDS: Report of three new cases and review of the literature. *Clinical Infectious Disease*. 1997; 25: 1397-400.

[76] Sartori, AMC, Ibrahim KY, Nunes Westphalen EV. et al. Manifestatons of Chagas disease (American trypanosomiasis) in patients with HIV/AIDS. *Ann. Trop. Med. Parasitol.* 2007; 101: 31-50.

[77] Benvenuti LA, Roggério A, Sambiase NV, et al. Polymerase chain reaction in endomyocardial biopsies for monitoring reactivation of Chagas' disease in heart transplantation. A case report and review of the literature. *Cardiovasc. Pathol.* 2005; 14: 265-268.

[78] Rosenbaum M. Nuevas observaciones sobre patogenia y tratamiento de la miocardiopatía chagásica e idiopática. in V jornadas Municipales de Cardiología. 1992. Buenos Aires, Argentina.

[79] Bustamante JM, Rivarola H, Fernández A, et al. Reinfections and Trypanosoma cruzi strains can determine the prognosis of the chronic chagasic cardiopathy in mice. *Parasitol. Res.* 2007; 100:1407-1410.

[80] Chagas, G.d.i.s.l.e.d. Aspectos clínicos de la enfermedad de Chagas. Informe de una revisión conjunta OMS/OPS de investigadores. *Bol. of Sanit. Panam.* 1974;77: 141-155.

[81] Theodoropoulos TAD, Bestetti RB, Ottaviano AP, et al. Predictors of all-cause mortality in chronic Chagas' heart disease in the current era of heart failure therapy. *Int. J. Cardiol.* 2008; 128: 22-29.

[82] Cardinalli-Neto A, Bestetti R, Cordeiro J, et al. Predictors of All-Cause Mortality for Patients with Chronic Chagas' Heart Disease Receiveing Implantable cardioverter Defibrillator Therapy. *Journal of Cardiovascular Electrophysiology.* 2007;18: 1236-1240.

[83] Rassi A Jr, Rassi A, Little WC, et al. Development and validation of a risk score for predicting death in Chagas' heart disease. *N. Engl. J. Med.* 2006; 355:799.

[84] Auger S, Storino R, Iglesias Ordoñez O, et al. Emergencies in patients with Chagas' disease in Buenos Aires city, Argentina. *Rev. Soc. Bras. Med. Trop.* 2002; 35: 609-619.

[85] Dias JCP. Doenca de Chagas em Bambui, Minas Gerais, Brasil. Estudo clínico empiedmiológico a partir da fase aguda entre 1940 e 1982. in Universidade Federal de Minas Gerais. 1982. Belo Horizonte.

[86] Linetzky B, Konfino J, Castellana N, et al. Risk of cardiovascular events associated with positive serology for Chagas: asystematic review. *International Journal of Epidemiology.* 2012; 41:1356–1366.

[87] Gonzalez J, Azzato F, Milei J, et al. La muerte súbita es infrecuente en la forma indeterminada de la enfermedad de Chagas: una revisión sistemática. *Rev. argent. cardiol.* 2012; 80: 242-249.

[88] Urbina J. A. Parasitological cure of Chagas disease: Is it possible? Is it relevant? *Mem. Inst. Oswaldo Cruz.* 1999; 94: 349-355.

[89] Urbina J. A. and Docampo R. Specific chemotherapy of Chagas disease: controversies and advances. *Trends in Parasitology.* 2003; 19: 495-501.

[90] Cançado J. R. Long Term evaluation of etiological treatment of Chagas disease with benznidazole. *Rev. Inst. Med. trop. S. Paulo.* 2002; 44: 29-37.

[91] Fabbro DL, Arias E, Streiger M, et al. Evolutive behaviour towards cardiomyopathy of treated (nifurtimox or benznidazole) and untreated chronic chagasic patients. *Rev. Inst. Med. trop. S. Paulo.* 2000; 42: 99-109.

[92] Fabbro DL, Streiger ML, Arias ED, et al. Trypanocide treatment among adults with chronic Chagas disease living in Santa Fe City (Argentina), over a mean follow-up of 21 years: parasitological, serological and clinical evaluation. *Rev. Soc. Bras. Med. Trop.* 2007; 40:1-10.

[93] Reyes P.A. and M. Vallejo. Trypanocidal drugs for late stage, symptomatic Chagas disease (Trypanosoma cruzi infection). Cochrane Database of Systematic Reviews, 2005. Issue 4. Art No.: CD004102.DOI: 10.1002/14651858.CD004102.pub2

[94] Braga MS, Lauria-Pires L, Arganaraz ER. et al. Persistent infections in chronic chagas disease patients treated with anti-trypanosoma cruzi nitroderivates. *Rev. Inst. Med. trop. S. Paulo.* 2000; 42:157-161.

[95] Lauria Pires L, Braga MS, Vexenat AC, et al. Progressive chronic Chagas heart disease ten years after treatment with anti-trypanosoma cruzi nitroderivatives. *Am. J. Trop. Med. Hyg.* 2000; 63: 111-118.

[96] Viotti R, Vigliano C, Lococo B, et al. Long-term cardiac outcomes of treating chronic Chagas disease with benznidazole versus no treatment. *Ann. Intern. Med.* 2006; 144:724-734.

[97] Sgambatti de Andrade AL, Zicker F, De Oliveira RM, et al. Randomised trial of efficacy of benznidazole in treatment of early Trypanosoma cruzi infection. *The Lanet.* 1996; 348: 1407-13.

[98] Solari A, Ortíz S, Soto A, et al. Treatment of Trypanosoma cruzi-infected children with nifurtimox: a 3 year follow up by PCR. *J. Antimicrob. Chemother.* 2001; 48: 515-9.

[99] Ferraz ML, Gazzinelli RT, Alves RO, et .al. The anti-trypanosoma cruzi activity of posaconazole in a murine model of acute Chagas' disease is less dependent on gamma interferon than that of benznidazole. *Antimicrobial agents and chemotherapy.* 2007; 51: 1359-1364.

[100] Berger B. J. and Fairlamb A. H. Interactions between immunity and chemotherapy in the treatment of trypanosomiases and leishmaniases. *Parasitology.* 1992; 105: 71-78.

[101] Targett G. A. Chemotherapy and the immune response in parasitic infections. *Parasitology.* 1985; 90: 661-673.

[102] Bern C, Montgomery S, Herwaldt B, et al. Evaluation and Treatment of Chagas Disease in the United States. *JAMA.* 2007; 298:2171-2181.

[103] Marin-Neto J, Rassi A., Morillo C, et al. Rationale and design of a randomized placebo-controlled trial assessing the effects of etiologic treatment in Chagas' cardiomyopathy: he BENznidazole Evaluation For Interrupting Trypanosomiasis (BENEFIT). *Am. Heart J.* 2008;156: 37-43.

[104] Botoni FA, Poole-Wilson PA, Ribeiro AL, et al. A randomized trial of carvedilol after renin-angiotensin system inhibition in chronic Chagas cardiomyopathy. *Am. Heart J.* 2007; 153: 544.

[105] Rassi A Jr, Rassi A, Marin-Neto JA. Chagas disease. *Lancet.* 2010; 375:1388.

[106] Andrade JP, Marin Neto JA, Paola AA, et al. I Latin American Guidelines for the diagnosis and treatment of Chagas' heart disease: executive summary. *Arq. Bras. Cardiol.* 2011; 96:434.

[107] Epstein AE, DiMarco JP, Ellenbogen KA, et al. ACC/AHA/HRS 2008 Guidelines for Device-Based Therapy of Cardiac Rhythm Abnormalities: a report of the American College of Cardiology/American Heart Association Task Force on Practice Guidelines (Writing Committee to Revise the ACC/AHA/NASPE 2002 Guideline Update for Implantation of Cardiac Pacemakers and Antiarrhythmia Devices): developed in collaboration with the American Association for Thoracic Surgery and Society of Thoracic Surgeons. *Circulation* 2008; 117:350.

[108] Benaim G, Paniz Mondolfi AE. The emerging role of amiodarone and dronedarone in Chagas disease. *Nat. Rev. Cardiol.* 2012; 9:605.

[109] Marin-Neto A, Maciel B, Simões M, et al. Treatment and prognosis of Chagas heart disease. *UpToDate* 2013.

[110] Rassi A Jr. Implantable cardioverter-defibrillators in patients with Chagas heart disease: misperceptions, many questions and the urgent need for a randomized clinical trial. *J. Cardiovasc. Electrophysiol.* 2007; 18:1241.

[111] Di Toro D, Muratore C, Aguinaga L, et al. Predictors of all-cause 1-year mortality in implantable cardioverter defibrillator patients with chronic Chagas' cardiomyopathy. *Pacing Clin. Electrophysiol.* 2011; 34:1063.

[112] Martinelli M, de Siqueira SF, Sternick EB, et al. Long-term follow-up of implantable cardioverter-defibrillator for secondary prevention in chagas' heart disease. *Am. J. Cardiol.* 2012; 110: 1040.

In: Recent Advances in Cardiology
Editors: José Milei and Giuseppe Ambrosio

ISBN: 978-1-63117-282-3

Chapter 6

Heparin-Induced Thrombocytopenia: Mechanisms and Management

Anna Vittoria Mattioli*
Department of Life Science, Lab of Cardiology and Angiology,
University of Modena and Reggio Emilia, Italy

Abstract

Heparin-induced thrombocytopenia (HIT) is an immune adverse drug-induced reaction characterized by thrombocytopenia and paradoxical thrombosis. HIT is induced by heparin dependent IgG antibodies that bind the PF4 factor and activate platelets. The pathophysiology of HIT is complex, involving platelet activation, the activation of coagulation cascade, and endothelial dysfunction. Clinical suspicion f HIT can be confirm by using two different types of laboratory assay: a platelet activation assays and immunoassays for detection of PF4-heparin antibodies. These latter are most frequently used in clinical practice due to their wide availability. The clinical picture includes severe thrombocytopenia, typically developing between days 4 to day 10 from the exposure to heparin, followed by venous or arterial thrombosis. The most frequent clinical presentations are deep venous thrombosis and pulmonary embolism, however patients affected by cardiovascular disease can develop embolic stroke, recurrent myocardial infarction and arterial thrombosis.

The management of HIT includes discontinuation of any kind of heparin drugs, including heparin flushes. Recent 2012 practice guidelines from the ACCP recommended the administration of directs thrombin inhibitors and factor Xa inhibitors in patients with acute HIT and in patients with heparin-induced antibodies even in absence of thrombocytopenia and thrombosis.

* Address for correspondence: Anna Vittoria Mattioli, MD PhD, FACC, FESC. Department of Life Science-University of Modena and R.E. Via del pozzo, 71, 41100 Modena (Italy). Phone: +39 59 4224043 Fax: +39 59 2055426, E-mail: annavittoria.mattioli@unimore.it.

Introduction

Heparin is one of the most commonly used drugs in patients that require therapeutic intervention for cardiovascular disease with million patients treated annually. The use of unfractionated heparin has some serious side effects and one of the most dramatic is heparin-induced thrombocytopenia (HIT) (table 1). HIT is an immune-mediated adverse drug-induced reaction characterized by thrombocytopenia and an increased incidence of thrombosis following subsequent exposure to heparin-like medications. [1, 2]. Two forms of thrombocytopenia are described: an early benign reversible non immune thrombocytopenia and a late more serious immunoglobulin G (IgG)-mediated immune thrombocytopenia and this latter will be described in the present chapter.

Frequency of HIT

HIT can be without any thromboembolic events (isolated HIT) or with associated thrombosis (HITT). Isolated HIT occurs in 1% to 5% of all patients receiving heparin, and 25% to 50% of these patients may develop HITT [3, 4]. Thrombosis affects large veins and arteries, however HITT can also involve microvascular thrombosis. Thrombosis usually occurs in association with great platelet count declines, which is consistent with platelet activation. Several risk factors are associated with HIT, most of them are related to heparin type, heparin preparation and duration of exposure.

HIT is more often seen with bovine heparin compared with porcine heparin, and with unfractionated heparin (UFH) compared with low-molecular-weight heparin (LMWH) and to patients treated with fondaparinux [5, 6]. Female gender is more likely to develop HIT antibodies during prophylaxis with heparin, however HIT is rare in pregnant women. Highest reported frequencies of HIT are in postsurgical thromboprophylaxis compared to medical treatment. [4, 7, 8]. Patients with cardiovascular disease and critically ill patients are at particular risk for the development of HIT antibodies. As many as 25% to 50% of patients who undergo cardiac surgery develop positive levels of anti heparin/PF4 antibodies postoperative. [8, 9, 10]. One of the most important risk factor is the duration of exposure to heparin.

Table 1. Heparin side effects

Bleeding (freq. 1% to 33%) • Type of heparin (UH or LMWH) • Dose of heparin • Mode of administration • Patients characteristics (i.e., concomitant use of aspirin or of antiplatelets drugs, age >60 years, concomitant serious disease, renal failure, hepatic disease, abuse of alcohol)
Osteoporosis
Alopecia
Necrotic skin lesion
Hyperaldosteronism
HIT with or without thrombosis

Table 2. Incidence of HIT according to patient population and type of heparin

Patient Population	Incidence of HIT %
Cardiovascular surgery patients	1-5
Postoperative patients: prophylactic dose of heparin	1-5
Postoperative patients: therapeutic dose of heparin	1-5
Postoperative patients: flushes of heparin	0.1-1
Postoperative patients prophylactic or therapeutic dose of LMWH	0.1-1
Medical patients: prophylactic or therapeutic dose of heparin	0.1-1
Medical patients: prophylactic or therapeutic dose of LMWH	0.6-08
Patients with cancer	1
Intensive care patients	0.4-08

A high number of cardiac surgery patients (19%) have already developed antibodies before surgery [2, 8, 11]. Most of these patients have a history of prior exposure to UFH, and the prevalence of antibodies detected after cardiac surgery in this heavily treated population is higher compared with patients who have no prior exposure to heparin suggesting a mechanism of anamnestic response [2].

HIT is a clinicopathologic syndrome; the diagnosis requires one or more clinical events (e.g., thrombocytopenia, thrombosis) bearing a temporal association with pathologic HIT antibodies formation [8, 12].

Pathogenesis

The pathophysiology of HIT is complex, involving the activation of platelet, of coagulation cascade and endothelial dysfunction [2, 13]. HIT is induced by heparin dependent IgG antibodies against platelets factor-4 (PF4)/heparin complex that activate platelets. PF4 is a member of the CXC chemokine family that plays important physiologic roles in processes of coagulation, inflammation, and tissue repair. It is stored in platelet alpha granules. They circulate in smaller amounts of accounting for approximately 2% to 3% of the total protein found in the platelets [14]. When the platelets are activated, PF4 is released in much larger concentrations from the alpha granules, especially in the proximity of vessel wall injury [15, 16]. During UFH infusion, PF4 levels increase 15- to 30-fold for several hours, by displacing PF4 from endothelial cell surfaces. PF4/heparin complexes bind to platelet surfaces. Complexes of CXCL4/PF-4 and heparin were found to circulate after heparin injection in most patients but without any clinical effect. However, some patients (1–5%) developed IgG specific antibodies against CXCL4/PF-4-heparin in close proximity to the platelet surface. These immune complexes are thought to activate platelets via the platelet Fc receptor FcγRII. [17] IgG antibodies recognize neoepitope sites on PF4, leading to formation of CXCL4/PF-4/heparin/IgG complexes on the platelet surface. Binding of the immune complex to Fc receptor of the platelets leads to platelet activation. Activated platelets release additional PF4 that induces a cycle of progressive platelet and coagulation activation. Binding of HIT-inducing antibodies to a complex PF4/heparin and this excess amount of PF4 can facilitate thrombosis by bringing together platelets and the endothelium and also by activating monocytes which carry tissue factor. The high frequency of HIT in patients undergoing cardiac surgery and orthopaedic procedures can also be explained by the 'adequate' tissue injury which occurs with these procedures. [16, 17] The release of large amounts of PF4 with tissue injury neutralises the negative charge on the platelets and endothelial surfaces allowing platelet–endothelial interaction necessary for thrombus formation either in veins and arteries.

Clinical Features

HIT is clinically considered when the platelet count falls by 50% or more of the baseline value (thrombocytopenia), occurring temporally between day 5 and 14 of therapy, and sometimes, followed by fatal paradoxical thrombotic events.

"Definite" HIT is established when a patient with possible HIT also has positive results of laboratory antigen assay for HIT-IgG typically between 5 and 10 days after a recent exposure to heparin as the immune system requires several days to produce sufficient amounts of antibodies (*Typical-onset HIT*).

The median platelet count nadir reported in HIT is about 60 $\pm$ 109/L [18, 19]. Most patients experienced a 50% or greater decrease in the platelet count. The most typical platelet count evolution associated with HIT is characterized by an unexpected fall that occurs at least 5 days after exposure to heparin. There are several potential explanations for thrombocytopenia in patients receiving heparin, especially in critically ill. The most frequent cause of thrombocytopenia in such patients is sepsis however several other conditions can cause thrombocytopenia and mimic HIT, i.e disseminated intravascular coagulation, intra-aortic balloon pump, multiorgan failure, heart failure, drugs such as glycoprotein IIb/IIIa (GpIIb/IIIa) inhibitors and very rarely aspirin, clopidogrel, and intravenous contrast dye [1, 2]. Early diagnosis is very important because patients with HIT have to interrupt heparin to stop the self-perpetuating mechanism that lead to increase PF4 release and to clinical thrombosis. Thrombocytopenia is a frequent postoperative event after cardiac surgery, either with or without cardiopulmonary bypass, and HIT is difficult to diagnose in this particular clinical setting. This transient thrombocytopenia can be triggered by haemodilution, hypothermia and platelet activation that results from the contact of blood with the extracorporeal circuit. Cardiopulmonary bypass induces strong platelet activation, with the release into the plasma of large amounts of PF4. In addition, patients are exposed to high doses of heparin and this probably explains why up to 50% of patients undergoing heart surgery develop antibodies to heparin–PF4 complexes. So that monitoring of the platelets count is therefore an important feature of postcardiac surgical care [19]. Interestingly the frequency of PF4/H antibody is the same among patients undergoing surgery with or without CPB [20].

Data from the CATCH study shows a higher incidence of thrombocytopenia among patients being treated with UFH or LMWH than previously reported [21]. Patients who develop thrombocytopenia has a lower baseline platelet count and a lower body mass index, and also are more likely to be admitted because of cardiovascular diseases: i.e., acute coronary syndrome or cardiovascular surgery. The CATCH investigators also find a direct and consistent relationship between the type, route, and duration of heparin therapy and the likelihood of thrombocytopenia.

Patients that receive UFH intravenously are at higher risk than those who receive UFH or LMWH subcutaneously. The risk increases with longer heparin exposure, 4% per 1-day increment beyond 4 days of heparin therapy. This observation has important implications for routine clinical practice.

Thrombocytopenia, in particular, a greater than 70% reduction in platelet count from baseline, is independently associated with adverse short-term clinical outcomes [22]. Thrombocytopenia is a common occurrence among ACS patients, and patients who develop even mild thrombocytopenia incur significantly higher risks of inhospital mortality and bleeding complications. Similarly there is evidence that the presence of antiheparin/PF4 antibodies is a risk factor for poor outcomes in certain populations, even in the absence of thrombocytopenia [23, 24, 25].

The timing of thrombocytopenia is influenced by the presence or absence of prior exposure to UFH.

In patients who have been exposed to UFH within the previous 3 weeks, the thrombocytopenia can begin at a median time of 10.5 hours after the initiation of heparin therapy. These patients already have circulating heparin-dependent antibodies developed during the previous treatment with UFH.

This clinical situation is named *rapid-onset HIT*. The onset of HIT in these cases is usually accompanied by fever, shivering, and skin lesions at the injection sites within 30 minutes after heparin administration [26]. Some patients also develop acute respiratory or cardiac dysfunction, or dyspnea. These manifestations may suggest pulmonary embolism because of the sudden pronounced platelet activation [26, 27].

Such a rapid and significant fall in the platelet count is very common during CPB, but the diagnosis of HIT is rarely evoked. Indeed, the platelets count quickly returns to normal values in the majority of cases after cardiac surgery although most patients have recently been exposed to heparin.

In rare circumstances, HIT may begin several days after heparin has already been stopped (*delayed-onset HIT*) and this is associated with high levels of anti-PF4/heparin antibodies and strongly positive tests for HIT antibodies. Delay onset HIT is very dangerous because it is always undiagnosed due to the delay in clinical manifestation [12]. As a result of lack of disease recognition, patients could receive additional heparin, resulting in a further decrease in platelet count and thrombosis complications. Heparin complications can become evident well after the initial heparin exposure is complete and the heparin is withdrawn.

Delay onset HIT can cause devastating venous thromboembolism or arterial clots, prolongs hospitalization, and increases costs. [27] Some patients experienced disseminated severe intravascular coagulation associated with depletion of fibrinogen. This is a rare complication of HIT but it seems to be more common in patients with delayed-onset HIT [27, 28].

Heparin induced antibodies persist in patients for a long period after cessation of heparin therapy (median time to a negative antigen assay of 90 days); we observe that in a number of patients antibodies persisted for many months after exposure, similarly to what happen to antibodies induced by other drugs i.e., sulfonamides. Importantly, the number of thrombotic events decreases over time in patients with persisting antibodies, but there remained a higher long-term risk of events. The presence of circulating antibodies is one of the possible mechanisms invoked to explain delay-onset HIT [8, 12].

Thrombotic Complications

Clinically, the majority of patients who develop HIT antibodies do not develop thrombocytopenia and thrombosis. However, HIT is associated with thrombotic complications in 30–70% of cases. These may develop without significant thrombocytopenia in 15% of patients [2, 4]. Thrombotic events occur around three days before the onset of thrombocytopenia in 40% of HIT patients. In HIT, the risk of thrombosis is 5% to 10% per day for the first 2 days after heparin is discontinued and may persist for weeks thereafter [29, 30].

In patients with symptomatic deep vein thrombosis (DVT) after initiation of heparin therapy, HIT cannot be excluded even in the absence of thrombocytopenia.

The most common thrombotic complications in patients with HIT include DVT (50%) and pulmonary embolism (25%) [31, 32]. Venous thrombosis is 4 to 10 times higher than arterial thrombosis [31, 33]. Other less common complications affected the arterial system and include limb artery thrombosis (10-15%), vascular stroke (5-8%), and myocardial infarction (5%). Other thrombotic events include sinus vein thrombosis, mesenteric venous or arterial occlusion, and skin necrosis [30, 33]. Adrenal hemorrhage associated with thrombosis of adrenal vein has been described.

Arterial thrombosis is more frequent in patients with cardiovascular disease and includes limb ischemia, thrombotic stroke, MI, loss of bypass conduits after coronary artery bypass graft surgery, mesenteric artery and renal artery thrombosis, distal aortic thrombosis, spinal artery thrombosis [30, 31, 33].

Thrombosis is more frequent during re-exposure to heparin in patients who had persisting anti-PF4/heparin antibodies. Recurrence of acute myocardial infarction (30 days after the first event) is more frequent in such patients even in the absence of thrombocytopenia. Persistent thrombin generation from the culprit lesion for up to 30 days after the acute event, along with antibody activation of platelets and endothelial surface in the vicinity of the plaque, could lead to recurrent thrombosis within the coronary artery [30, 31, 34].

The occlusion rate of saphenous venous grafts compared with arterial grafts is significantly increased in HIT patients [35].

Necrotizing skin lesions at heparin injection sites are specific for HIT. Erythematous plaques or skin necrosis at heparin injection sites may be seen in 5% to 10% of HIT patients. Heparin-induced skin lesions are strongly associated with formation of HIT antibodies even in the absence of thrombocytopenia [36].

About 10%–20% of patients who have HIT have disseminated intravascular coagulation. Regardless of therapy, the mortality rate of HIT patients developing thrombosis is very high (8% to 20%) [37].

A clinical score has been developed for evaluation of patients for possible HIT [38]. This scoring system allows stratifying patients based on the probability of HIT (unlikely, likely, and very likely). The 4 Ts Score, evaluates Thrombocytopenia, its Timing, the presence of Thrombosis (or other sequelae of HIT), and whether oTher plausible (Table 3).

Patients with low pretest scores (< 4 points) are unlikely to be positive for HIT antibodies (0 to 1.6%), whereas patients with intermediate (4–5 points) and high (> 5 points) scores are more likely to test positive (21.4% to 100%). The 4Ts Score has a high-negative predictive value. However the positive predictive value varies in different clinical settings.

Table 3. 4T score

Parameter	Point 2	Point 1	Point 0
Thrombocytopenia	Platelet count fall >50% or platelet nadir ≥20	Platelet count fall 30–50% or platelet nadir 10–19	Platelet count fall <30% or platelet nadir <10
Timing	Clear onset between days 5–14 or Platelet fall ≤1 day (prior heparin exposure within 30 days)	Consistent with days 5–10 fall, but not clear or Onset after day 10days; or Fall ≤1 day (prior heparin exposure 30–100 days ago)	Platelet count fall <4 days without recent heparin exposure
Thrombosis	New thrombosis or skin necrosis (at site of injection)	Progressive/recurrent thrombosis or Suspected thrombosis	None
Other plausible causes of thrombocytopenia	None apparent	Possible other cause	Definite other cause

Modified from Lo [38].

In critically ill patients, the Warkentin 4-T scoring system lacks specificity. It has been suggested that the Warkentin 4-T in the ICU might assist in ruling out HIT for a 4-T score <4; an intermediate to high score (>4) necessities more specific testing [39].

Laboratory Tests

Two general types of laboratory assay are used to confirm the diagnosis: platelet activation assays such as the serotonin release assay (SRA) and immunoassays such as the enzyme-linked immunosorbent assay (ELISA) for detection of PF4-heparin antibodies.

Activation assays, the platelet SRA, detect HIT-IgG on the basis of their ability to activate platelets. The SRA is considered to be the gold standard for a laboratory diagnosis of HIT. The SRA measures the platelet-activation response to the anti–PF4- heparin complex as opposed to solely determining the presence of antibody however the test is performed by few laboratories [40, 2].

Commercial antigen assays, the enzyme-linked immunosorbent assay (ELISA) for detection of PF4-heparin antibodies is easier to find in clinical practice [40, 41].

Commercially available ELISAs are highly sensitive in the detection of PF4-heparin–Ig G antibodies; however, nonpathologic, non– platelet-activating antibodies are also detected by these assays. As such, available polyspecific ELISAs have poor diagnostic specificity for PF4-heparin platelet-activating antibodies as many patients exposed to heparin develop detectable antibodies even in the absence of clinical HIT.

A reason for low diagnostic specificity is the detection of the cutoff values in optical density (OD) units that define positive test results, cutoff values were determined using blood derived from normal individuals who have presumably not been exposed to heparin. In contrast, diagnostic testing is almost always performed in patients who have been exposed to heparin. Thus, the OD distribution of heparin-exposed patients without HIT could differ considerably from the distribution of normal individuals. A second reason is that not all the antibodies detected by the ELIZA test are able to activated platelets and consequently not all antibodies are pathogenic [42].

Moreover these commercial assays cannot detect antibodies against heparin-dependent antigens other than PF4. However the enzyme-immuno assays test is wide available and highly sensitive (about 99.5%) for detecting heparin-dependent platelet-activating antibodies, so that it is ideal for ruling out HIT. A negative EIA result usually indicates that further assessment with a functional assay is not indicated [42].

However, because HIT antibodies can be transient, it is important the timing for serum or plasma tests [42, 8]. Anti heparin/PF4 antibodies persist for a relatively long period, and this persistence is associated with a high risk of HIT and HIT-thrombosis. Patients in whom heparin/PF4 antibodies are already detectable before surgery as a result of previous exposure to heparin has an even greater increase of titer after surgery and a more prolonged persistence of positivity during follow-up. These patients are also more likely to have thrombotic events during follow-up [8, 43].

Treatment

The association between HIT and thrombosis and the tendency for thrombotic events to occur early, mean that many patients have symptomatic thrombosis at the time that HIT is diagnosed. Moreover due to the high frequency of late thrombotic events in patients with HIT antibodies suggests that such patients should be treated with an alternative nonheparin anticoagulant even in absence of evident thrombosis.

To prevent thrombosis and HIT, recent "2012 practice guidelines from the ACCP for the treatment of HIT" include recommendations for platelet count monitoring for patients with a minimum heparin exposure of at least 4 days [44].

Recommendations for frequency of platelet count monitoring vary according to the estimated risk of HIT and depend on both the population and type of heparin therapy considered. The guidelines advocate as a Grade 2C recommendation platelet count monitoring every 2–3 days from days 4 through 14 or until cessation of heparin, whichever occurs first, in patients with >1 % risk of HIT (i.e., cardiac surgery patients and any postoperative patient without recent heparin exposure treated with therapeutic- or prophylactic-dose UFH). In contrast, patients in whom the risk of HIT is considered <1 % (i.e., medical and obstetrical patients, and non-cardiac surgery postoperative patients receiving LMWH or heparin flushes) should not have platelet counts routinely monitored (Grade 2C) [44].

The first step in treatment of HIT is discontinuation of all heparin products, including heparin flushes and heparin-coated catheters. In addition to heparin cessation, appropriate non-heparin anticoagulants should be started immediately, even if in the absence of thrombosis. In fact, the 30-day risk for subsequent thrombosis in isolated HIT after heparin cessation has been estimated to be as high as 55.5 %.

Current treatment is focused on reduction of thrombin generation via direct thrombin inhibition (e.g., bivalirudin, argatroban, lepirudin) or indirect factor Xa inhibition (e.g., fondaparinux or danaparoid) [44]. Treatment with direct thrombin inhibitors is strongly recommended in patients with HIT. While both direct thrombin inhibitors (DTIs) and factor Xa inhibitors have been used to treat patients with HIT, few data on randomized trials are available so that guidelines focused on historical control studies.

For patients with HITT, ACCP guidelines recommend use of argatroban, lepirudin and danaparoid (no longer available in the U.S.) over continuation of heparin products or use of vitamin K antagonist therapy (Grade 1C) or other non-heparin anticoagulants (Grade 2C). [44].

Inhibition of thrombin generated by HITT can be achieved with DTIs, such as lepirudin (recombinant hirudin), desirudin (recombinant hirudin), argatroban, or bivalirudin, or indirect factor Xa inhibitors, such as danaparoid or fondaparinux [45, 46, 47, 48, 49, 50, 51].

All of these agents have been used to treat patients with HITT, but there are no high-quality prospective head-to-head trials comparing one agent with another [44].

In patients with HITT who have normal renal function, guidelines suggest the use of argatroban or lepirudin or danaparoid over other nonheparin anticoagulants (Grade 2C). While in patients with HITT and renal insufficiency, is indicated the use of argatroban over other nonheparin anticoagulants (Grade 2C). Argatroban and lepirudin have been directly compared in small retrospective cohort studies. However, comparison across these studies is problematic because the primary outcome measure differed, and the outcomes we have identified as important were not consistently reported [52, 53, 54].

In patients with acute HIT (thrombocytopenia and HIT antibody positive) or subacute HIT (platelets recovered, but still HIT antibody positive) who require urgent cardiac surgery, guidelines suggest the use of bivalirudin over other nonheparin anticoagulants and over heparin plus antiplatelet agents (Grade 2C).

In patients with acute HIT who require nonurgent cardiac surgery, it is recommend delaying the surgery (if possible) until HIT has resolved and HIT antibodies are negative (Grade 2C).

Patients with a past history of HIT can theoretically be re-exposed to heparin, in specific circumstances, because of several properties of HIT antibodies. First, the HIT antibody is known to be transient, with a median time to disappearance of 50 to 80 days (depending on the assay performed). [8, 43, 44] Second, there is no evidence to suggest that patients with a prior history of HIT (who are currently HIT antibody negative) will have an amnestic immune response on re-exposure to heparin (i.e., sensitization does not occur with , 4 days of exposure to heparin and the level of response is not stronger than with the initial episode of HIT).

Because there are no clinical trials evaluating the safety of this premise guideline recommendation are based on the incidence of recurrent HIT or re-emergence of HIT antibodies following intentional (or accidental) re-exposure to heparin or LMWH in observational studies.

The ACCP guidelines for treatment of HIT also include recommendations for use of platelet transfusions. The risk of bleeding in patients with HIT is very low, and platelet transfusions has been reported to increase the risk of thrombosis in HIT patients [55]. Thus, platelet transfusions are only recommended in patients with bleeding or as a prophylactic measure in patients undergoing an invasive procedure with high risk of bleeding (Grade 2C).

VKA therapy is typically used for longer-term anticoagulation, according to Guidelines initial treatment of HIT should not include this agent as its use may exacerbate hypercoagulability due to faster depletion of protein C than prothrombin [56]. ACCP guidelines advocate both waiting to start VKA in patients with strongly suspected or confirmed HIT until platelets have recovered (>150, 000/ μL) and starting VKA at low doses (maximum of 5 mg warfarin) as Grade IC recommendations.

These guidelines are easily applicable to regular HIT but the late diagnosis of delay-onset HIT could cause a prolongation of heparin treatment with life-threatening complications.

With the availability of nonheparin anticoagulants, the potential risk of reexposing previous heparin-induced thrombocytopenia patients to long courses of heparin appears unwarranted.

Conclusion

In conclusion, HIT is a serious adverse drug reaction with potentially fatal consequences. Due to wide variability in the clinical presentation and limitations of laboratory testing, the diagnosis can be difficult. Treatment of HIT and of thrombosis associated with HIT can also be difficult.

Despite the availability of several non-heparin anticoagulant therapeutic options, very little data support the use of these drugs in patients with HIT. In terms of prevention of HIT in patients undergoing surgery a recent analysis found that there was a lower incidence of HIT and HIT complicated by VTE in postoperative patients undergoing thromboprophylaxis with LMWH compared with UFH. This observation supports the current clinical use of LMWH over UFH as front-line heparin therapy [57]. However due to the wide use of unfractionated heparin in patients with cardiovascular disease the monitoring of platelet count is mandatory in such patients.

References

[1] Das P; Ziada K; Steinhubl SR; et al. Heparin-induced thrombocytopenia and cardiovascular diseases. *Am. Heart J.* 2006; 152: 19-26.

[2] Mattioli AV. Prevalence of Anti-PF4/Heparin Antibodies and the HIT Syndrome in Cardiovascular Medicine. *Seminars in Thrombosis and Hemostasis* 2004; 30: 291- 295.

[3] Spencer FA. Heparin-induced thrombocytopenia: patient profiles and clinical manifestations. *J. Thromb. Thrombolysis* 2000;10: S21- 5.

[4] Warkentin TE., Heparin induced thrombocytopenia. *Hematol. Oncol. Clin. N. Am.* 2007; 21, 589–607.

[5] Martel N; Lee J; Wells PS. Risk for heparin-induced thrombocytopenia with unfractionated and low-molecular-weight heparin thromboprophylaxis: a meta-analysis. *Blood* 2005; 106:2710 –5.

[6] Greinacher A; Farner B; Kroll H; et al. Clinical features of heparin-induced thrombocytopenia including risk factors for thrombosis. A retrospective analysis of 408 patients. *Thromb. Haemost*. 2005;94:132–5.

[7] Warkentin TE; Sheppard JI; Siguoin CS; et al. Gender imbalance and risk factor interactions in heparin-induced thrombocytopenia. *Blood* 2006;108(9):2937–41.

[8] Mattioli AV; Bonetti L; Zennaro M; et al. Heparin/PF4 Antibodies Formation After Heparin Treatment: Temporal Aspects and Long-term Follow-up. *Am. Heart J.* 2009; 157:589-95.

[9] Hourigan LA; Waters DI; Keck SA; et al. Heparin induced thrombocytopenia: a common complication in cardiac transplant recipients. *J. Heart Lung Transplant.* 2002;21: 1283–9.

[10] Warkentin TE; Sheppard JI; Sun JC; et al. Anti-PF4/heparin antibodies and venous graft occlusion in postcoronary artery bypass surgery patients randomized to postoperative unfractionated heparin or fondaparinux thromboprophylaxis. *J. Thromb. Haemost.* 2013;11:253-60. doi: 10.1111/jth.12098.

[11] Warkentin TE; Greinacher A. Heparin-induced thrombocytopenia and cardiac surgery. *Ann. Thorac. Surg.* 2003;76:2121– 31.

[12] Mattioli AV. Heparin-induced thrombocytopenia: a misdiagnosed clinical syndrome. Boletim da SPHM 2012; 27: 5-10.

[13] Rauova L; Zhai L; Kowalska MA; et al. Role of platelet surface PF4 antigenic complexes in heparin-induced thrombocytopenia pathogenesis: diagnostic and therapeutic implications. *Blood* 2006;107(6):2346–53.

[14] Holt JC; Niewiarowski S. Biochemistry of alpha granule proteins. *Semin. Hematol.* 1985;22:151–63.

[15] Lane DA; Ireland H; Wolff S; et al. Detection of enhanced in vivo platelet alpha-granule release in different patient groups: comparison of beta thromboglobulin, platelet factor 4 and thrombospondin assays. *Thromb. Haemost.* 1984;52:183–7.

[16] Thachil J. The prothrombotic potential of platelet factor 4. *European Journal of Internal Medicine* 2010;21:79–83.

[17] Vandercappellen J; VanDamme J; Struyf S. The role of the CXC chemokines platelet factor-4(CXCL4/PF-4) and its variant (CXCL4L1/PF-4var)in inflammation, angiogenesis and cancer. *Cytokine Growth Factor Rev.* 2011 Feb;22(1):1-18. doi: 10.1016/j.cytogfr.2010.10.011. Epub 2010 Nov 26.

[18] Warkentin TE; Kelton JG. A 14-year study of heparin-induced thrombocytopenia. *Am. J. Med.* 1996;101(5):502–7.

[19] Pouplard C; May MA; Regina S et al. Changes in platelet count after cardiac surgery can effectively predict the development of pathogenic heparin-dependent antibodies. *British Journal of Haematology* 2005;128: 837–841.

[20] Paparella D; Scrascia G; Galeone A et al. Formation of anti–platelet factor 4/heparin antibodies after cardiac surgery: Influence of perioperative platelet activation, the inflammatory response, and histocompatibility leukocyte antigen status. *The Journal of Thoracic and Cardiovascular Surgery* 2008;136:1456- 1463.

[21] Oliveira and the CATCH study group. Incidence and Prognostic Significance of Thrombocytopenia in Patients Treated With Prolonged Heparin Therapy. *Arch. Intern. Med.* 2008;168:94-102

[22] Wang TY; Ou FS; Roe MT et al. Incidence and Prognostic Significance of Thrombocytopenia Developed During Acute Coronary Syndrome in Contemporary Clinical Practice. *Circulation* 2009;119;2454-2462.

[23] Selleng K; Warkentin TE; Greinacher A: Heparin-induced thrombocytopenia in intensive care patients. *Crit. Care Med.* 2007; 35:1165–1176.

[24] Matsuo T; Tomaru T; Kario K; et al. Incidence of heparin-PF4 complex antibody formation and heparin-induced thrombocytopenia in acute coronary syndrome. *Thromb. Res.* 2005;115:475– 481.

[25] Pena de la Vega L; Miller RS; Benda MM; et al. Association of heparin-dependent antibodies and adverse outcomes in hemodialysis patients: a population based study. *Mayo Clin. Proc.* 2005;80:995–1000.4–6.

[26] Lubenow N; Kempf R; Eichner A; et al: Heparin induced thrombocytopenia: temporal pattern of thrombocytopenia in relation to initial use or reexposure to heparin. *Chest* 2002; 122:37–42.

[27] Warkentin TE; Kelton JG. Delayed-onset heparin-induced Thrombocytopenia and thrombosis. *Ann. Intern. Med.* 2001;135: 502-506.

[28] Rice L; Attisha WK; Drexler A et al. Delayed-Onset Heparin-Induced Thrombocytopenia. *Ann. Intern. Med.* 2002;136:210-215.

[29] Greinacher A; Farner B; Kroll H; et al. Clinical features of heparin-induced thrombocytopenia including risk factors for thrombosis. A retrospective analysis of 408 patients. *Thromb. Haemost.* 2005; 94:132–135.

[30] Mattioli AV; Bonetti L; Zennaro M; et al. Thrombotic Events in Patients with Anti-Platelet Factor 4/Heparin-Antibodies**.** *Heart* 2009; Aug;95(16):1350-4. Epub 2009 May 28.

[31] Mattioli AV; Bonetti L; Sternieri S; et al. Heparin-induced thrombocytopenia in patients treated with unfractionated heparin: prevalence of thrombosis in a 1 year follow-up. *Italian Heart Journal* 2000; 1:39-42.

[32] Mattioli AV; Bonetti L; Tampieri F. Embolia polmonare in un paziente sottoposto a By pass aorto coronarico in trattamento con eparina non frazionata: un caso di trombosi associata a trombocitopenia eparino-indotta. (Pulmonary embolism: a case report). La cardiologia nella pratica clinica 2003:10; 263-270.

[33] Pohl C; Klockgether T; Greinacher A; et al. Neurological complications in heparin-induced thrombocytopenia. *Lancet* 1999; 353:1678–1679.

[34] Williams RT; Damaraju LW; Mascelli MA et al. Anti-Platelet Factor 4/Heparin Antibodies An Independent Predictor of 30-Day Myocardial Infarction After Acute Coronary Ischemic Syndromes. *Circulation.* 2003;107:2307-2312.

[35] Liu JC; Lewis BE; Steen LH; et al. Patency of coronary artery bypass grafts in patients with heparin-induced thrombocytopenia. *Am. J. Cardiol.* 2002;89:979- 81.

[36] Warkentin TE; Roberts RS; Hirsh J; et al. Heparin-induced skin lesions and other unusual sequelae of the heparin-induced thrombocytopenia syndrome. A nested cohort study. *Chest* 2005;127:1857-6.

[37] Lewis BE; Wallis DE; Berkowitz SD; et al. ARG-911 Study Investigators. Argatroban anticoagulant therapy in patients with heparin induced thrombocytopenia. *Circulation* 2001;103:1838–43.

[38] Lo GK; Juhl D;Warkentin TE; et al. Evaluation of pretest clinical score (4 T's) for the diagnosis of heparin-induced thrombocytopenia in two clinical settings. *J. Thromb. Haemost.* 2006; 4:759–65.

[39] Selleng K; Warkentin TE; Greinacher A. Heparin-induced thrombocytopenia in intensive care patients. *Crit. Care Med.* 2007;35:1165–1176.

[40] Kelton JG; Sheridan D; Santos A, et al. Heparin-induced thrombocytopenia: laboratory studies. *Blood* 1988;72(3):925–30.

[41] Greinacher A; Ittermann T; Bagemühl J et al. Heparin-induced thrombocytopenia: towards standardization of platelet factor 4/heparin antigen tests. *J. Thromb. Haemost.* 2010;8:2025-31. doi: 10.1111/j.1538-7836.2010.03974.

[42] Greinacher A; Juhl D; Strobel U et al. Heparin-induced thrombocytopenia: a prospective study on the incidence, platelet-activating capacity and clinical significance of antiplatelet factor 4/heparin antibodies of the IgG, IgM, and IgA classes. *J. Thromb. Haemost.* 2007; 5: 1666–73.

[43] Mattioli AV. Heparin-induced thrombocytopenia: clinical implications. *Giornale Italiano di Cardiologia* 2006; 7: 675-683

[44] Linkins LA; Dans AL; Moores LK; et al. Treatment and prevention of heparin-induced thrombocytopenia: antithrombotic therapy and prevention of thrombosis, 9th ed: American College of Chest Physicians Evidence-Based Clinical Practice Guidelines. *Chest* 2012 141:e495S–e530S.

[45] Mattahi Wh. Treatment of heparin-induced thrombocytopenia in cardiovascular patients. *Exper. Opinion Pharmacother.* 2006; 7: 267-276.

[46] Dang CH; Durkalski VL; Nappi JM. Evaluation of treatment with direct thrombin inhibitors in patients with heparin-induced thrombocytopenia . *Pharmacotherapy* 2006; 26: 461– 468.

[47] Lubenow N; Eichler P; Lietz T; et al. Lepirudin for prophylaxis of thrombosis in patients with acute isolated heparin-induced thrombocytopenia: an analysis of 3 prospective studies. *Blood.* 2004; 104: 3072- 3077.

[48] Kiser TH; Burch JC; Klem PM; et al. . Safety, efficacy, and dosing requirements of bivalirudin in patients with heparin-induced thrombocytopenia. *Pharmacotherapy* 2008; 28: 1115 – 1124.

[49] Salem M; Elrefai S; Shrit MA; et al. Fondaparinux thromboprophylaxis-associated heparin-induced thrombocytopenia syndrome complicated by arterial thrombotic stroke. *Thromb. Haemost.* 2010; 104: 1071–1072.

[50] Lewis BE; Wallis DE; Hursting MJ ; et al. .Effects of argatroban therapy, demographic variables, and platelet count on thrombotic risks in heparin-induced thrombocytopenia. *Chest* 2006; 129: 1407 – 1416.

[51] Greinacher A; Janssens U; Berg G; et al; for the Heparin associated Thrombocytopenia Study (HAT) Investigators . Lepirudin (recombinant hirudin) for parenteral anticoagulation in patients with heparin-induced thrombocytopenia. Heparin-Associated Thrombocytopenia Study (HAT) investigators. *Circulation* 1999; 100: 587 – 593.

[52] Kiser TH; Jung R; MacLaren R; et al. Evaluation of diagnostic tests and argatroban or lepirudin therapy in patients with suspected heparin-induced thrombocytopenia. *Pharmacotherapy* 2005; 25:1736-1745.

[53] Smythe MA; Stephens JL; Koerber JM; et al. . A comparison of lepirudin and argatroban outcomes. *Clin. Appl. Thromb. Hemost.* 2005;11:371-374.

[54] Curzio KM; Cheng-Lai A; Kheyfets V; et al. A comparison of direct thrombin inhibitors in the treatment of Heparin-Induced Thrombocytopenia: a single institution experience. *J. Thromb. Thrombolysis* 2009; 28: 117-12.

[55] Babcock RB; Dumper CW; Scharfman WB Heparin induced immune thrombocytopenia. *N. Engl. J. Med.* 1976; 295:237–241. doi:10.1056/NEJM197607292950501

[56] Warkentin TE; Elavathil LJ; Hayward CP; et al. The pathogenesis of venous limb gangrene associated with heparin-induced thrombocytopenia. *Ann. Intern. Med.* 1997;127:804–812.

[57] Junqueira DR; Perini E; Penholati RR et al. Unfractionated heparin versus low molecular weight heparin for avoiding heparin-induced thrombocytopenia in postoperative patients. *Cochrane Database Syst. Rev.* 2012 12;9:CD007557. doi:10.1002/14651858.CD007557.pub2.

In: Recent Advances in Cardiology
Editors: José Milei and Giuseppe Ambrosio
ISBN: 978-1-63117-282-3

Chapter 7

Diagnostic Use of Echostress

Marina Deljanin Ilic*
Institute of Cardiology, Niska Banja,
Faculty of Medicine, University of Nis, Serbia

Abstract

Stress echocardiography is technique which combines echocardiographic imaging with exercise testing, pharmacological or electrical stress. Among different stresses exercise is the most used, dobutamine is the best test for viability, and dipyridamole the safest and simplest pharmacological stress. Stress echocardiography is frequently used for the diagnosis of coronary artery disease, for risk stratifying patients with known or suspected coronary artery disease, for detecting myocardial hibernation after myocardial infarction or in heart failure, as well as in quantitative assessment of right and left ventricular function in valvular heart diseases. The diagnostic end point for the detection of myocardial ischemia is the induction of a transient worsening in regional function during stress. Stress echocardiography is as effective as myocardial perfusion imaging for the stratification of risk in patients with coronary artery disease but at a lower cost. The future of stress echocardiography will be determined by better training, use of contrast agents, technical developments and improvement of quantitative approaches such as strain and real-time 3D echocardiography.

Introduction

Stress echocardiography (SE) is a popular cardiac imaging technique which combines 2D echocardiographic imaging with exercise, pharmacologic stress, or cardiac pacing [1]. In 1970, Kraunz and Kennedy [2] made ultrasonic determination of left ventricular wall motion in normal individuals at rest and during exercise. In the late 1970s, many investigators used M-mode echocardiography in combination with exercise stress for the detection of ischemia-

* Correspondence: Prof. Marina Deljanin Ilic, Faculty of Medicine, Bul. Zorana Djindjica 81, 18000 Nis, Serbia. Tel 381-18-4570029; Fax 381-18- 238 770; E-mail: marinadi@open.telekom.rs.

induced wall motion abnormalities [3]. Enhanced interest in SE came in the mid 1980s, with the introduction of two-dimensional echocardiography and development of digital image processing [4]. Early studies used supine exercise, handgrips, upright bicycles and cold pressor tests [5]. Subsequently, cardiac pacing has also been used to induce ischemic wall motion abnormalities. However, the evolution of SE largely progressed with the use of pharmacological agents to induce ischemia.

Two-dimensional echocardiographic imaging performed during or immediately after stress is used primarily to detect the presence and extent of ischemia via assessment of regional wall motion, and to estimate overall ventricular systolic function. In addition, Doppler echocardiographic imaging performed during or immediately after exercise stress allows evaluation of valvular function, pulmonary artery pressure, and left ventricular diastolic function. During the past decades, SE has developed from a technique initially performed in a few tertiary care centers to a widely applied technique for evaluation of patients with known or suspected ischemic heart disease [6].

Pathophysiology. Exercise and inotropic stress normally induce increased regional wall motion and thickening, with an increase of ejection fraction. Ischemia typically manifests as new or worsening wall motion abnormalities, delayed contraction, or development of left ventricular enlargement or a decrease in ejection fraction [7]. Myocardial ischemia results in a typical 'cascade' of events, in which the various markers are ranked in a well-defined sequence [8]. Regional systolic changes generally precede the development of ST segment changes and chest pain, but follow the initial development of abnormalities of diastolic function and regional malperfusion. The concept of the ischemic cascade is translated clinically into a gradient of sensitivity of different available clinical markers of ischemia, with chest pain being the least and regional malperfusion the most sensitive [9]. In case of microvascular disease or left ventricular hypertrophy, in the absence of coronary artery disease, coronary flow reserve (CFR) can be reduced, and during stress angina ST-segment changes may occur with regional perfusion changes, however in the absence of regional wall motion abnormalities. Therefore, wall motion abnormalities are more specific than CFR and/or perfusion changes for the diagnosis of coronary artery disease [10, 11].

Methodology

Standardized protocols for SE are required to conduct a safe study with optimal diagnostic accuracy, therefore SE study should be performed according to the stress echocardiography expert consensus statement [9, 12].

Ischemic stressors. The most common stressors are exercise, or administration of dobutamine or dipyridamole. Patients who are able to exercise should undergo exercise stress testing, which is the prototype of demand-driven ischemic stress and the most widely used when coupled with ECG to detect ischemia. Exercise stress testing can be performed on a treadmill, with images obtained within one minute from cessation of exercise. Upright or supine bicycle exercise permits imaging during exercise, and assessment of the ischemic threshold, and it avoids the possibility that ischemia resolves between the end of exercise and the start of imaging-which may reduce sensitivity [7].

The primary indications for pharmacological stress are inability to exercise, or the desire to identify viable myocardium (which does not require inducing ischemia). Pharmacological stressors also minimize factors (e.g. hyperventilation, tachycardia, hypercontraction of normal walls, and excessive chest wall movements) which reduce image quality in SE and lead to higher interobserver variability and lower diagnostic accuracy [9].

Dobutamine infusion upscaling to a peak dose of 40 μg/kg/min (plus atropine in doses 0.25 mg up to a maximum of 1mg, if no endpoint is reached) is the most commonly used pharmacological stressor, which primarily increases myocardial oxygen demand through increase in inotropic state, heart rate, and blood pressure [13, 14]. Protocols with lower dobutamine dose or longer duration of increments, as well as protocols with higher peak dosage of dobutamine (up to 60 μg/kg/min), seem to have no advantages compared to standard dobutamine protocol [9].

Enoximone echocardiography. The clinical use of dobutamine SE may be limited in patients with chronic heart failure by the substantial proportion of such patients treated with beta-blockers, since the inotropic response to adrenergic stimulation is known to be attenuated in patients receiving beta-adrenoceptor blockers [15]. Enoximone, a nonglycoside, noncatechol, positive inotropic agent at the dose of 1, 5 mg/kg over 10 min proved to be as useful as low-dose dobutamine in evaluating left ventricular contractile reserve and functional recovery after revascularization in chronically beta-blocked heart failure patients [16].

Vasodilator agents (dipyridamole to 0.84 mg/kg or adenosine to 0.18 mg/kg/min) mainly act through reduced subendocardial flow supply subsequent to inappropriate arteriolar vasodilation and steal phenomena [17]. Atropine may be added if the response to dipyridamole is negative [18], and other protocols involve combination of dobutamine with a vasodilator [19].

Ergometrine. The diagnosis of coronary vasospasm is often complicated. Ergometrine SE has demonstrated excellent accuracy for the diagnosis of coronary vasospasm, compared with the invasive provocation tests [20]. The protocol consists of an injection of ergometrine (50 μg) administered intravenously at 5 min intervals until a positive response is obtained or a total dose of 0.35 mg is reached [9]. Ergometrine SE is a safe, well tolerated in the majority of cases, and it is a useful technique for orientating the ischemia mechanism if patients are appropriately selected on the basis of either previous normal coronary angiography, normal exercise electrocardiography or pharmacological stress test, contributing to a more complete differential diagnosis of chest pain [21].

Initial reports of *atrial pacing* by transesophageal stimulation during echocardiographic imaging for detection of ischemic heart disease hold promising results. However, the technique has not gained widespread use because of its semi-invasive nature and the poor tolerability in many patients [6]. Lee et al. reported findings in 100 patients undergoing atrial pacing and dobutamine stress echocardiography (DSE) and found pacing to be tolerated in most patients and echocardiographic findings to be comparable to DSE [22]. These findings suggest that pacing echocardiography may be used, particularly in patients with contraindication to exercise or dobutamine infusion.

Imaging techniques. SE is performed using transthoracic harmonic imaging, usually in the two parasternal and three apical views. Transoesophageal imaging is occasionally used in the setting of poor image quality, but has been superceded by use of contrast agents for left ventricular opacification [7]. Number of studies have documented that intravenous transpulmonary contrast agents can improve endocardial delineation at rest and with stress

[23, 24]. Myocardial perfusion imaging using ultrasound contrast agents now allows simultaneous assessment of both function and perfusion, [25, 26] with an improvement in diagnostic accuracy for the detection of coronary disease [27].

Digital imaging is very important for stress echo-mostly for side-by-side comparison of regional function at rest and stress, however review of the videotape is sometimes still of value [7].

Interpretation. The standard approach to interpretation is qualitative, based on visual analysis of thickening and motion before, during, and after stress. Assesment of thickening is very important, because motion may be influenced by traslation or tethering. A semiquantitative approach includes regional wall motion (WM) scoring and calculation of wall motion score index (WMSI) and ejection fraction at rest and stress. Four fundamental SE responses can be established: normal (rest=stress=normal function); ischaemia (rest=normal; stress=abnormal); necrotic (rest=stress=abnormal); and viability (rest=abnormal; stress=normal or biphasic) [9].

A quantitative approach may overcome some of the limitations of the qualitative approach, and a number of techniques for the measurement of radial or longitudinal function have been studied. The main quantitative approaches include the centreline technique or automated border recognition methods, and longitudinal velocity, displacement or strain. Tissue Doppler imaging permits the quantitative assessment of myocardial velocity at rest and stress [28-30], and in the MYocardial Doppler In Stress Echocardiography (MYDISE) study was found that tissue velocities were predictive of angiographic disease [31]. Changes in systolic tissue velocity during dobutamine stress identify viable myocardium [32], predict outcomes in patients with an ischemic response [33] after a myocardial infarction, [34] and may help identify false-positive WM abnormalities [35].

The newly occurring post-systolic shortening during stress echo, known sign of regional ischemia, can be recognized with Tissue Doppler imaging as well as deformation imaging and used for diagnosing ischaemia [36, 37].

Changes in strain precede those in WM or tissue velocity during dobutamine stress [38] and can differentiate stunned from ischemic myocardium [39]. Strain rate may be better than strain, and both are likely superior to tissue velocity in detecting coronary artery disease via SE [40]. Also, it has been showed that strain-rate response during low-dose dobutamine is superior to WM analysis and tissue velocity for identification of viable myocardium, [41] and strain-rate data improve the sensitivity for prediction of functional recovery after revascularization [42].

However, there is no easy solution as to which quantitive techique to use because of traslational motion, tethering, torsional movement, and image quality, and so on [43]. Recent introduction of real-time 3D echocardiography opened a new horizon for quantitative approach in stress echocardiography. Initial studies with 3D echocardiography during stress have been encouraging [44, 45]; however, no data are available on the additional value of this technique over conventional WM interpretation.

Diagnostic accuracy. A great number of studies have showed that exercise [46-52], dobutamine [53-63], and dipyridamole SE [64-70], all have similar accuracy and similar sensitivity [70, 71]. The sensitivity for the detection of coronary artery disease is 85%, 80% and 78% for exercise, dobutamine and dipyridamole SE, respectively, with corresponding specificity of 77%, 86% and 91%, respectively [7, 72]. The addition of atropine augments sensitivity of dipyridamole stress echocardiography.

Ergonovine SE has demonstrated excellent accuracy in orientating the diagnosis of coronary vasospasm, compared with the invasive provocation test, with a sensitivity of 93%, specificity of 96%, positive predictive value of 96% and negative predictive value of 86% [73, 74].

Prognostic value of stress echocardiography. A normal SE gives an annual risk of 0.4-0.9% based on a total of 9, 000 patients, [75-78] similar to that of a normal stress myocardial perfusion scan [79]. This also holds true for patients with diabetes [80] Thus, in patients with suspected coronary artery disease, a normal stress echocardiogram confers an excellent prognosis. By contrast, an abnormal stress echocardiogram is associated with a far higher risk of events, which is directly related to the extent of the WM abnormality in patients with [80] and without diabetes [75]. Information derived from exercise echocardiography [75] is incremental and independent of clinical data, Duke score and resting left ventricular function. In a study of 3, 156 patients followed for nine years [81], ischemia and the extent of abnormal WM were independent predictors of cardiac death. Patients with resting left ventricular dysfunction and additional ischemia had a worse outcome than those with ischemia alone. In another study involving 7,333 patients [77] undergoing pharmacological SE, an abnormal response provided independent and incremental value over and above clinical data.

Myocardial infarction. Despite thrombolysis or primary PTCA, many patients are left with significant residual left ventricular dysfunction, either due to post-ischemic stunning or myocardial necrosis. Post-ischemic stunning implies a good prognosis, as patients almost always recover left ventricular function in the absence of residual infarct-related artery stenosis, and low dose DSE demonstrates increased contractility in these dysfunctional segments [82]. Several studies have confirmed the ability of DSE to discriminate between stunned and necrotic myocardium after acute myocardial infarction [83, 84] with similar sensitivity but higher specificity compared to radionuclide perfusion imaging [79]. Absence of dobutamine-induced contractile response is a more accurate marker of a poor prognosis than angiography or clinical variables, with or without subsequent revascularization [85, 86]. SE can also stratify risk by demonstrating wall motion abnormalities in remote areas, thus implying multi-vessel disease [85]. It has been shown that the extent of non-viable myocardium was the only predictor of cardiac events after revascularization, while in medically-treated patients both the extent of non-viable myocardium and stress echocardiographic indicators of non-viable myocardium and remote ischemia were independent predictors of cardiac events [85, 86].

Patients with ischemic left ventricular dysfunction and a significant amount of viable myocardium (at least five segments or a WMSI 0.25) [87-90] have lower perioperative mortality, greater improvements in regional and global left ventricular function, fewer heart failure symptoms, and improved long-term survival after revascularization than patients with large areas of non-viable myocardium. It has been also shown that in patients with ischaemic cardiomyopathy, LV diastolic filling may largely improve after revascularization, and this improvement of diastolic dysfunction is related to the amount of viable tissue [91].

Detection of hibernating myocardium. Hibernation implies myocardium which fails to contract normally but which may recover after revascularisation. It occurs in the presence of either repetitive stunning or a chronically sustained low level of blood flow [82, 92].

It has been showed that revascularisation is effective in heart failure only in patients with hibernating (and, hence viable) myocardium [93]. The sensitivity and specificity of low-dose DSE for predicting recovery of regional function following revascularisation is 84% and 81%, respectively, comparable to more expensive techniques [94-96].

The sensitivity, specificity and overall accuracy of enoximone stress echocardiography in predicting reversible dysfunction after myocardial infarction were respectively 93%, 85% and 88% [97]. Study used enoximone echocardiography to predict functional recovery after myocardial revascularisation, found that it was more sensitive and had a greater negative predictive value than dobutamine, and also induced fewer hemodynamic alterations [98]. Finally, enoximone may be combined with very low-dose dobutamine in order to detect myocardial viability in the infarcted myocardium of patients with severe heart failure and life-threatening arrhythmias [99].

Indications for stress echocardiography. SE should not be used as a first-line technique for diagnostic and prognostic purposes in subjects with known or suspected coronary artery disease, but only when exercise ECG stress test is either non-diagnostic or non-interpretable. The American College of Cardiology together with a number of other organizations, including the American Society of Echocardiography, has issued appropriateness criteria for stress echocardiography [100]. The main indications for SE are patients who either cannot exercise or exercise submaximally (who should undergo pharmacologic stress) and patients with an uninterpretable ECG caused by repolarisation abnormalities. Main indications for SE are in table 1 [9, 101].

Contraindications. The choice of one test over the other is mostly determined by local experience and relative contraindications. DSE is a better choice for patients with asthma and conduction disturbances, while dipyridamole stress is preferable in patients with severe hypertension or serious atrial or ventricular arrhythmias.

Table 1. Indications for stress echo

- Ischaemic heart disease
Ischaemia identification
Prognostic stratification
Viability evaluation
- Preoperative risk assessment
- Evaluation of revascularization
- Exertional dispnea
- Heart valve disease

Table 2. Selection of stress echocardiography test

	Inability to exercise	Asthma	Tachy arrhytmia	Brady arrhythmia	Severe Hypertension	Hypo tension
Exercise	-	+	+	++	-	++
Dypiridamole	++	-	++	-	++	-
Dobutamine	++	++	-	++	-	++
Pacing	+	+	+	+	+	+

A poor acoustic window makes any form of SE unfeasible to perform. However, with use of harmonic imaging, as well as intravenous contrast agents, optimal endocardial border delineation can be achieved in the vast majority of patients. Specific contraindications and test selection are listed in table 2.

Safety of stress echocardiography. Minor but limiting side effects preclude the achievement of maximal pharmacological stress in <5% of patients with dipyridamole stress [102, 103] and in <10% of patients with DSE [104-106]. In order to assess frequency of complications during stress echocardiography, Varga and colleagues performed a study, using a simple written questionnaire which was distributed to echocardiography laboratories across the world known to perform SE. Out of 85,997 patient examinations, exercise was used in 26,295 cases, dobutamine in 35,103, and dipyridamole in 24,599 cases. Life-threatening events occurred in 86 cases: during exercise in 4 patients, during dobutamine infusion (small dose for viability and/or large dose for ischemia) in 63 patients, and during dipyridamole stress testing in 19 patients. Of the 86 patients with complications, 5 died during DSE and one after dipyridamole testing. Authors concluded that SE is a safe method in the real world, however serious complications may occur. Exercise seems safer than pharmacologic stress and dipyridamole safer than dobutamine [107].

Use in non-coronary artery disease. Exercise Doppler echocardiography is useful in patients with valvular heart diseases, as it allows the evaluation of symptoms and exercise capacity and the assessment of the hemodynamic consequences of valve disease on left ventricular (LV) function, on valve function itself, and on pulmonary arterial pressure. The interpretation of all these parameters can help to optimize the timing of surgery versus guiding medical therapy [108]. The European Society of Cardiology (ESC) and the American College of Cardiology/American Heart Association (ACC/AHA) recommend prompt surgical treatment of patients with symptomatic severe valvular heart diseases or low ejection fraction [109, 110]. However, there are asymptomatic patients with severe valvular heart diseases or with high surgical risk for whom disease management is more difficult. One of the main role of SE in this setting is to identify patients with unrecognized symptoms or with latent LV dysfunction. SE may provide important information for the management of patients who are still in a grey zone between valve surgery and medical treatment after echocardiography at rest.

DSE has been poorly studied in the case of asymptomatic severe aortic stenosis (AS) with preserved LV ejection fraction (LVEF) [111], while exercise stress testing, which is more physiologic, has been demonstrated to be safe in asymptomatic AS [112]. Exercise echocardiography has demonstrated an additive prognostic value over clinical findings, rest Doppler echocardiography and exercise test alone [113]. An increase of at least 18 mmHg in mean transaortic gradient (MTAG) with exercise predicts an increased risk of cardiac events in asymptomatic patients with an aortic valve area (AVA) less than 1 cm^2. The presence of contractile reserve is important to identify high-risk patients, and it was showed that patients with AS who do not increase LVEF with exercise have a poor prognosis [114, 115].

Patients with AS and LV dysfunction (LVEF <40%) frequently exhibit low MTAG (between 30 and 40 mmHg) and the distinction between pseudosevere and true severe AS remains challenging. DSE has been demonstrated to be useful in differentiating relative AS versus true severe AS in patients with LV dysfunction [116]. DSE is also helpful to demonstrate the presence and the extent of contractile reserve, and thus it provides comprehensive surgical risk stratification [117, 118]. In this setting, DSE is used with a low-to-moderate dose of dobutamine (2.5 up to 20 μg/kg/min) to obtain an increase in heart rate of 10-20 bpm. There are three types of response with DSE in patients with severe AS and LV dysfunction: 1. Patients who demonstrate a significant increase in peak transaortic gradient (PTAG) and MTAG and/or an AVA of less than 0.6 cm^2/m^2. These patients have true fixed severe AS and should be referred for surgery; 2. Patients with relative severe AS show an increase in AVA (≥0.3 cm^2) with few modifications of transaortic gradients. The prevalence of relative AS range from 5 to 30% [116], and the medical treatment seems to be the most appropriate solution in this case [116, 117, 119]; and 3. Patients who do not exhibit functional reserve and do exhibit an increase of stroke volume less than 20%. These patients are said to have an indeterminate type of AS and have a poor prognosis with a surgical risk of 32% [117].

The main indication of performing exercise stress test in aortic regurgitation (AR) is to elicit symptoms in patients with subjective exercise limitation or before participation in an athletic activity (class II-A) [110]. By coupling Doppler echocardiography with exercise stress test, identification of a limited rise in LVEF at exercise may help to identify patients who will not demonstrate an increase in LVEF after surgery [120].

The ACC/AHA guidelines recommended exercise Doppler echocardiography testing (class I-C) in patients with mitral stenosis (MS) when there is a discrepancy between symptoms, clinical evaluation and echocardiographic findings at rest [110]. A complete echocardiogram should be performed before the test focusing on the MVA, mean transmitral gradient (MTMG) and transtricuspid pressure gradient (TTG) for estimation of systolic pulmonary arterial pressure. Exercise Doppler echocardiography is the preferred mode of evaluation, however DSE can also be used , although measurement of pulmonary artery pressure will not be helpful by this method. Percutaneous valvuloplasty may be performed in patients with MS who exhibit systolic pulmonary pressure more than 60 mmHg or a mean transaortic gradient (MTAG) of more than 15 mmHg at exercise [121]. It can also be considered in patients with an MVA of more than 1.5 cm^2 with objective limited exercise capacity and previously described echocardiographic criteria. When using DSE, a MTMG of more than 18 mmHg may be used as a cutoff value to predict symptoms or consider surgery [122].

Exercise echocardiography remains the best stress modality in patients with ischemic mitral regurgitation (MR). Estimation of MR, systolic pulmonary pressure by the TTG, as well as the ratio of E:Ea at rest and at exercise are important [123]. Evaluation of WM and myocardial viability are also essential components of the exam. In ischemic MR, an effective regurgitant orifice of 20 mm^2 or more at rest is considered severe and increases cardiac mortality [124]. Furthermore, an effective regurgitant orifice (ERO) increase of at least 13 mm^2 at exercise is associated with a poor outcome [125].

Exercise Doppler echocardiography is a class II-A (ACC/AHA guidelines) recommendation in patients with asymptomatic severe MR to assess exercise capacity and the effect of exercise on pulmonary artery pressure [110]. The echocardiogram should focus on the evaluation on LV function, diameter and volumes, quantitation of MR with the proximal isovelocity surface area and Doppler volumetric methods, and the estimation of systolic arterial pulmonary pressure. Surgery may be considered in patients with exercise-induced systolic pulmonary arterial pressure more than 60 mmHg, as well as, in patients with limited contractile reserve at exercise. Previous reports have demonstrated that an exercise-induced increase of LVEF or less than 4% [126, 127] can identify patients with latent LV dysfunction.

More recently, limited exercise LV longitudinal contractile recruitment assessed by speckle-tracking method has been shown to predict postoperative LV dysfunction in patients with degenerative organic MR [128].

Stress echocardiography in the emergency department. Patients presenting to emergency departments (ED) with atypical chest pain are a dilemma whenever their ECG and biomarkers are nondiagnostic [129]. Exercise stress testing to further define risk is not effective in many patient populations, including some women, patients with mobility problems, and patients with underlying conduction issues such as pre-excitation syndromes, left bundle branch blocks, and ventricular pacemakers. Stress echocardiography is a reasonable alternative for such patients [130].

SE allows the identification of resting wall motion abnormalities, which have been reported to be more sensitive than the initial ECG for detecting cardiac events (91% vs 40%) [131]. Studies have also shown that patients with acute chest pain who have resting wall motion abnormalities are at much higher risk for cardiac events than those who do not [132]. Trippi et al. evaluated 163 low-risk ED patients presenting with chest pain who underwent dobutamine echocardiography. The negative predictive value was 98.5%. [133]. In another study by Stomel et al., only 11 of 455 patients followed for one year after negative SE in a chest pain center had further evidence of CAD (negative predictive value = 97.6%) [134]. Colon and colleagues followed 108 patients after SET reported no cardiac events (negative predictive value = 100%) [135]. One of the advantages of SE is that the results are immediately available, which allows prompt decision by the emergency physician; a further advantage of SE is low cost and availability [136, 137].

Comparison With Other Imaging Techniques. Perfusion scintigraphy is the main diagnostic alternative to SE, and it has a sensitivity > 90% for the detection of coronary artery disease [7]. Previous reports of a specificity of only 70%, and the problems of false positives have been reduced by recent developments including gated single photon emission computed tomography (SPECT). In a meta-analysis [138] based on 44 studies in patients without prior acute myocardial infarction or known ischaemic heart disease, SE had a sensitivity of 85% (95% CI, 83-87%) with a specificity of 77% (95% CI, 74-80%), while SPECT had a sensitivity of 87% (95% CI, 86-88%) with a specificity of 64% (95% CI, 60-68%). Review of both techniques in this meta-analysis showed that the superior sensitivity of SPECT is balanced by a greater specificity with SE, so that the accuracy of both techniques was comparable. In a study by Nagel et al., [139] cardiac magnetic resonance was found to be superior to SE for the diagnosis of coronary artery disease but only in patients with suboptimal echocardiography imaging.

In choosing one technique over the other we have to consider indication and contraindication, as well as advantages and disadvantages of each technique. Echocardiography is universally available and relatively inexpensive while magnetic resonance and SPECT are less available and more expensive. Echocardiography does not involve ionising radiation and has the important advantage of being portable so that it can be taken to patients in emergency departments or coronary care units. All techniques require training. In the case of SE, a training set of 100 studies is recommended under the supervision of an expert reader and maintenance of competence requires at least 100 SE exams per year [9].

Real time three dimensional imaging applied to stress echocardiography. Real time three dimensional (RT-3D) SE is a growing and exciting field with several advantages over 2D-SE.

At the present time, it is applied as an adjunctive technique to 2D stress, but rapid improvement in technology should appropriately make it a superior and an independent technique in the evaluation of ischemia [140]. Validation by large multicenter studies, improvements in both spatial and temporal resolution, acquisition of good quality full volume of the LV during a single cardiac beat, faster image analysis, and automated side-by-side display of baseline and stress images are needed to establish RT-3D SE as the reference technique in the evaluation of patients with coronary artery disease [141], as well as for assessment of diastolic function during stress [142].

Cost-effectiveness of stress echocardiography. Stress imaging has superior diagnostic and prognostic accuracy to exercise electrocardiography, which is expected to lead to fewer normal coronary angiograms and fewer coronary events. Thus, SE is likely to be more cost-effective than exercise electrocardiography [82]. Marwick et al. [143] studied 7, 656 patients undergoing exercise testing, half of whom undergoing SE. Compared to exercise electrocardiography, SE classified more patients as low risk (24% vs 51%) and fewer as intermediate (51% vs 27%) and high risk (25% vs 22%). Survival was greater in low- and intermediate-risk and less in high-risk patients and was better classified by SE than exercise electrocardiography. Although initial procedural costs were greater, exercise echocardiography was associated with a greater incremental life-expectation (0-2 years) and a lower cost of additional diagnostic procedures when compared with exercise electrocardiography. Exercise echocardiography was therefore more cost-effective than exercise electrocardiography. Similar results were obtained in a study of patients presenting with chest pain to an emergency department [144] and in patients with asymptomatic diabetes mellitus [145].

Conclusion

Stress echocardiography combines 2D echocardiographic imaging with exercise, pharmacologic stress or cardiac pacing. Multiple controlled trials have established stress echocardiography as an accurate, cost-effective non-invasive tool not only for the diagnosis of coronary artery disease but also for risk assessment in patients with known or suspected coronary disease and for detecting myocardial hibernation after myocardial infarction or in heart failure. It is as effective as myocardial perfusion imaging for the stratification of risk in patients with coronary artery disease. SE improves evaluation of valvular heart disease and provides important information for the management of patients who are still in a grey zone between valve surgery and medical treatment after echocardiography at rest. The future of SE will be determined by technical developments and improvement of quantitative approaches such as strain and real-time 3D echocardiography.

References

[1] Picano E. Stress Echocardiography. 4th ed. Heidelberg, Germany: Springer Verlag; 2003.

[2] Kraunz RF, Kennedy JW. An ultrasonic determination of left ventricular wall motion in normal man: studies at rest and after exercise. *Am. Heart J.* 1970;79:36– 43.
[3] Mason SJ, Weiss JL, Weisfeldt ML, Garrison JB, Fortuin NJ. Exercise echocardiography: detection of wall motion abnormalities during ischemia. *Circulation* 1979;59:50– 9.
[4] Armstrong WF, O'Donnell J, Dillon JC, McHenry PL, Morris SN, Feigenbaum H. Complementary value of two-dimensional exercise echocardiography to routine treadmill exercise testing. *Ann. Intern. Med.* 1986;105:829–35.
[5] Feigenbaum H. The evolution of stress echocardiography. *Cardiol. Clin.* 1999;17:443–6.
[6] Lewis JF. Current Status of Stress Echocardiography. *Clin. Cardiol.* 2000; 23:242– 6.
[7] Marwick TH. Stress echocardioghraphy. *Heart* 2003;89:113–8.
[8] Picano E. Dipyridamole-echocardiography test: historical background and physiologic basis. *Eur. Heart J.* 1989;10:365–76.
[9] Sicari R, Nihoyannopoulos P, Arturo Evangelista A, et al. Stress echocardiography expert consensus statement. European Association of Echocardiography (EAE) (a registered branch of the ESC). *Eur. Journal of Echocardiography* 2008; 9: 415–37.
[10] Nihoyannopoulos P, Kaski J-C, Crake T, Maseri A. Absence of myocardial dysfunction during stress in patients with syndrome X. *J. Am. Coll. Cardiol.* 1991;18:1463–70.
[11] Picano E, Palinkas A, Amyot R. Diagnosis of myocardial ischaemia in hypertensive patients. *J. Hypertens.* 2001;19:1177–83.
[12] Pellikka PA, Nagueh SF, Elhendy AA, et al. American Society of Echocardiography: Recommendations for performance, interpretation, and application of stress echocardiography. *J. Am. Soc. Echocardiogr.* 2007, 20:1021-4.
[13] Geleijnse ML, Fioretti PM, Roelandt JR. Methodology, feasibility, safety and diagnostic accuracy of dobutamine stress echocardiography. *J. Am. Coll. Cardiol.* 1997; 30:595–606.
[14] Ilić S, Deljanin Ilić M, Lović B, Kocić R. Dobutamine stress echocardiography in detection of silent and supersilent myocardial ischemia in diabetic patients. *Cardiovasc. Imag.* 1999; 11: 115-8.
[15] Stefano Ghio S, Cristina Constantin C, Claudia Raineri C, et al. Enoximone echocardiography: a novel test to evaluate left ventricular contractile reserve in patients with heart failure on chronic beta-blocker therapy. *Cardiovascular Ultrasound* 2003; 1:13, at http://www.cardiovascularultrasound.com/content/1/1/13
[16] Senior R, Kaul S, Lahiri A. Lu C, Carlino M, Fragasso G, et al. Enoximone echocardiography for predicting recovery of left ventricular dysfunction after revascularization. A novel test for detecting myocardial viability. *Circulation* 2000;101:1255-60.
[17] Picano E. Stress echocardiography. From pathophysiologic toy to diagnostic tool. *Circulation* 1992;85:1604–12.
[18] Pingitore A, Picano E, Colosso MQ, et al. The atropine factor in pharmacologic stress echocardiography. Echo Persantine (EPIC) and Echo Dobutamine International Cooperative (EDIC) Study Groups. *J. Am. Coll. Cardiol.* 1996;27:1164–70.
[19] Borges AC, Richter WS, Witzel M, et.al. Combined dipyridamole and dobutamine echocardiography in myocardial hibernation: comparison with thallium uptake in

patients after percutaneous transluminal coronary revascularization under circulatory support. *J. Am. Soc. Echocardiogr.* 2001;14:1057-64.

[20] Song JK, Park SW, Kang DH, et al. Safety and clinical impact of ergonovine stress echocardiography for diagnosis of coronary vasospasm. *J. Am. Coll. Cardiol.* 2000;35:1850–56.

[21] Cortell A, Marcos-Alberca P, Almería C, et al. Ergonovine stress echocardiography: Recent experience and safety in our centre. *World J. Cardiol.* 2010; 2: 437–42.

[22] Lee CY, Pellikka PA, McCully RB, et al. Nonexercise stress transthoracic echocardiography: Transesophageal atrial pacing versus dobutamine stress. *J. Am. Coll. Curdiol.* 1999;33:506-11.

[23] Crouse LJ, Cheirif J, Hanly DE, et al. Opacification and border delineation improvement in patients with suboptimal endocardial border definition in routine echocardiography: results of phase III Albunex multicenter trial. *J. Am. Coll. Cardiol.* 1993; 22:1494–500;

[24] Ikonomidis I, Holmes E, Narbuvold H, et al. Left ventricular wall motion assessment and endocardial border delineation after intravenous injection of InfosonTM during dobutamine stress echocardiography. *Coron Artery Dis.* 1998;9:567–76.

[25] Shimoni S, Zoghbi WA, Xie F. Real-time assessment of myocardial perfusion and wall motion during bicycle and treadmill exercise echocardiography: comparison with single photon emission computed tomography. *J. Am. Coll. Cardiol.* 2001;37:741-7.

[26] Senior R, Lepper W, Pasquet A et al. Myocardial perfusion assessment in patients with medium probability of coronary artery disease and no prior myocardial infarction: comparison of myocardial contrast echocardiography with 99mTc-SPECT. *Am. Heart J.* 2004;147:1100-05.

[27] Moir S, Haluska BA, Jenkins C et al. Myocardial contrast stress echocardiography for the assessment of coronary artery disease: incremental benefit of qualitative and quantitative approaches. *Circulation* 2004;110:1108-13.

[28] Deljanin Ilic, M., Ilic, S., Lovic, B. Detection of myocardial ischemia during dipyridamole stress echocardiography using pulsed wave Doppler tissue imaging. *Cardiovasc. Imag.* 1999; 11:119-22.

[29] Deljanin Ilić M, Ilić S, Lović B, et al. Tissue Doppler imaging –value of regional myocardial function quantification in stress echocardiography testing. *Acta Facultatis Medicae Naissensis* 2000;17:42-6.

[30] Deljanin Ilić M, Ilić S, Lović B. Detection of viable myocardium during dobutamine echocardiography using Doppler myocardial imaging in patients with recent myocardial infarction. *Facta Universitatis* 2001;8:31-4.

[31] Madler CF, Payne N, Wilkenshoff U, et al. Non-invasive diagnosis of coronary artery disease by quantitative stress echocardiography: optimal diagnostic models using off-line tissue Doppler in the MYDISE study. *Eur. Heart J.* 2003; 24:1584–94.

[32] Bountioukos M, Schinkel AF, Bax JJ, et al. Pulsed-wave tissue Doppler quantification of systolic and diastolic function of viable and nonviable myocardium in patients with ischemic cardiomyopathy. *Am. Heart J.* 2004;148: 1079–84.

[33] Marwick TH, Case C, Leano R, et al. Use of tissue Doppler imaging to facilitate the prediction of events in patients with abnormal left ventricular function by dobutamine echocardiography. *Am. J. Cardiol.* 2004;93: 142–6.

[34] Cain P, Khoury V, Short L, Marwick TH. Usefulness of quantitative echocardiographic techniques to predict recovery of regional and global left ventricular function after acute myocardial infarction. *Am. J. Cardiol.* 2003;91: 391–6.

[35] Altinmakas S, Dagdeviren B, Turkmen M, et al. Usefulness of pulse-wave Doppler tissue sampling and dobutamine stress echocardiography for identification of false positive inferior wall defects in SPECT. *Jpn. Heart J.* 2000; 41: 141–52.

[36] Voigt JU, Lindenmeier G, Exner B, et al. Incidence and characteristics of segmental postsystolic longitudinal shortening in normal, acutely ischemic, and scarred myocardium. *J. Am. Soc. Echocardiogr.* 2003;16: 415–23.

[37] Celutkiene J, Sutherland GR, Laucevicius A, et al. Is post-systolic motion the optimal ultrasound parameter to detect induced ischaemia during dobutamine stress echocardiography? *Eur. Heart J.* 2004; 25: 932–42.

[38] Armstrong G, Pasquet A, Fukamachi K, et al. Use of peak systolic strain as an index of regional left ventricular function: comparison with tissue Doppler velocity during dobutamine stress and myocardial ischemia. *J. Am. Soc. Echocardiogr.* 2000;13:731–7.

[39] Derumeaux G, Ovize M, Loufoua J, et al. Assessment of nonuniformity of transmural myocardial velocities by color-coded tissue Doppler imaging: characterization of normal, ischemic, and stunned myocardium. *Circulation* 2000;101:1390–5.

[40] Weidemann F, Jamal F, Kowalski M, et al. Can strain rate and strain quantify changes in regional systolic function during dobutamine infusion, B-blockade, and atrial pacing? Implications for quantitative stress echocardiography. *J. Am. Soc. Echocardiogr.* 2002; 15: 416–24.

[41] Hoffmann R, Altiok E, Nowak B, et al. Strain rate measurement by Doppler echocardiography allows improved assessment of myocardial viability inpatients with depressed left ventricular function. *J. Am. Coll. Cardiol.* 2002; 39: 443–9.

[42] Hanekom L, Jenkins C, Jeffries L, et al. Incremental value of strain rate analysis as an adjunct to wall-motion scoring for assessment of myocardial viability by dobutamine echocardiography: a follow-up study after revascularization. *Circulation.* 2005;112: 3892–900.

[43] Sicari R. Relevance of tissue Doppler in the quantification of stress echocardiography for the detection of myocardial ischaemia in clinical practice. *Cardiovasc. Ultrasound* 2005;3:2, at http://www.cardiovascularultrasound.com/content/3/1/2

[44] Ahmad M, Xie T, McCulloch M, et al. Real-time threedimensional dobutamine stress echocardiography in assessment stress echocardiography in assessment of ischaemia: comparison with twodimensional dobutamine stress echocardiography. *J. Am. Coll. Cardiol.* 2001;37:1303–9.

[45] Hung J, Lang R, Flachskampf F, et al. ASE. 3D echocardiography: a review of the current status future directions. *J. Am. Soc. Echocardiogr.* 2007;20:213–33.

[46] Pozzoli MM, Salustri A, Sutherland GR, et al. The comparative value of exercise echocardiography and 99 m Tc MIBI single photon emission computed tomography in the diagnosis and localization of myocardial ischaemia. *Eur. Heart J.* 1991;12:1293–9.

[47] Marwick TH, Nemec JJ, Pashkow FJ, et al. Accuracy and limitations of exercise echocardiography in a routine clinical setting. *J. Am. Coll. Cardiol.* 1992;19:74–81.

[48] Marwick TH, Anderson T, Williams MJ, et al. Exercise echocardiography is an accurate and cost-efficient technique for detection of coronary artery disease in women. *J. Am. Coll. Cardiol.* 1995;26:335–41.

[49] Dagianti A, Penco M, Agati L, et al. Stress echocardiography: comparison of exercise, dipyridamole and dobutamine in detecting and predicting the extent of coronary artery disease. *J. Am. Coll. Cardiol.* 1995;26:18–25.

[50] Bjornstad K, Aakhus S, Hatle L. Comparison of digital dipyridamole stress echocardiography and upright bicycle stress echocardiography for identification of coronary artery stenosis. *Cardiology* 1995;86:514–20.

[51] Luotolahti M, Saraste M, Hartiala J. Exercise echocardiography in the diagnosis of coronary artery disease. *Ann. Med.* 1996;28:73–7.

[52] Lancellotti P, Hoffer EP, Pierard LA. Detection and clinical usefulness of a biphasic response during exercise echocardiography early after myocardial infarction. *J. Am. Coll. Cardiol.* 2003;41:1142–7.

[53] Mazeika PK, Nadazdin A, Oakley CM. Dobutamine stress echocardiography for detection and assessment of coronary artery disease. *J. Am. Coll. Cardiol.* 1992;19: 1203–119.

[54] Pingitore A, Picano E, Colosso MQ, et al. The atropine factor in pharmacologic stress echocardiography. Echo Persantine (EPIC) and Echo Dobutamine International Cooperative (EDIC) Study Groups. *J. Am. Coll. Cardiol.* 1996;27:1164–70.

[55] Salustri A, Fioretti PM, McNeill AJ, et al. Pharmacological stress echocardiography in the diagnosis of coronary artery disease and myocardial ischaemia: a comparison between dobutamine and dipyridamole. *Eur. Heart J.* 1992;13:1356–62.

[56] Martin TW, Seaworth JF, Johns JP, et al. Comparison of adenosine, dipyridamole and dobutamine in stress echocardiography. *Ann. Intern. Med.* 1992;116:190–6.

[57] Segar DS, Brown SE, Sawada SG, et al. Dobutamine stress echocardiography: correlation with coronary lesion severity as determined by quantitative angiography. *J. Am. Coll. Cardiol.* 1992;19: 1197–202.

[58] Baudhuin T, Marwick T, Melin J, et al. Diagnosis of coronary artery disease in elderly patients: safety and efficacy of dobutamine echocardiography. *Eur. Heart J.* 1993; 14:799–803.

[59] Marwick T, D'Hondt AM, Baudhuin T, et al. Optimal use of dobutamine stress for the detection and evaluation of coronary artery disease: combination with echocardiography scintigraphy or both? *J. Am. Coll. Cardiol.* 1993;22:159–67.

[60] Afridi I, Quinones MA, Zoghbi WA, et al. Dobutamine stress echocardiography: sensitivity, specificity, and predictive value for future cardiac events. *Am. Heart J.* 1994;127:1510–5.

[61] Sahin M, Karakelleoglu S, Alp N, et al. Diagnostic value of dobutamine stress echocardiography in coronary artery disease. *Thorac. Cardiovasc. Surg.* 1994;42:285–9.

[62] Schroder K, Voller H, Dingerkus H, et al. Comparison of the diagnostic potential of four echocardiographic stress tests shortly after acute myocardial infarction: submaximal exercise, transesophageal atrial pacing, dipyridamole, and dobutamine–atropine. *Am. J. Cardiol.* 1996;77:909–14.

[63] Hennessy TG, Codd MB, McCarthy C, et al. Dobutamine stress echocardiography in the detection of coronary artery disease in a clinical practice setting. *Int. J. Cardiol.* 1997;62:55–62.

[64] Picano E, Lattanzi F, Masini M, et al. High dose dipyridamole echocardiography test in effort angina pectoris. *J. Am. Coll. Cardiol.* 1986;8:848–54.

[65] Salustri A, Fioretti PM, McNeill AJ, et al. Pharmacological stress echocardiography in the diagnosis of coronary artery disease and myocardial ischaemia: a comparison between dobutamine and dipyridamole. *Eur. Heart J.* 1992;13:1356–62.

[66] Picano E, Pingitore A, Conti U, et al. Enhanced sensitivity for detection of coronary artery disease by addition of atropine to dipyridamole echocardiography. *Eur. Heart J.* 1993;14:1216–22.

[67] Deutsch HJ, Schenkel C, Klaer R, et al. Comparison of ergometer and dipyridamole echocardiography in patients with suspected coronary heart disease. *Z. Kardiol.* 1994;83:446–53.

[68] Sochowski RA, Yvorchuk KJ, Yang Y, et al. Dobutamine and dipyridamole stress echocardiography in patients with a low incidence of severe coronary artery disease. *J. Am. Soc. Echocardiogr.* 1995;8:482–7.

[69] San Roman JA, Vilacosta I, Castillo JA, et al. Dipyridamole and dobutamine–atropine stress echocardiography in the diagnosis of coronary artery disease. Comparison with exercise stress test, analysis of agreement, andimpact of antianginal treatment. *Chest* 1996;110:1248–54.

[70] De Albuquerque Fonseca L, Picano E. Comparison of dipyridamole and exercise stress echocardiography for detection of coronary artery disease (a meta-analysis). *Am. J. Cardiol.* 2001;87:1193–6.

[71] Picano E, Molinaro S, Pasanisi E. The diagnostic accuracy of pharmacological stress echo: a meta-analysis. *Cardiovasc. Ultrasound* 2008;6:30, at Ultrasound 2008;6:30, at http://www.cardiovascularultrasound.com/content/6/1/30

[72] Beleslin BD, Osojic M. Djordjevic-Dikic A et al. Integrated evaluation of relation between coronary lesion features and stress echocardiography results: the importance of coronary lesion morphology. *J. Am. Coll. Cardiol.* 1999;33:717-26.

[73] Song JK, Park SW, Kim JJ, et al. Values of intravenous ergonovine test with two-dimensional echocardiography for diagnosis of coronary artery spasm. *J. Am. Soc. Echocardiogr.* 1994;7:607–15.

[74] Song JK, Park SW, Kang DH, et al. Safety and clinical impact of ergonovine stress echocardiography for diagnosis of coronary vasospasm. *J. Am. Coll. Cardiol.* 2000; 35:1850–6.

[75] Marwick TH, Case C, Vasey C, et al. Prediction of mortality by exercise echocardiography. A strategy for combination with the Duke treadmill score. *Circulation* 2001;29:2566-71.

[76] McCully RB, Roger VL, Mahoney DW et al. Outcome after normal exercise echocardiography and predictors of subsequent cardiac events: follow-up of 1, 325 patients. *J. Am. Coll. Cardiol.* 1998;31:144-9.

[77] Sicari R, Pasanisi E, Venneri L et al. Stress echo results predict mortality: a large-scale multicenter prospective international study. *J. Am. Coll. Cardiol*. 2003;41:589-95.

[78] Chung G, Krishnamani R, Senior R. Prognostic value of normal stress echocardiogram in patients with suspected coronary artery disease - a British general hospital experience. *Int. J. Cardiol.* 2004;94:181-6.

[79] Geleijnse ML, Elhendy A. Can stress echocardiography compete with perfusion scintigraphy in the detection of coronary artery disease and cardiac risk assessment? *Eur. J. Echocardiography* 2000;1:12-21.

[80] Elhendy A, Arruda AM, Mahoney et al. Prognostic stratification of diabetic patients by exercise echocardiography. *J. Am. Coll. Cardiol.* 2001; 37:1551-7.

[81] Marwick TH, Case C, Sawada S et al. Prediction of mortality using dobutamine echocardiography. *J. Am. Coll. Cardiol.* 2001;37:754-60.

[82] Senior R, Chambers J. Stress Echocardiography - Current Status. *Br. J. Cardiol.* 2007;14:90-97.

[83] Pierard L, De Landsheere CM, Berthe C, et al. Identification of viable myocardium by echocardiography during dobutamine infusion in patients with myocardial infarction after thrombolytic therapy: comparison with positron emission tomography. *J. Am. Coll. Cardiol.* 1990;15:1021-31.

[84] Barilla F, Gheorghiade M, Alam M et al. Low dose dobutamine in patients with acute myocardial infarction identifies viable but not contractile myocardium and predicts the magnitude of improvement in wall motion abnormalities in response to coronary revascularisation. *Am. Heart J.* 1991;122:1522-31.

[85] Carlos ME, Smart SC, Wynsen JC, et al. Dobutamine stress echocardiography for risk stratification after myocardial infarction. *Circulation* 1997;95:1402-10.

[86] Swinburn J, Senior R. Extent of non-viability, not ischaemia, predicts mortality after myocardial infarction. *Heart* 2004;90(suppl II): A35.

[87] Sicari R, Ripoli A, Picano E, et al. The prognostic value of myocardial viability recognized by low dose dipyridamole echocardiography in patients with chronic ischaemic left ventricular dysfunction. *Eur. Heart J.* 2001;22:837–44.

[88] Sicari R, Picano E, Cortigiani L, et al. Prognostic value of myocardial viability recognized by low-dose dobutamine echocardiography in chronic ischaemic left ventricular dysfunction. *Am. J. Cardiol.* 2003;92:1263–6.

[89] Meluzin J, Cerny J, Spinarova L, et al. Prognosis of patients with chronic coronary artery disease and severe left ventricular dysfunction. The importance of myocardial viability. *Eur. J. Heart Fail.* 2003;5:85–93.

[90] Carluccio E, Biagioli P, Alunni G, et al. Patients with hibernating myocardium show altered left ventricular volumes and shape, which revert following revascularization: Evidence that dysynergy may directly induce cardiac remodeling. *J. Am. Coll. Cardiol.* 2006; 47:969-977.

[91] Carluccio E, Biagioli P, Alunni G, et al. Effect of revascularizing viable myocardium on left ventricular diastolic function in patients withischaemic cardiomyopathy. *European Heart Journal* 2009; 30:1501–09.

[92] Ambrosio.G. The elusive difference between hibernation and stunning in patients. *Basic Res. Cardiol.* 1995;90:297-9.

[93] Allman KC, Shaw LJ, Hachamovitch R, et al. Myocardial viability testing and impact of revascularization on prognosis in patients with coronary artery disease and left ventricular dysfunction: a meta-analysis. *J. Am. Coll. Cardiol.* 2002;39:1151-8.

[94] Bax JJ, Wijns W, Cornel JH et al. Accuracy of currently available techniques for prediction of functional recovery after revascularisation in patients with left ventricular dysfunction due to chronic disease: comparison of pooled data. *J. Am. Coll. Cardiol.* 1997;30:1451-60.

[95] Myocardial viability on echocardiography predicts long term survival after revascularisation in patients with ischaemic congestive heart failure. *J. Am. Coll. Cardiol.* 1999;33:1848-54.

[96] Afridi I, Grayburn PA, Panza JA et al. Myocardial viability during dobutamine echocardiography predicts survival in patients with coronary artery disease and severe left ventricular dysfunction. *J. Am. Coll. Cardiol.* 1998;32:921-6.
[97] Natale E, Minardi G, Wang F, et al. Identification of viable myocardium early after acute myocardial infarction under beta-blockade by enoximone echocardiography. *G. Ital. Cardiol.* 1997, 27:342-8.
[98] Lu C, Carlino M, Fragrasso G, et al. Enoximone echocardiography for predicting recovery of left ventricular dysfunction after revascularization. A novel test for detecting myocardial viability. *Circulation* 2000, 101:1255-60.
[99] Mangieri E, Alessandri N, Tanzilli G, et al. Enoximone coupled to very low dose dobutamine echocardiography detects myocardial viability in akinetic and dyskinetic post-myocardial infarcted areas. *Am. J. Cardiol.* 1999; 84:264-9.
[100] ACCF/ASE/ACEP/AHA/ASNC/SCAI/SCCT/SCMR appropriateness criteria for stress echocardiography. *J. Am. Coll. Cardiol.* 2008;51:1127-47.
[101] Pellikka PA, Nagueh SF, Elhendy AA, et al. American Society of Echocardiography: Recommendations for performance, interpretation, and application of stress echocardiography. *J. Am. Soc. Echocardiogr.* 2007, 20:1021-41.
[102] Picano E, Marini C, Pirelli S, et al. Safety of intravenous high-dose dipyridamole echocardiography. The Echo-Persantine International Cooperative Study Group. *Am. J. Cardiol.* 1992;70:252–8;
[103] Lette J, Tatum JL, Fraser S, et al. Safety of dipyridamole testing in 73, 806 patients: the Multicenter Dipyridamole Safety Study. *J. Nucl. Cardiol.* 1995;2:3–17.
[104] Picano E, Mathias W Jr, Pingitore A, et al. Safety and tolerability of dobutamine–atropine stress echocardiography: a prospective, multicentre study. Echo Dobutamine International Cooperative Study Group. *Lancet* 1994;344:1190–2.
[105] Secknus MA, Marwick TH. Evolution of dobutamine echocardiography protocols and indications: safety and side effects in 3, 011 studies over 5 years. *J. Am. Coll. Cardiol.* 1997;29:1234–40.
[106] Mathias W Jr, Arruda A, Santos FC, et al. Safety of dobutamine-atropine stress echocardiography: A prospective experience of 4, 033 consecutive studies. *J. Am. Soc. Echocardiogr.* 1999;12:785–91.
[107] Varga A, Garcia MA, Picano E. Safety of Stress Echocardiography (from the International Stress Echo Complication Registry). *Am. J. Cardiol.* 2006;98:541–3.
[108] O'Connor K, Lancellotti P, Piérard L. Stress Doppler Echocardiography in Valvular Heart Diseases: Utility and Assessment. *Future Cardiol.* 2010;6:611-25.
[109] Vahanian A, Baumgartner H, Bax J et al.: Guidelines on the management of valvular heart disease: The Task Force on the Management of Valvular Heart Disease of the European Society of Cardiology. *Eur. Heart J.* 2007; 28: 230–68.
[110] Bonow RO, Carabello BA, Kanu C et al.: ACC/AHA 2006 guidelines for the management of patients with valvular heart disease: a report of the American College of Cardiology/American Heart Association Task Force on Practice Guidelines (writing committee to revise the 1998 guidelines for the management of patients with valvular heart disease) developed in collaboration with the Society of Cardiovascular Anesthesiologists: endorsed by the Society for Cardiovascular Angiography and Interventions and the Society of Thoracic Surgeons. *Circulation* 2006;114:84–231.

[111] Das P, Rimington H, Smeeton N, Chambers J: Determinants of symptoms and exercise capacity in aortic stenosis: a comparison of resting haemodynamics and valve compliance during dobutamine stress. *Eur. Heart J.* 2003; 24:1254–63.

[112] Amato MC, Moffa PJ, Werner KE, et al. Treatment decision in asymptomatic aortic valve stenosis: role of exercise testing. *Heart* 2001;86:381–386.

[113] Lancellotti P, Lebois F, Simon M, et al. Prognostic importance of quantitative exercise Doppler echocardiography in asymptomatic valvular aortic stenosis. *Circulation* 2005;112(Suppl. 9):377–82.

[114] Marechaux S, Ennezat PV, LeJemtel TH et al.: Left ventricular response to exercise in aortic stenosis: an exercise echocardiographic study. *Echocardiography* 2007;24:955–9.

[115] Lancellotti P, Karsera D, Tumminello G et al.: Determinants of an abnormal response to exercise in patients with asymptomatic valvular aortic stenosis. *Eur. J. Echocardiogr.* 2008; 9: 338–43.

[116] Bermejo J, Yotti R: Low-gradient aortic valve stenosis. Value and limitations of dobutamine stress testing. *Heart* 2007; 93: 298–302.

[117] Monin JL, Quere JP, Monchi M et al.: Low-gradient aortic stenosis: operative risk stratification and predictors for long-term outcome: a multicenter study using dobutamine stress hemodynamics. *Circulation* 2003;108:319–24.

[118] Blais C, Burwash IG, Mundigler G et al.: The projected valve area at normal flow rate improves the assessment of stenosis severity in patients with low flow aortic stenosis: the multicenter TOPAS (Truly or Pseudo Severe Aortic Stenosis) study. *Circulation* 2006;113:711–21.

[119] Nishimura RA, Grantham JA, Connolly HM et al.: Low-output, low-gradient aortic stenosis in patients with depressed left ventricular systolic function: the clinical utility of the dobutamine challenge in the catheterization laboratory. *Circulation* 2002;106: 809–13.

[120] Wahi S, Haluska B, Pasquet A, t al.: Exercise echocardiography predicts development of left ventricular dysfunction in medically and surgically treated patients with asymptomatic severe aortic regurgitation. *Heart* 2000; 84:606–14. .

[121] Pierard LA, Lancellotti P: Stress testing in valve disease. *Heart* 2007;93:766–772.

[122] Reis G, Motta MS, Barbosa MM, et al. Dobutamine stress echocardiography for noninvasive assessment and risk stratification of patients with rheumatic mitral stenosis. *J. Am. Coll. Cardiol.*2004;43:393–401.

[123] Podolec P, Rubis P, Tomkiewicz-Pajak L, et al. Usefulness of the evaluation of left ventricular diastolic function changes during stress echocardiography in predicting exercise capacity in patients with ischemic heart failure. *J. Am. Soc. Echocardiogr.* 2008; 21:834–40.

[124] Grigioni F, Enriquez-Sarano M, Zehr KJ, et al. Ischemic mitral regurgitation. long-term outcome and prognostic implications with quantitative Doppler assessment. *Circulation* 2001;103:1759–64.

[125] Lancellotti P, Troisfontaines P, Toussaint AC, et al. Prognostic importance of exercise-induced changes in mitral regurgitation in patients with chronic ischemic left ventricular dysfunction. *Circulation* 2003;108: 1713–17.

[126] Leung D, Griffin B, Stewart W, et al. Left ventricular function after valve repair for chronic mitral regurgitation: predictive value of preoperative assessment of contractile reserve by exercise echocardiography. *J. Am. Coll. Cardiol.* 1996;28:1198–1205.

[127] Lee R, Haluska B, Leung DY, et al. Functional and prognostic implications of left ventricular contractile reserve in patients with asymptomatic severe mitral regurgitation. *Heart* 2005;91:1407–12.

[128] Lancellotti P, Cosyns B, Zacharakis D et al. Important of left ventricular longitudinal function and functional reserve in patients with degenerative mitral regurgitation: assessment by 2-D speckle tracking. *J. Am. Soc. Echocardiogr.* 2008; 21: 1331–1336.

[129] Ambrosio G, Mandorla S. Chest pain and a non-diagnostic ECG: trying not to be frustrated. *Eur. Heart J.* 2000; 21 (17):1403-5.

[130] Bucshbaum M, Marshall E, Levine B, et al. Emergency Department Evaluation of ChestPain Using Exercise Stress Echocardiography. *Academic Emerg. Med.* 2001; 8:196–9.

[131] Kontos MC, Arrowood JA, Paulsen WH, et al. Early echocardiography can predict cardiac events in emergency department patients with chest pain. *Ann. Emerg. Med.* 1998; 31:550–7.

[132] Kontos MC, Arrowood JA, Jesse R, et al. Comparison between 2-dimensional echocardiography and myocardial perfusion imaging in the emergency department in-patients with possible myocardial ischemia. *Am. Heart J.* 1998; 136: 724–33.

[133] Trippi JA, Lee KS, Kopp G, et al. Dobutamine stress tele-echocardiography for evaluation of emergency department patients with chest pain. *J. Am. Coll. Cardiol.* 1997; 30:627–32.

[134] Stomel R, Grant R, Eagle KA. Lessons learned from a community hospital chest pain center. *Am. J. Cardiol.* 1999; 83:1033–7.

[135] Colon PJ, Guarisco JS, Murgo J, Cheirif J. Utility of stress echocardiography in the triage of patients with atypical chest pain from the emergency department. *Am. J. Cardiol.* 1998; 82: 1282–4.

[136] Marine JE, Freedberg KA, Davidoff R. Cost-effectiveness of stress-echocardiography. *Cardiol. Clin. North Am.* 1999; 17:583–95.

[137] Kuntz KM, Fleischmann KE, Hunink MG, et al. Cost-effectiveness of diagnostic strategies for patients with chest pain. *Ann. Intern. Med.* 1999; 130: 709–18.

[138] Fleischmann KE, Hunink MGM, Kuntz KM et al. Exercise echocardiography or exercise SPECT imaging? A meta-analysis of diagnostic test performance. *JAMA* 1998;280:913-20.

[139] Nagel E, Lehmkuhl HB, Bocksch W et al. Noninvasive diagnosis of ischemia-induced wall motion abnormalities with the use of high-dose dobutamine stress MRI: comparison with dobutamine stress echocardiography. *Circulation* 1999;99:763-70.

[140] Ahmad M: Real-time three-dimensional dobutamine stress echocardiography: A valuable adjunct or a superior alternative to two-dimensional stress echocardiography? *J. Am. Soc. Echocardiogr.* 2009;22:443–4.

[141] Abusaid G, Ahmad M. Real Time Three-Dimensional Stress Echocardiography Advantages and Limitations. *Echocardiography* 2012;29:200-6.

[142] Kort S, Mamidipally S, Madahar P, Real Time Three-Dimensional Stress Echocardiography: A New Approach for Assessing Diastolic Function. *Echocardiography* 2011;28:676-83.

[143] Marwick TH, Shaw L, Case C et al. Clinical and economic impact of exercise electrocardiography and exercise echocardiography in clinical practice. *Eur. Heart J.* 2003;24:1153-63.

[144] Jeetley P, Burden L, Senior R. Superior risk stratification by stress echocardiography compared with exercise electrocardiography in troponin negative acute chest pain - a prospective randomised trial. *Heart* 2004;90 (suppl II):A33.
[145] Hayashino Y, Nagata-Kobayashi S, Morimoto T, et al.Cost-effectiveness of screening for coronary artery disease in asymptomatic patients with type 2 diabetes and additional atherogenic risk factors. *J. Gen. Int. Med.* 2004;19:1181-91.

In: Recent Advances in Cardiology
Editors: José Milei and Giuseppe Ambrosio

ISBN: 978-1-63117-282-3

Chapter 8

Hypertension in the Elderly

***Claudio A. Bellido*[1] *and Eduardo J. Rusak*[2]**
[1]Cardiologist (UBA), Hypertension Specialist (SAHA),
Professor of Internal Medicine (University of Buenos Aires),
Department of Internal Medicine Hospital de Clínicas "José de San Martín"
[2] Cardiologist (SAC), Hypertension Specialist (SAHA),
Magister in Vascular Mechanics and Hypertension (Universidad Austral),
Head of the National Career in Arterial Hypertension
of The Argentine Society of Hypertension (SAHA)

Abstract

Management of hypertension in the elderly is quite different in comparison with the younger population. Hypertension - especially in its isolated systolic (ISH) form - is an important risk factor for cardiovascular and cerebrovascular events, as well as for cognitive impairment and dementia among elderly patients.

Aortic arterial stiffness is the main cause for the development of IS. Nowadays it is well known that- among the elderly- antihypertensive treatment leads to an improvement of prognosis with a modest fall in systolic blood pressure (SBP). Nevertheless, treatment should be carefully applied to avoid dangerous fall in diastolic blood pressure (DBP). For this reason, recent guidelines are prone to support a SBP goal at approximately 150 mmHg.

Abbreviations

ISH	Isolated systolic hypertension
SBP	Systolic blood pressure
DBP	Diastolic blood pressure
PP	Pulse pressure
BP	Blood pressure
CV	Cardiovascular

DBT	Diabetes
CKD	Chronic kidney disease
LVH	Left ventricular hypertrophy
PWV	Pulse wave velocity
TOD	Target organ damage
WCH	White coat hypertension
RAAS	Renin angiotensin aldosterone system

Isolated systolic hypertension was considered a normal consequence of arterial aging without clinical relevance among elderly people for many years. Nevertheless, it represents a result of increased arterial stiffness with direct effects on cardiovascular and brain disease in this period of life. Moreover, this subtype of hypertension is the most commonly seen in the elderly hypertensives; it is defined by a SBP over 140 mmHg and DBP below 90 mmHg [1]. Interestingly, most patients who develop ISH –more than 60 per cent- never had systolic and/or diastolic hypertension previously in their lives; they have ISH *de novo*. [2]

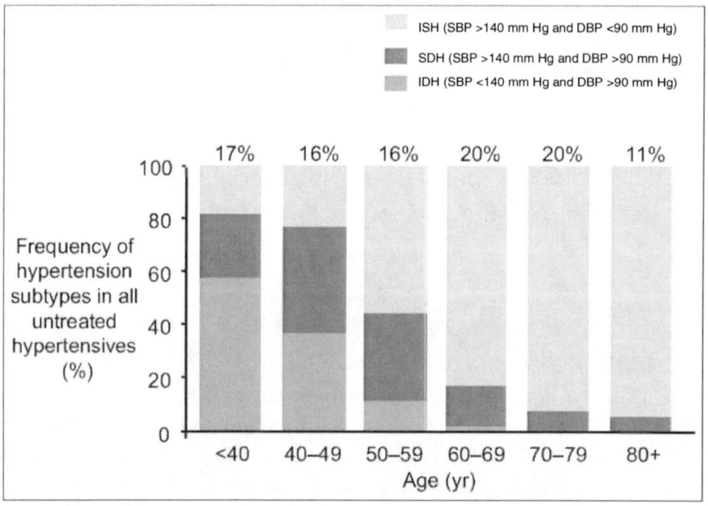

Figure 1. Frequency distribution of untreated hypertensive individuals by age and hypertension subtype. Numbers at the top of the bars represent the overall percentage distribution of all subtypes of untreated hypertension in the age group (National Health and Nutrition Examination Survey III, 1988–1994). SBP=systolic blood pressure; DBP=diastolic blood pressure. Reproduced with permission from J. Clin Hypertens. 2006;8:444-449.

Aortic arterial stiffness is a major pathological change in the aging process, both among hypertensive and normotensive subjects in the middle age, generally over 65 years old. [3] Arterial wall stiffness is produced by progressive degeneration and rupture of elastic fibers in the middle layer of the vessel, and their replacement with collagen. [4,5] These changes lead to rising of SBP and PP. At brachial level PP is directly related to SBP and to the fall in DBP, [3] and predicts future CV events, especially the development of heart failure. [6]

Even among very old hypertensive patients –over 80 years old- hypertension is an important CV risk factor, and its treatment prolongs life and prevents brain attacks (stroke) and heart failure. In this group of patients prevalence of hypertension is more than 60 per cent. [7] It is important to consider that among younger people, or in those who have healthy arterial structure, vessel elasticity produces a cushion effect in the pulsatile activity related to ventricular systolic ejection. [8] This cushioning protects organs from the pulsatility of an intermittent blood flow and produces a more continuous one. Aging process leads to enhanced stiffness with a lack of cushioning as a result. The consequence is a more pulsatile flow with the risk of heart failure and myocardial ischemia.

The arterial wave amplification along the vascular tree produces higher BP at brachial level than in central aorta. On the other hand, central BP represents a more confident predictor index to CV risk. The lowering of DBP associated with rising of SBP could be considered as a mark of aging. This aging change is sometimes found in other pathological situations than hypertension such as obesity, DBT, CKD, among several others. Moreover, some old people with ISH and a very low DBP below 70 mmHg -about 30 per cent of ISH patients without treatment-, have a higher prevalence of diabetes and CV disease, in comparison with those exhibiting DBP over these levels. [9,10]

Stiffness is associated with an early reflection of pulse wave in every branch or bifurcation of the arterial system in the elderly population. This reflection leads to a rise in aortic central pressure in late systole with a subsequent elevation of left ventricular afterload. This pressure load produces LVH. [11] This hemodynamic impairment is known as ventricular-arterial uncoupling. Early arterial stiffness is another pathological process resulting from lack of treatment or not well controlled hypertension. An accelerated aging of elastic arteries results in developing of LVH and an enhanced risk of CV events similar to those produced by coronary artery disease, stroke, vascular dementia and CKD. [2]

Carotid-femoral PWV measurement is an accurate method to indirectly evaluate aortic stiffness. It is a non invasive easy procedure with a very good coefficient of repetition intra and inter observer. [12] In addition, PWV changes are more evident in patients older than 50, also among normotensive subjects. This fact suggests that PWV measurement is a very sensitive marker of arterial stiffness in older people, compared to the younger population. [10]

It is very important to consider the frequent baroreflex failure seen among elderly people closely related to arterial stiffness and also a low sensitivity to catecholamines. These are the main reasons why the elderly are more prone to orthostatic hypotension and a wide changes in BP, both spontaneously and pharmacologically induced by antihypertensive treatment.

In summary, among people in their fifties and older SBP rises; meanwhile DBP reaches a plateau and after this decreases as a result of arterial stiffness, in spite of a continuous elevation of peripheral resistance. A wide PP is seen as a result. Both PWV and aortic central pressure elevations–the latter as a result of a former- are important markers of TOD and their correction should be the main therapeutic objective.

- PP is an arterial stiffness index of great (elastic) arteries
- Great (elastic) arteries stiffness is a main factor for SBP rising and DBP fall, and hence for ISH in the elderly (from the sixties afterwards)
- Hypertension not accurately treated accelerates arterial stiffness and the rigidity leads more hypertension (vicious circle). [13]

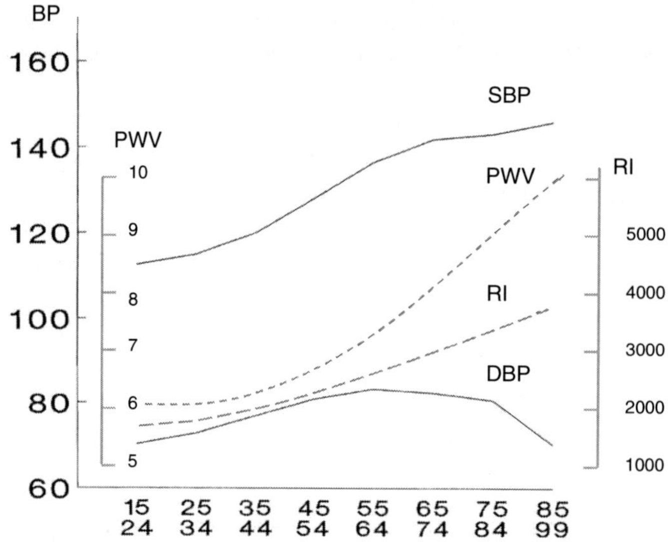

Figure 2. Diagram of changes over different ages of systolic blood pressure (SBP), diastolic blood pressure (DBP), resistence index (RI in dynas per cm2) and arterial stiffness, represented by pulse wave velocity (PWV in meters per second).

Another factor to take into consideration is that aging (more than 85 years old) could be associated with very low BP, both SBP and DBP. In regard to this, SBP below 120 mmHg and DBP below 60 mmHg could be markers of a severe impairment of left ventricular function. Moreover, this finding is very common among patients aggressively treated. [9,14]

Then, differences between elderly and younger hypertensive patients are based on the following data:

1. Older hypertensive subjects have a higher ISH prevalence, and this subtype of hypertension in more difficult to control
2. It exists enhanced arterial stiffness mainly in great elastic vessels (aorta and main branches)
   - PP widening and DBP fall with elevation of CV risk
   - Ventricular-arterial uncoupling, heart failure, organ damage due to a more pulsatile flow, dementia and CKD
   - Baroreflex failure, orthostatic hypotension, high BP variability and white coat effect
3. High CV risk before antihypertensive treatment mainly because aging is a powerful independent and additive risk factor
4. There is an important benefit to treat healthy older hypertensive patients
5. There is less benefit for the treatment of more frail patients. Low BP can increase mortality and frequently indicate left ventricular dysfunction. On the other hand, it is very common to find orthostatic hypotension. It is also important to consider co-morbidities and disabling diseases.

Multiple benefits are seen to endorse pharmacological management of ISH (SBP > 140 mmHg and DBP < 90 mmHg) it exists a burden of evidence about the benefits. The treatment reduces the incidence of CV adverse events and prolongs survival in the elderly. Nevertheless, among very old patients (over 80 years old), several studies found that the treatment reduced the incidence of stroke and heart failure without prolongation of life. In regard to this, the HYVET study found, in addition to less heart failure and stroke, an increase in survival rate.

ISH in the elderly is due especially to arterial stiffness. The aging process is also aggravated by other coexisting factors as atherosclerosis, diabetes, smoking, etc.; consequently management of this subtype of hypertension is difficult compared to DBP of younger people.

Diagnosis of Hypertension and Target Organ Damage in the Elderly

Among the elderly, due to an increasing arterial stiffness, may occur frequently problems in relation to diagnosis.

It is very common to suspect pseudo-hypertension in those subjects, who, in spite of exhibit high BP, have few vascular changes - for example, lack of arteriolar narrowing in the funduscopic exam. Other patients have symptomatic postural hypotension, despite being under very careful treatment. In these and other situations the diagnosis is difficult to confirm and arises discrepancies between the recorded pressures with the conventional cuff sphygmomanometer -falsely high- and intra-arterial pressures. [15] The Osler maneuver, characterized by the digital palpation of the radial artery, even after compression of the brachial artery with the blood pressure cuff above systolic pressure, allows us to suspect this situation.

On the other hand, in older patients, BP are highly variable, so it is advisable to repeat the measurement not less than three which should be applied with the patient in a sitting position and also standing. It is very frequent -usually more than 30 percent- to find more than 20 mmHg fall in standing position (orthostatic hypotension), in patients with systolic pressures above 160 mmHg. In these cases, the pressure in the standing position should be the one that is taken into account for therapeutic decisions.

Ambulatory Monitoring (ABPM) and Home Blood Pressure Measurement (HBPM)

Recent guidelines give enough knowledge about the utility of ABPM, both in regard to how and also when this procedure may be important for the diagnosis and management of hypertension. [16,17] It is well known that ambulatory blood pressure predicts CV morbidity and other adverse events independently and better than office BP measurement in older people than in middle aged and younger subjects. [18,19] This fact is especially relevant in relation with ISH.

WCH, i.e., office elevation of BP with normotension in ABPM is generally more pronounced and more frequent among elderly patients. [20] The opposite of WCH is masked hypertension, characterized by normal BP at the office and elevated BP in the ABPM. This subtype of hypertension is also seen in older people with evidence of TOD. The presence of TOD evidence (narrowing of funduscopic arteries, LVH, microalbuminuria, etc.) without high BP at the office is an indication for ABPM to rule out masked hypertension.

However, there has been concern about reproducibility and, for that reason, the clinical significance of WCH and white coat effect. Moreover, WCH has been considered to be a benign condition that does not require antihypertensive treatment and, for this reason this finding –by means of ABPM or HBPM, both of them out of the office setting- is very important to avoid unnecessary and aggressive treatments. [21] On the other hand, in recent HYVET's sub-study, it has been estimated that 50 per cent of the patients had WCH in the main study, and the reduction in total mortality with indapamide sustained release with or without perindopril found after an average follow-up of 13 months is a strong indication to treat this patients. [22]

BP fall during the sleep period is also less pronounced among the elderly and, interestingly, it disappears in centenarians. Older people, on the other hand, have higher average ABP, due to high SBP, a characteristic of these patients. [23,24]

Data about HBPM in the elderly are scarce. This type of measurement has acquired especial relevance and now is considered an accurate method to register BP because is better tolerated than ABPM. In addition, HBPM is more cost-effective in comparison with ABPM.

Ohasama study considers HBP data better than office BP to predict mortality and brain attacks (stroke). Nevertheless, there are limitations for the wide use of HBPM among the elderly patients, mainly due to cognitive impairment of many of them, and also due to the uncertain accuracy of measurements done by relatives. [25]

Blood Pressure Management in the Elderly. CV Risk Evaluation and Time to Begin Antihypertensive Treatment

The classic concept about treatment of hypertension in the elderly had been to apply the same indications than in younger people. Although, this approach has important limitations and has been the matter of discussions and revisions. In regard to this, it is especially relevant to consider the patient's individual risk according to hypertension guidelines. [2, 26-28] In addition to other CV risks, the finding of an elevated SBP with a discordantly low DBP, leading to the development of ISH, [29] is a valuable predictor of CV and brain damage. In the Framingham cohort after adjustment for age, sex and other variables, coronary heart disease risk correlated inversely with DBP at any SBP level. This is the reason why PP should be considered a better predictor of CV disease than SBP and/or DBP alone.

The HYVET study results have demonstrated that a subtle SBP fall in patients older than 80 years –from 170-180 to 140-150 mmHg- reduced mortality, stroke and heart failure. Though, among the very old hypertensive patients the treatment should be limited to those healthier –characteristic of the enrolled in this study- and to those with SBP above 160 mmHg (Hypertension grade 2 according to JNC-7). [30]

Lifestyle changes and pharmacological treatment are indicated in those patients with BP above 140 mmHg without other co-morbidities compelling lower BP levels, as diabetes or

CKD. Several guidelines, including the JNC-7, indicated the necessity of lower SBP –less than 130 mmHg- in these patients. However, nowadays, this indication is under discussion. The ADVANCE study did not demonstrate benefit to lower SBP below 140 mmHg among diabetic patients. [31]

In summary, in very old patients it should be especially careful in lowering BP because these patients are prone to co-morbidities and frailty; they can also suffer falls due to baroreflex insufficiency. It is important to keep in mind that the frailty of many old patients should be a limitation for an aggressive treatment.

An accurate intervention on lifestyle is able to reduce the needs of a more intensive pharmacological treatment and also contributes favorably to modify several of the risk factors commonly hypertension related. Although, few treated elderly hypertensive patients reach the BP goals –in regard to BP levels- but modest decrease in BP lead to important benefit on the outcomes –significant less CV events-. The Systolic Hypertension in the Elderly Program (SHEP) published more than 20 years ago, showed that a subtle fall in SBP –a little bit below 160 mmHg- led a near 46 per cent decrease in stroke incidence. The more recent HYVET study also demonstrated an important reduction in events rate and also mortality. The decrease in mortality under pharmacological treatment in the very old subjects was demonstrated for the first time in this trial. However, BP decrease in this study seems to be insufficient in accordance with the hypertension guidelines.

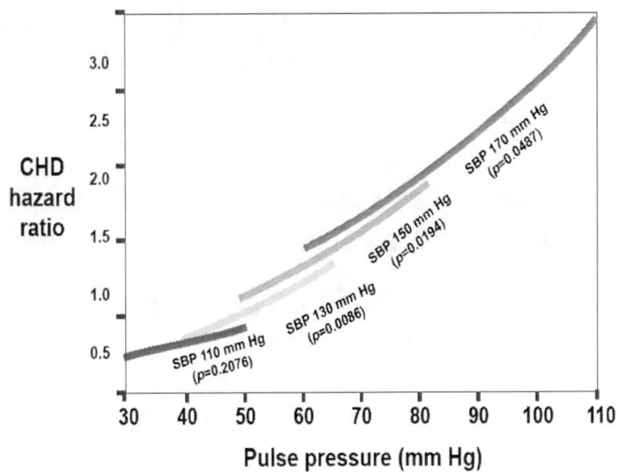

Figure 3. Joint influences of systolic blood pressure (SBP) and pulse pressure on coronary heart disease (CHD) risk, from the Framingham Heart Study. CHD hazard ratio was determined from level of pulse pressure within SBP groups. Hazard ratios were set to a reference value of 1.0 for SBP values of 110, 130, 150, and 170 mm Hg, respectively. All estimates were adjusted for age, sex, body mass index, cigarettes smoked per day, glucose intolerance, and total cholesterol/high-density lipoprotein Reproduced with permission from J. Clin Hypertens. 2006;8:444-449.

On the other hand, to reach the goal in regard to BP levels it is necessary to prescribe pharmacological combinations, generally adding a diuretic. This is very important in case of severe and/or resistant hypertension. Older patients receiving diuretics need frequent electrolyte control because it is very frequent the development of hyponatremia.

Frailty is a frequent problem among very old people. Most of these subjects present orthostatic hypotension, with a subsequent risk of falls and fractures. It is important to consider that there is a "J" curve in the elderly, both to SBP as DBP. An intensive antihypertensive pharmacological therapy to treat SBP also descends DBP, and when the latter falls below 75 mmHg, mortality rises again. SBP follows a different pattern with persistence of "J" curve: mortality generally increases when SBP falls below 120 mmHg in very old people. This fact is especially relevant among patients with coronary heart disease. According to recent observations, it is important to keep in mind that SBP between 145-155 mmHg is associated with a healthy condition in older patients, in comparison with lesser SBP levels considered optimum in younger people.

Finally, the goal of antihypertensive therapy in the elderly should focus in the reduction of arterial stiffness and the early pulse wave reflection. The latter leads to an elevation of central aortic blood pressure and left ventricular overload. The most accurate treatment is RAAS blockade, commonly in association with low dose diuretics or calcium channel blockers. The new developed beta blockers with vasodilator properties can be also considered. These pharmacological agents are capable to reduce central aortic blood pressure, while classic selective beta blockers (ej. Atenolol) do not reduce central pressure.

Arterial stiffness is the leading cause for the development of ISH and PP elevation in addition to LV afterload rising and subsequent LVH. The latter is a multiplier factor for CV disease and mortality. These are the reasons why the focus of treatment needs to be directed to them. The aim of the treatment is to revert, if possible, or at least to delay, the arterial aging.

Brachial BP usually does not represent central aortic BP. It is very important the election of an antihypertensive drug capable to lower the latter, especially in those patients who exhibit enhanced arterial stiffness. This condition is the rule among elderly people as a result of arterial wall aging and also due to other factors that modify the normal arterial wall architecture. Cardioselective beta blockers, as atenolol and metoprolol, do not produce effective central aortic BP fall, in spite of their antihypertensive effect al brachial level, in comparison with other antihypertensive agents such as calcium channel blockers (CCB), diuretics (Diur) and angiotensin converting enzyme inhibitors (ACE-i).

The Conduit Artery Function Evaluation (CAFÉ) study, a sub-study of Anglo Scandinavian Cardiac Outcomes Trial (ASCOT) showed that amlodipine-perindopril combination was better to significantly descend central aortic BP than atenolol-thiazide therapeutic schedule. Although, both combinations produced the same antihypertensive effect at brachial level.

The Preterax in Regression of Arterial Stiffness in a Controlled Double-blind study (REASON) demonstrated that ACEi-Diur combination was also similar to descend brachial BP with a more significant fall in SBP and PP. However, central aortic BP fall was more pronounced with the first antihypertensive regimen. [32] In addition, in a subgroup of patients receiving ACEi-Diur combination there was LV mass regression.[33]

In another trial, valsartan-amlodipine combination also produced central aortic BP fall more important than amlodipine-atenolol with the same levels of achieved brachial BP. [34]

Besides this, all the antihypertensive agents acting against RAAS have shown success to delay and also revert arterial stiffness progression.

Carotid-femoral PWV is an accurate marker of arterial stiffness and, in a short cohort of hypertensive patients successfully treated and controlled, descended continuously, more than expected along five years of follow up. All of these patients were receiving drugs acting on RAAS (ACEi or ARBs) and BP control was achieved after few weeks of antihypertensive treatment. These outcomes represent an improvement of arterial elasticity induced by a prolonged RAAS blockade. [35] In addition, there are studies suggesting that two drugs with different mechanisms but with the same antihypertensive benefit on brachial BP can result in different effect on PWV due to the possibility or not to affect central aortic BP, independently of brachial BP. In regard to this observation, in diabetic patients valsartan-amlodipine combination reduced PWV more than amlodipine-hydrochlothiazide. These findings suggest that RAAS blockade acts also on arterial structure. [36] In very old patients, it is well known since more than twenty years ago [37] that SBP descend reduces adverse cardiac events incidence, especially stroke, heart failure and CKD without modifying total mortality. Almost all of these papers represented hypertensive patients cohorts treated with diuretics and another drug to achieve BP control, if necessary, but not with more than two drugs in the elderly.[38] A meta-analysis of several studies agreed with other previously published, and also with the results of HYVET.[39-41] Antihypertensive treatment in older subjects diminishes the adverse events incidence compared to placebo or no treatment. Nevertheless, total mortality reduction was only seen in the HYVET study. This difference between HYVET and previous studies in regard to mortality in the elderly treated hypertensive patients could be explained by the characteristic of patients enrolled in this trial. Patients in HYVET study were healthier than those of other cohorts and also to the usual older hypertensive patients in real life. Then, it is difficult to extrapolate results for using in clinical practice. It is especially interesting to mention that approximately 30 per cent of HYVET patients were Chinese. Basal characteristics of those subjects were markedly different from those enrolled in other countries because Chinese elderly patients had lower body mass index, lower total cholesterol levels, higher HDL-cholesterol, and better renal function. These patients also had less myocardial infarctions and heart failure incidence at the beginning of the study. The difference in mortality observed in this trial could be related to the diuretic used in the therapeutic schedule. [28,34] Long acting diuretics as indapamide slow release in comparison with other diuretics could also explain differences in mortality. However, this seems improbable because four out of six other studies also used this type of diuretics.

It is important to consider that regression analysis suggests a possible association between total mortality and intensity of treatment, as well as the level of BP achieved. In other words it means that a aggressive treatment does not produce outcome benefits in these patients.

JATOS study included patients between 65 and 85 years old; the conclusion was that tight BP control did not result in more benefit than an achievement of less optimal level of BP. [42]

Objectives of BP and Benefits Achieved with the Addition of Aspirin and Statins

The Hypertension Optimal Treatment (HOT) study, done almost 20 years ago, was the last trial in which DBP level was the goal of treatment, with three progressive objectives: <90, <85, and <80 mmHg, comparing them with morbidity and mortality in hypertensive patients. This study also considered the effects of low dose aspirin (75 mg daily) on the outcomes. Felodipine, an dihydropiridine CCB, was selected as a first drug prescribed and then, if necessary, adding other antihypertensive agents to achieve the goal of DBP. HOT study included many patients older than 65 years old. [43] A significant conclusion of the study was that aspirin added to the antihypertensive therapy diminished significantly the incidence of CV events, especially myocardial infarction. On the other hand, there were no differences in the frequency of stroke or serious bleeding.

ASCOT study also added atorvastatin to the antihypertensive drugs in a subgroup of patients. In older people of this cohort, atorvastatin was at least similar in efficacy to the younger people in lowering cholesterol levels. [44]

In conclusion, older hypertensive patients obtain significant benefit with antihypertensive treatment. There is an evident reduction of stroke and heart failure incidence. However, there is concern about the reduction in total mortality because only HYVET study showed real decrease of death in treated patients.

Randomised and controlled trials against placebo or no antihypertensive treatment both in systolic and diastolic hypertension used diuretics or beta blockers as initial drug to treat patients. In those studies including ISH patients, drugs selected primarily were diuretics or CCB (dihydropiridine). All of these trials demonstrated benefit from active drug therapy compared to placebo or no treatment. Other class antihypertensive drugs were only used in combination in comparative studies. In regard to this, ACEi and ARBs also showed efficacy in older patients. On the other hand, the onset of treatment in the elderly should follow usual guidelines considering mainly TOD and comorbidities.

BP goal level should be set carefully, especially in very old patients. It is very important to keep in mind that there are more evident pathophysiological changes in people older than 80 years. Recognizing these changes allows a better management of hypertension in the elderly.[45] Endothelial dysfunction is present in almost all elderly patients, mainly due to prolonged exposure to oxidative stress in the lifespan. This fact leads to progressive arterial smooth muscle hypertrophy. In addition, arteries become stiffer, leading to less vasodilatation as a response to nitric oxide secretion. Moreover, nitric oxide synthesis and secretion are markedly diminished in the very old subjects. Other morbid conditions, such as autonomic dysfunction and baroreflex failure also need to be considered at the time to treat hypertensive old patients. Many of them have frailty and other diseases, including CKD. It is well known that glomerular filtration rate falls, approximately 8 mL/min/1.73 m^2 body surface by decade after 40 years old. For this reason pharmacological dosage needs to be adjusted in older patients.

Management of hypertensive patients aged 65-75 years old –named younger old people- is different to the applied in subjects older than 80 years. Moreover, in this group, the treatment of those healthy patients is different and could be more aggressive than in frail patients, in order to achieve benefit. This is the characteristic of patients enrolled in HYVET study. On the contrary, frailty patients or those with co-morbidities should be treated carefully with at low dose of antihypertensive drugs.

In summary, antihypertensive treatment in older patients has to consider not only CV risk but also a clinical condition of patients. Younger old patient treatment does not differ from treatment in the middle aged subjects. In the oldest it is important to consider clinical conditions such as frailty.

The prevention of orthostatic hypotension, closely related to baroreflex insufficiency and autonomic dysfunction, is very important in the oldest patients. This disability may lead to frequent and dangerous falls, with severe consequences as hip fractures, a very common accident among the elderly.

References

[1] Chaundhry, SI; Krumholz, HM; Foody, JM. Systolic hypertension in older persons. *JAMA*, 2004, 292, 1074-80.

[2] Franklin, SS. Elderly hypertensives: How are they different? *J Clin Hypertens (Greenwich)*, 2012, 14, 779-786.

[3] Franklin, SS. Hypertension in older people: part 1. *J Clin Hypertens*. 2006, 8, 444-49.

[4] Cockcroft, J; Mancia, G. Vascular aging: shifting the paradigma of risk assessment and reduction in hypertension. *J Hypertens*, 2012, 30 (Suppl 1), S1-S2.

[5] Laurent, S. Defining vascular aging and cardiovascular risk. *J Hypertens*, 2012, 30 (Suppl 1), S3-S8.

[6] Haider, AW; Larson, MG; Franklin, SS; et al. Systolic blood pressure, and pulse pressure as predictors of risk for congestive heart failure in the Framingham Heart Study. *Ann Intern Med*, 2003, 138, 10-16.

[7] Harris, T; Cook, EF; Kannel, WB; et al. Blood pressure experience and risk of cardiovascular disease in the elderly. *Hypertension*, 1985, 7, 118-124.

[8] Cockroft, J; Mancia, G. Vascular aging, shifting the paradigma of risk assessment and reduction in hypertension. *J Hypertens*, 2012, 30 (Suppl 1), S1-S2.

[9] Franklin, SS; Chow, VH; Mori, A; et al. The significance of low DBP in US adults with isolated systolic hypertension. *J Hypertens*, 2011, 29, 1101-8.

[10] Franklin, SS; Levy, D. Aging. Blood Pressure, and Heart Failure. What are the connections. *Hypertension*, 2011, 58, 760-62.

[11] McEniery, CM; Hall, IR; Qasem, A; et al. ACCT Investigators. Normal vascular aging, differential effects on wave reflection and aortic pulse wave velocity: The Anglo-Cardiff, Collaborative Trial (ACCT) *J Am Coll Cardiol*, 2005, 46, 1753-60.

[12] Laurent, S; Cockcroft, J; Van Bortel, L; et al. European Network for Noininvasive Investigation of Large Arteries. Expert consensus document on arterial stiffness: methodological issues and clinical applications. *Eur Heart J*, 2006, 27, 2588-2605.

[13] Franklin, SS; et al. Hemodynamic patterns of age-related changes in blood pressure. The Framingham Heart Study. *Circulation*, 1997, 96, 308-15.

[14] Satish, S; Zhang, DD; Goodwin, JS. Clinical significance of falling BP among older adults. *J Clin Epidemiol*, 2001, 54, 961-7.

[15] Zweifler, AJ; Tariq Shahab, S. Pseudohypertension, a new assessment. *J Hypertens*, 1993, 11, 1-6.

[16] O'Brien, E; Asmar, R; Beilin, L; et al. European Society of Hypertension recommendations for conventional, ambulatory, and home blood pressure measurement. *J Hypertens*, 2003, 21, 821-848.

[17] Guías de la Sociedad Argentina de Hipertensión Arterial para el diagnóstico, estudio, tratamiento y seguimiento de la hipertensión arterial. 2011, pág 19-21.

[18] Björklund, K; Lind, L; Zethelius, B; et al. Prognostic significance of 24-h ambulatory blood pressure characteristics for cardiovascular morbidity in a population of elderly men. *J Hypertens*, 2004, 22, 1691-97.

[19] Stassen, J; Lutgarde, T; Fagard, R; et al. Predicting cardiovascular risk using conventional vs ambulatory blood pressure in older patients with systolic hypertension. *JAMA*, 1999, 282, 539-46.

[20] Wiinberg, N; Höegholm, A; Christensen, HR; et al. 24-h ambulatory blood pressure in 352 normal Danish subjects, related to age and gender. *Am J Hypertens*, 1995, 8, 978-86.

[21] Wing, LMH; Brown, MA; Beilin, LJ; et al. Reverse White coat hypertension in older hypertensives. *J Hypertens*, 2002, 20, 636-44.

[22] Bulpitt, CJ; Beckett, N; Peters, R; et al. Does white coat hypertension require treatment over age 80? Results of the Hyperetension in the Very Elderly Trial Ambulatory Blood Pressure Side Project. *Hypertension*, 2013, 61, 89-94.

[23] Bertineri, G; Grassi, G; Rossi, P; et al. 24-hour blood pressure profile in centenarians. *J Hypertens*, 2002, 20, 1765-69.

[24] O'Sullivan, C; Duggan, J; Atkins, N; et al. Twenty-four hour ambulatory blood pressure in community dwelling elderly men and women, aged 60-102 years. *J Hypertens*, 2003, 21, 1641-47.

[25] Okhubo, T; Asayama, K; Kikuya, M; et al. How many times should blood pressure be measured at home for better prediction of stroke risk? *Ten-years follow-up results from the Ohasama study*, 2004, 22, 1099-1104.

[26] Thijs, L; Fagard, R; Lijnen, P; et al. A meta análisis of outcome trials in elderly hypertensives. *J Hypertens*, 1992, 10, 1103-1109.

[27] Lever, AF; Ramsay, LE. Treatment of hypertension in the elderly. *J Hypertens*, 1995, 13, 571-79.

[28] Franklin, S; Hypertesion in older people. Part 2. *J. Clin Hypertens*, 2006, 8 521-6. Guidelines Committee. The 2003 European Society of Hypertension – European Society of Cardiology Guidelines for the Management of arterial hypertension. *J Hypertens*, 2003, 21, 1011-53.

[29] Beckett, NS; Peters, R; Fletcher, AE; et al. The HYVET Study Group. Treatment of hypertension in patients 80 years of age and older. *N Engl J Med*, 2008, 358, 1887-98.

[30] The ADVANCE Collaborative Group. Intensive Blood Glucose Control and Vascular Outcomes in Patients with Type 2 Diabetes. *N Engl J Med*, 2008, 358, 2560-72.

[31] Asmar, RG; London, GM; O'Rourke, ME; et al. Improvment in blood pressure, arterial stiffness and wave reflections with a very low dose perindopril-indapamide combination in hypertensive patients: A comparison with atenolol. *Hypertension*, 2001, 38, 922-926.

[32] De Luca, N; Asmar, RG; London, GM; et al. Selective reduction of cardiac mass and central blood pressure on low dose combination perindopril-indapamide in hypertensive subjects. *J Hypertens*, 2004, 22, 1623-30.

[33] Boutouyrie, P; Achouba, A; Trunet, P; et al. Amlodipine-Valsartan combination decreases central systolic blood pressure more effectively than the amlodipine-atenolol combination: The EXPLOR Study. *Hypertension*, 2010, 55, 1314-22.

[34] Bellido, CA; Iavicoli, OR; Rusak, EJ; et al. Continuous improvement of arterial compliance beyond blood pressure decrease alter 5 years of anihypertensive treatment. *J Clin Hypertens*, 2006, 8, 555-60.
[35] Karalliedde, J; Smith, A; De Angelis, L; et al. Valsartan improves arterial stiffness in type 2 diabetes independently of blood pressure lowering. *Hypertension*, 2008, 51, 1617-23.
[36] SHEP Cooperative Research Group. Prevention of stroke by antihypertensive drug treatment in older persons with isolated systolic hipertensión: final results of the Systolic Hipertensión in the Elderly Program. *JAMA*, 1991, 265, 3255-64.
[37] Bejan-Angoulvant, T; Saadatan-Elahi, M; Wright, JM; et al. Treatment of hypertension in patients 80 years and older: the lower the better? A meta-analysis of randomized controlled trials. *J Hypertens*, 2010, 28, 1366-72.
[38] Gueyffier, F; Bulpitt, C; Boissel, JP; et al. Antihypertensive drugs in very old people: a subgroup meta-analysis of randomised controlled trials. INDANA Group. *Lancet*, 1999, 353, 793-96.
[39] Collins, R; Peto, R; MacMahon, S; et al. Blood pressure, stroke, and coronary heart disease. Part 2, short-term reductions in blood pressure: overview of randomized drug trials in their epidemiological context. *Lancet*, 1990, 335, 827-38.
[40] Beckett, NS; Peters, R; Fletcher, AE; et al. Treatment of hypertension in patients 80 years of age or older. *N Engl J Med*, 2008, 358, 1887-98.
[41] JATOS Trial Group. Principal results of the Japanese trial to assess optimal systolic blood pressure in elderly hypertensive patients (JATOS). *Hypertension Res.*, 2008, 31, 2115-27.
[42] Kjeldsen, SE; Kolloch, RE; Leonetti, G; et al. Influence of gender anda ge on preventing cardiovascular disease by antihypertensive treatment and acetyl salicylic acid. The HOT study. *J Hypertens*, 2000, 18, 629-42.
[43] Sever, PS; Dahlöf, B; Poulter, NR; et al. The ASCOT investigators. Prevention of coronary and stroke events with atorvastatin in hypertensive patients who have average or lower than average cholesterol concentrations, in the Anglo-Scandinavian Cardiac Outcomes Trial-Lipid Lowering Arm (ASCOT-LLA): a multicentre randomized controlled trial. *Lancet*, 2003, 361, 1149-58.
[44] Tabriziani, H; Steiner, J; Papademetriou, V; Dilemmas in treating hypertension in octogenarians. *J Clin Hypertens (Greenwich)*. 2012, 14, 711-17.

In: Recent Advances in Cardiology
Editors: José Milei and Giuseppe Ambrosio

ISBN: 978-1-63117-282-3

Chapter 9

Current Advances in the Chronobiology of Blood Pressure

Matilde E. Otero-Losada ***and J. Milei***
Instituto de Investigaciones Cardiológicas "Prof. Dr. Alberto C. Taquini"
University of Buenos Aires– National Res. Council (ININCA UBA– CONICET),
Buenos Aires, Argentina

Abstract

Biologic rhythms are viewed as adaptive adjustments of our ancestors to cyclic changes in their environment during the 24-h day, the month, and the year. Cycles of day and night resulting from the earth's rotation movement around its axis have clearly influenced all life forms. Most organisms have evolved to synchronize their activities with it as an adaptive response bringing them an evolutive advantage. Some have chosen day or night, while others escaped daily temporal constraints altogether by living in constant conditions such as deep in the oceans or in natural caves [1]. Many organisms have developed biological clocks to time their metabolic processes rather than simply responding to the daily light-dark transitions.

Rhythmic patterns have been observed in most biological functions and oscillations with a peak and trough have been demonstrated for many bodily functions, including arterial blood pressure, heart rate, vascular tone, coagulation, and fibrinolysis among many others [2]. Depending on cycle length, these oscillations can be circadian, infradian, ultradian, circannual or seasonal.

Chronobiology adds a new dimension, namely, biologic time, to medicine. Improper blood pressure control throughout the entire 24 h can increase the risk of end-organ injury and cardiovascular events. Shallow declines in nocturnal compared with diurnal blood pressure (dipping) have been associated with cardiovascular disease [3]. A tendency of progression in the visual field defect in patients with primary open-angle glaucoma or normal-tension glaucoma has been observed in nondipper and extreme dipper subjects [4]. These observations imply that true 24-h blood pressure control should involve not only attenuation of the morning blood pressure rate of rise (morning surge) but also normalization of both daytime blood pressure levels and sleep-time blood pressure patterns [5,6].

* Corresponding author: Email: mol@fmed.uba.ar.

The mechanisms controlling circadian rhythms of blood pressure and heart rate have been actively investigated health and disease. Crucial factors such as smoking [7], obesity [8] and diabetes [9,10] have been studied in relation with the chronobiology of hypertension. Interestingly, considering the growing incidence of metabolic syndrome, a lack of nocturnal shift in blood pressure (dipping) has been reported in untreated hypertension associated with metabolic syndrome [11].

The chronobiology of blood pressure has been updated [12,13] and reviewed in this chapter including additional comments on clinical observations obtained at our laboratory not long ago [14].

Introduction

Biological clocks developed early in life as an evolutive behavior pertaining to the adaptation of organisms, nearly from algae to mammals, to the cycles of day and night that result from earth´s rotation around its axis. The ubiquity and importance of chronobiological regulation is such that similar mechanisms that govern central clocks are thought to be functional at the cell level in peripheral organs. In that way peripheral clocks may be able to synchronize the activity of the organ with the central ´master´ clock by receiving and sending (feed-back) information.

Nearly all behaviors and physiology appear to be somewhat adjusted to the process. Almost all organisms display circadian rhythms, indicating an evolutionary benefit to enable coping with the cyclic nature of the environment.

Every day is a new twist on the question of how biological clocks work. Evidence-based experience shows that biological clocks help organize a vertiginous array of biochemical processes in the body. Yet, despite a number of hypotheses, exactly how the microscopic pacemakers in every cell in the body exert such a widespread influence still remains a mystery.

High variability in response to a wide variety of stimuli that characterizes blood pressure challenges the reliability of cardiovascular morbidity and mortality predictions based on isolated measures. Only multiple measures over time are acceptable in order to reach meaningful and reliable conclusions according to the present knowledge status.

Topics in this review

- Circadian rhythm. Various studies including some of ours [5,6,15,16] are commented. Discussion revolves around the goal of identifying reliable predictors of risk for cardiovascular disease development.
- Infradian rhythms. Reports by Pérez-Lloret and colleagues working in our Institute [16] and others [17-19] are contrasted.
- Chronobiology of blood pressure regulation is discussed in the light of the theory of chaos and fractal mathematics. The physical structure of the vascular tree, the His-Purkinje network of the heart and heart rate variability are only some of the large list of processes and anatomical structures bearing fractal structure. Fractal analysis of blood pressure variability broadens our comprehension cardiovascular time-dependent behavior.

- Chronotherapeutics´ advantages in the management of hypertension are commented and compared with the therapeutic response to the conventional once-a-day administration of antihypertensive drugs.

'There is an appointed time for everything.
And there is a time for every event under Heaven.
A time to give birth, and a time to die.
A time to plant and a time to uproot what was planted.'

Ecclesiastes 3:1-2

Circadian Rhythms

Circadian [from 'circa'—about; 'dies'—a day] clocks are among the best characterized biological clocks, and they time biological events that occur once a day. Even in the absence of environmental time cues, these clocks maintain a period close to 24h, which remains stable within physiologically tolerable temperature range [20]. Circadian clocks regulate different aspects of metabolism, physiology, and behavior, in a wide variety of organisms. Although it is not clear how and why clocks with an approximately 24h period evolved in a cyclic environment of an exactly 24h period, a careful analysis would make it clear that it provides optimal stability to its expression under natural light-dark cycles [1,21].

Human beings inherit, by genetic transmission, unique biologic clock mechanisms. The main pacemaker clock of circadian rhythms is located in the anterior hypothalamus, more specifically in the suprachiasmatic nuclei [22-25]. The inherited period of the human circadian clock is not precisely 24 h; in most people it is slightly longer while it is slightly shorter in some others [26,27]. The light–dark and other cyclic environmental and societal time cues entrain the period of the suprachiasmatic nuclei to precisely 24 h, and stage the peaks and troughs of circadian rhythms to support the diurnal activity–nocturnal sleep routine characteristic of humans [28,29]. The same environmental time cues also are responsible for adjusting the phasing of 24-h rhythms when the sleep–activity routine is suddenly altered, for example, in workers who rotate between day and night shifts and in travelers who are rapidly displaced by jet aircraft across several time zones [30-32].

The timing of the peaks and troughs of circadian rhythms is quite predictable from one day to the next in the majority of people who adhere to a fairly regular sleep–activity schedule. However, the staging of 24-h rhythms in those who work rotating shift schedules or follow variable rest–activity routines is less predictable. This has clinical importance. The activity–sleep routine determines when the peaks and troughs of circadian rhythms occur with reference to the 24-h time scale. The phasing of the circadian time structure in turn determines when the symptoms of diseases are likely to flare, and they can affect responses to diagnostic tests and therapeutic interventions according to their timing, as discussed below.

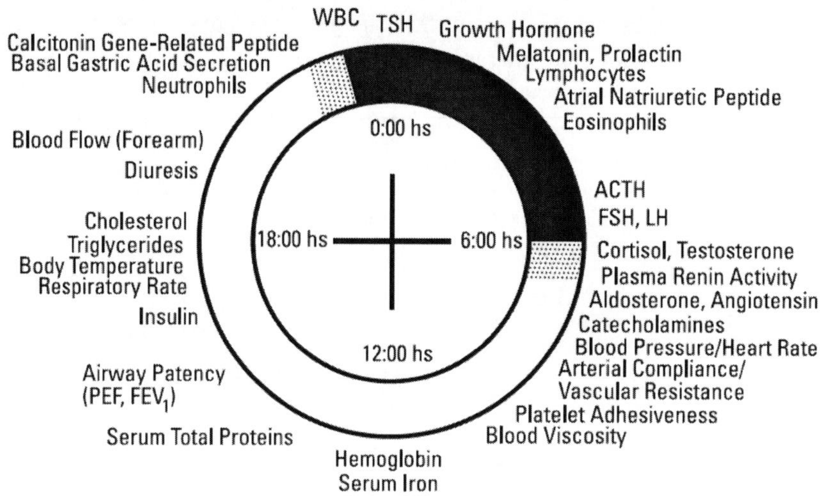

Figure 1. Human circadian time structure. Shown is the approximate peak time of circadian [24-h] rhythms of selected biological variables in persons adhering to a normal routine of daytime activity [6–7 a.m. to 10–11 p.m.] alternating with nighttime sleep. The activity in light-sleep in darkness daily routine determines the phasing of all circadian rhythms. Modified from Devdhawala & Seth [33].

The peak in basal gastric acid secretion, white blood cell count, calcitonin gene–related protein and atrial natriuretic peptides is late at night or early in sleep [Figure 1]. Interestingly both calcitonin gene–related protein and atrial natriuretic peptides exert blood pressure–lowering effects [33]. The circadian rhythms of white blood count, thyroid stimulating hormone [TSH], growth hormone, melatonin, prolactin, atrial natriuretic peptide, and eosinophil and lymphocyte cell numbers in blood peak between bedtime and the early hours of sleep. Circadian rhythms in the blood level of adrenocortical tropic hormone, follicle stimulating hormone, luteinizing hormone, testosterone, cortisol, catecholamines, renin activity, aldosterone, and angiotensin peak near the end of nighttime sleep or start of daytime activity [33]. The morning peak of the rhythm in vaso-active entities contributes to the morning peak time of the circadian rhythms in heart rate, blood pressure, arterial compliance, and vascular resistance in normotensive and uncomplicated essential hypertension persons, and the morning peak of the circadian rhythm in blood catecholamines gives rise to the morning peak of the circadian rhythm in platelet aggregation [33]. Circadian rhythms of hemoglobin and serum iron peak around mid-day and total serum proteins and airway caliber — peak expiratory flow rate and forced expiratory volume in 1 s—peak in the afternoon. Circadian rhythms of body temperature and respiratory rate and blood insulin, cholesterol, and triglycerides peak late in the afternoon, while those of urine production, forearm blood flow, neutrophils, basal gastric acid production, and calcitonin gene related peptide [vasodilator] peak late in the activity span [33]. Together, the phasing [peak time] of these and numerous other 24-h rhythms in biological processes and functions make up the circadian time structure of human beings, giving rise today–night patterns in disease activity, with the potential for varying-in-time requirements for pharmacotherapy, as well as administration-time differences in the kinetics and dynamics of medications. Clearly, the biochemistry and physiology of human beings are not constant; rather, they are variable in a predictable manner during the 24-h period [33].

Nitric oxide [NO] is involved in the regulation of blood pressure and local blood flow. Its biological activity is impaired in hypertension and atherosclerosis. Bode-Böger and others studied 8 healthy volunteers, 8 patients with essential hypertension, and 8 patients with peripheral arterial occlusive disease. They found circadian variation in urinary nitrate and cyclic GMP excretion rates, two markers for systemic NO production, in healthy humans [34]. Production of NO was increased in the morning, along with the morning rise in blood pressure, indicating that NO may buffer blood pressure increase. Diurnal variation in nitrate and cyclic GMP excretion was absent in hypertension, pointing to impaired NO formation. The major change in peripheral arterial occlusive disease was increased nitrate/cyclic GMP ratio, which pointed to increased oxidative inactivation of NO in this disease. Therefore disturbed formation and activity of NO may contribute to blood pressure alterations in cardiovascular disease [34].

Regardless of potential mechanisms, there is little doubt that the peak time for cardiovascular events - myocardial infarction, stroke, sudden death, and hypertensive crises - is in the hours between 6 am and noon, although the exact location of the peak varies across studies [26,34-36]. Heart rate, blood pressure, neurohumoral vasoactive factors, such as plasma norepinephrine levels and renin activity, and probably also contractility are increased in the morning hours [37]. Ludka and collaborators evaluated the circadian variability of plasma big endothelin and N-terminal pro-brain natriuretic peptide level in patients with severe heart failure. Mean plasma level of big endothelin [1.25 to 1.71 pmol/L] had diurnal variability [normal values < 0.7 pmol/L]. Mean plasma level of N-terminal pro-brain natriuretic peptide [782 to 934 pmol/L] had no diurnal variability [normal values <350 pmol/L]. Plasma level of N-terminal pro-brain natriuretic peptide proved to be stable during 24 hours and showed no circadian variability. Plasma big endothelin showed a morning peak after a systematic increase during bed rest [37].

Hypertensive patients with altered circadian blood pressure rhythms are prone to morbid cardiovascular events and end-organ damage [38,39]. In fact, we have observed differences between diurnal and nocturnal blood pressure variability associated with geometrical patterns of left ventricle remodelling in elder patients [5,6].

The involvement of the renin-angiotensin system in blood pressure variability has been indicated by studying the overactive renin-angiotensin system studies in transgenic hypertensive rats. These rats manifest inversion of the circadian rhythm of blood pressure [40,41], resembling secondary forms of human hypertension ["nondipping"]. Baltatu and others demonstrated inversion of the circadian rhythm of blood pressure induced by angiotensin II [42]. The angiotensin II-induced shift on blood pressure circadian rhythm was not related to alterations in the 24-h rhythmicity of heart rate or locomotor activity, indicating that circadian variability of blood pressure and heart rate were differentially regulated. The brain renin-angiotensin system was found to modulate angiotensin II-induced hypertension and cardiac hypertrophy [43]. Brain areas connected with the suprachiasmatic nucleus that regulate circadian rhythms include the pineal gland and paraventricular nucleus, all expressing renin-angiotensin system components [44,45].

Circadian rhythms are controlled by an internal autonomous oscillator system in the brain that coordinates the rhythms of peripheral oscillators [46]. Campos and others investigated the possible involvement of brain renin-angiotensin system in the adaptation of the circadian rhythms of blood pressure to light cycle shifts in transgenic rats with low levels of brain angiotensinogen. They observed that the brain renin-angiotensin system was not involved in the maintenance of the internal circadian rhythms of blood pressure and heart rate and the brain renin-angiotensin system might play an important role in mediating the effects of light cycle shifts on the circadian variation of blood pressure and heart rate [47].

Light is considered as the major environmental stimulus to entrain the internal circadian biological rhythms. The only known mammalian oscillators that can be entrained by light are located in the hypothalamic suprachiasmatic nucleus [46]. This indicates the existence of a hierarchical model of internal oscillators, in which the suprachiasmatic nucleus represents the master clock (zeitgeber) linking the environmental stimuli (e.g., light) and the internal circadian clocks [46]. Neural outputs from the suprachiasmatic nucleus may affect the cardiovascular system through hormonal, sympathetic, or parasympathetic signals [48,49]. Transgenic rats with low levels of brain angiotensinogen used in the study by Campos et al. [47] have low levels of the pineal melatonin [49]. One possible mechanism on the modulatory effect of melatonin on the circadian rhythms of blood pressure and heart rate is through its influence on the autonomic nervous system [50].

Continuous exposure to light suppresses the circadian rhythm of blood pressure and heart rate in rats [51]. Differently from environmental light stimuli, nonphotic stimuli, such as angiotensin II, may induce a dichotomy in the circadian rhythms of blood pressure and heart rate. Angiotensin II acts as a hormonal modulator and induces a light independent inversion of the circadian rhythm of blood pressure but not of the heart rate [42]. Thus photic (environmental) and nonphotic (hormonal) stimuli induce different mechanisms of the central clock circuitry to alter blood pressure or heart rate circadian rhythms. The brain renin-angiotensin appears to be involved in the effects of both types of stimuli.

Blood pressure in both healthy normotensives and hypertensives (essential hypertension) is subjected to diurnal rhythm with higher daily values and lower nocturnal values. Differently, patients with secondary hypertension show disrupted circadian rhythm of blood pressure [52,53]. Among dialyzed patients nocturnal blood pressure reduction is blunted [54-57]. Abnormal circadian rhythm of blood pressure appears to correlate with high incidence of cardiovascular disease morbidity and mortality among patients with chronic kidney disease [54,55,58]. Baranowicz-Gąszczyk and collaborators evaluated the correlation of diurnal rhythm of blood pressure and diurnal heart rate variability, with adrenergic activity measured by levels of catecholamines, among normotensive patients treated with continuous ambulatory peritoneal dialysis [8 patients] and hemodialysis [13 patients]. Diurnal blood pressure was blunted in 80% of hemodialized patients during the day of hemodialysis, 70% during the day without hemodialysis and in 50% in patients undergoing continuous ambulatory peritoneal dialysis [59]. Baseline noradrenaline as well as noradrenaline post cold pressure test levels were higher among hemodialised patients and patients with continuous ambulatory peritoneal dialysis compared with controls [59].

Abnormalities in circadian blood pressure variability are risk factors for cardiovascular disease and premature death [60,61]. Prediabetes has been associated with abnormal circadian blood pressure variability [62].

Normal circadian blood pressure variability for systolic blood pressure and diastolic blood pressure over a 24-hour span is shown in Figure 2.

Gupta and others tested the hypothesis that changes in circadian blood pressure variability and endothelial function may be early correlates of cardiometabolic disorders [8]. Obese participants with circadian blood pressure variability abnormalities (Mesor-hypotension, circadian hyper amplitude tension, elevated pulse pressure) had attenuated flow-mediated brachial artery dilatation at 78, 52, and 56% of resting reference diameter respectively. MESOR Hypotension (M-Hypotension) or MESOR Hypertension (M-Hypertension) in this system was defined as a blood pressure MESOR below the lower 5% or above the upper 95% prediction limit of peers matched by age and gender. Mesor-Hypertension for systolic blood pressure and diastolic blood pressure is shown in Figure 3 [8].

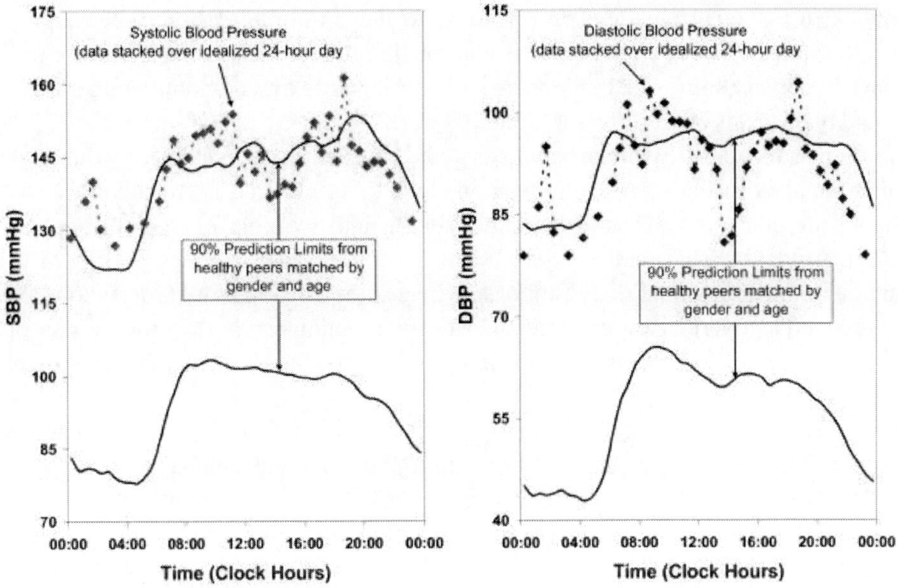

Figure 2. Normal circadian blood pressure variability. From Gupta et al. [62].

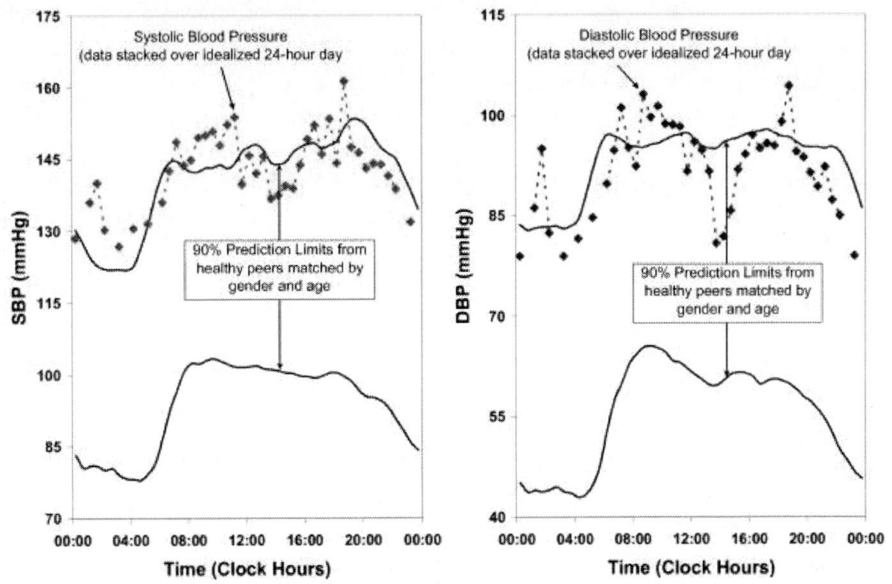

Figure 3. MESOR-hypertension .From Gupta et al. [8].

Systolic blood pressure and diastolic blood pressure vary considerably during the 24 h [35,63]. With the beginning of morning activity, systolic blood pressure rises rapidly typically by 20 to 25 mm Hg and diastolic blood pressure by 10 to 15 mm Hg. Both systolic blood pressure and diastolic blood pressure are highest late in the afternoon. In the evening they tend to decline, attaining lowest levels during sleep. This variation is attributable to temporal patterns in activity, stress, and posture during the 24 h, as well as to circadian rhythms in autonomic nervous and endocrine systems [64]. The temporal picture of blood pressure in uncomplicated essential hypertension is similar to that in normotension; however, the 24-h mean and/or and amplitude of variation is abnormally elevated. The blood pressure profile of secondary hypertension, for example in renal insufficiency, dysautonomia, mineral corticoid excess and diabetes, is often different [63,65-67].

In contrast to other rhythmic parameters, the diurnal blood pressure rhythm is largely dependent on activity and sleep rather than on clock time. This has been demonstrated by the blood pressure characteristics after shifted sleeping and working phases, during transition from sleep to wakefulness, and by the influence of sleep and activities on the 24-h blood pressure curve during normal daily routines. Whereas the circadian rhythm of blood pressure is predominantly governed by external time triggers, endogenous rhythmicity can only be detected by time accurate analysis or in conditions where effects of external time triggers are almost excluded [64].

Heart rate, blood pressure and autonomic nervous system activity vary diurnally, with a reduction in heart rate and blood pressure, and a shift to vagal dominance during the dark phase. However, the cause of these changes, particularly the relative influence of sleep and circadian mechanisms, remains uncertain. Carrington and others reported that night-time decrease in heart rate was due to both sleep onset and a circadian influence, with the circadian component being more prominent [68]. In contrast, the fall in blood pressure was largely due to a sleep onset effect. Increased vagal activity, as reflected in the high frequency component and a shift to vagal dominance in the low/high frequency ratio, appeared to be primarily a function of the sleep system, while sympathetic activity, as assessed by pre-ejection period, evidenced a circadian influence [68].

Even during sleep stages, like non-REM sleep, characterized by an overall vagal predominance, phases of sustained sympathetic activation do occur that resemble that occurring during REM. Throughout the overnight sleep period, the arterial baroreflex acts to buffer surges of sympathetic activation by means of rapid changes in cardiac vagal circuits [69].

Typically, there is a blunting of the nocturnal decline or even an increase in blood pressure during sleep relative to the daytime level. The extent of the circadian variation plus the differential phasing of the blood pressure rhythms in primary compared to secondary hypertension can complicate the accurate assessment of blood pressure and make difficult the clinical differentiation of hypertension from normotension. In-home blood pressure measurements made at different times of the day and night and 24-h ambulatory monitoring are useful strategies to complement office assessments, especially in those who display a "white coat" effect [63,67].

A diurnal variation in the onset of cardiac events and stroke is well recognized [70]. Cardiovascular events usually peak in the early morning and forenoon [71].

The non–24-h sleep–wake syndrome is characterized by complaints of difficulty in initiating and terminating sleep at consistent clock times every day. Diagnostic studies show that sleep onset and offset times are progressively delayed by 2 to 3 h from day to day. The period of the inherited biologic clock controlling the sleep–wake cycle is abnormal, being as long as 26 or 27 h. Other medical conditions, such as seasonal affective mood disorder, premenstrual dysphoric disorder and even regular depression, at least to some extent, might result from abnormalities in circadian time-keeping [26].

Pérez-Lloret and others working in our laboratory, characterized gender differences in age-related variation of nocturnal elevation of blood pressure, as well as of diurnal and nocturnal systolic blood pressure and diastolic blood pressure. A large sample of untreated subjects [n=1689] underwent 24h ambulatory blood pressure monitoring [72].

Men were found to be more hypertensive than women, in both the awake and asleep blood pressure measurements. The frequency of nocturnal elevation of blood pressure was similar in elderly men and women (50% for both), but was lower in females of age less than 30 years as compared to men of the same age (0% vs. 20% respectively) (Figure 4) [72].

Women and men showed differences in the decennial progression rate. In men, the frequency of nocturnal elevation of blood pressure increased by 4.2±0.7% per decade, whereas women showed a higher progression rate (7.3±1.0%). Diurnal and nocturnal systolic blood pressure increased with age by 15% and 25% in females and by 3% and 8% in males. Diurnal and nocturnal diastolic blood pressure were lower in females of all age groups (Figure 5) [72]. The results indicated a lower prevalence of nocturnal elevation of blood pressure among young women compared to young men that was not detected between aged men and women. Higher progression rate of nocturnal elevation of blood pressure with advancing age in women was suggested. Accordingly, a steeper age-related increment in the frequency of nocturnal elevation of blood pressure was observed in women compared to men, likely resulting in worse cardiovascular prognosis in aged women. Proper evaluation and control of nocturnal elevation of blood pressure was finally recommended for the elderly population, especially for women [72].

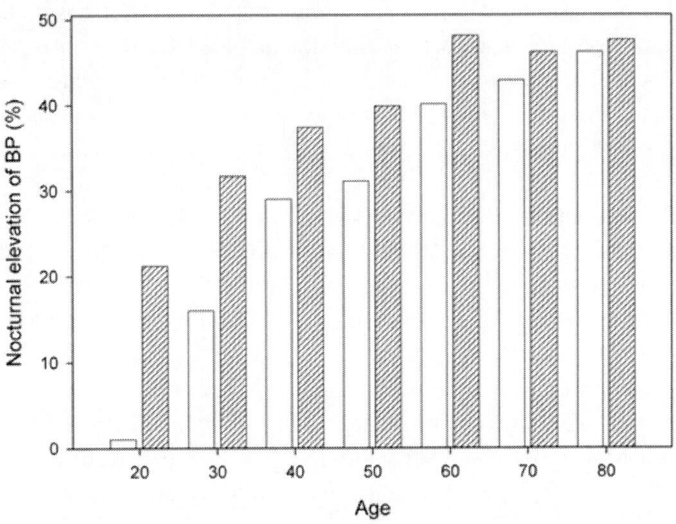

Figure 4. Age-related variations in the percentages of males (hatched bars) and females (open bars) classified as nocturnal hypertensives. A significant difference was noticed in the younger groups ($p < 0.001$) but not in the groups with aged subjects. Taken from Pérez-Lloret S et al. [72].

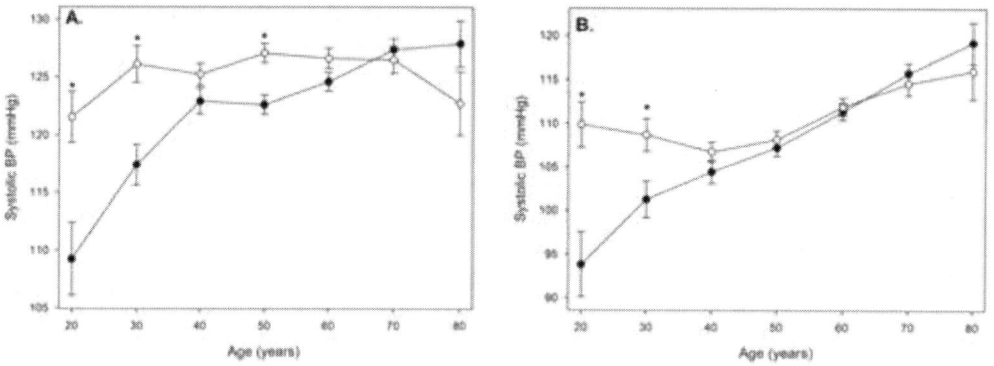

Figure 5. Age-related variations in mean values of awake (panel A) and asleep (panel B) systolic blood pressures in males [○] and females [●].*p < 0.05 vs. females.Taken from Pérez-Lloret S et al. [72].

Infradian Rhythms

Blood pressure shows 24-h rhythms (circadian) embedded in larger cycles with seasonal fluctuation (infradian: cycling *less* than daily)) [16,73,74].

Seasonal blood pressure variations [75] and seasonal differences in cardiovascular and non-cardiovascular mortality rates are reported [76-78]. Blood pressure rises in winter and decreases in summer [7].

Ischemic heart disease and stroke as well as respiratory diseases have been reported to cause more deaths in winter than in summer [77]. Likewise, infradian daytime blood pressure rhythms have been observed in young and older adults [7,79-86]. Kristal-Boneh and others found that seasonal changes in blood pressure were related to body mass index, as a result of high thermoregulatory requirements of lean individuals [80].

Sinha and others studied seasonal variation in hypertension prevalence among females (n=275, 18-40 years of age) in an Indian urban location. The prevalence of hypertension based on systolic blood pressure (SBP) was 12.72% in summer and increased to 22.22% in winter [73]. Using diastolic blood pressure (DBP) criteria, prevalence of hypertension increased to more than double (summer vs. winter: 11.27% vs. 26.59%). Overall prevalence of hypertension (i.e., SBP ≥ 140 or DBP ≥ 90 mm of Hg) was 1.9 times in winter compared to summer. Prevalence of hypertension increased with aging [73].

Nakajima and others evaluated factors affecting seasonal variation in blood pressure in 38 men and 57 women with essential hypertension who stayed almost entirely indoors in a stable environmental temperature and who took a calcium channel blocker during the study which was conducted during the summer and winter. The subjects spent virtually the entire day (average > 22h) indoors in both summer and winter (prospective study). During the waking hours, the systolic/diastolic blood pressures were significantly higher in winter than in summer. The differences were 8±9/4±5 mmHg in men and 5±11/2±6 mmHg in women and no gender difference was found. No seasonal differences in blood pressure during the sleeping hours were noted. There was no between-seasons difference in urinary sodium excretion or in physical activity. Only body height was correlated with the winter increase in waking blood pressure regardless gender. Body height was a determinant of the winter increase in waking blood pressure in hypertensive patients living almost entirely indoors [18].

Iwabu and collaborators examined the relationships between home blood pressure and atmospheric temperature in 20 treated-hypertensive patients [74]. Morning and evening blood pressure and atmospheric temperature were correlated. For morning SBP, the maximal seasonal difference was 13.2 mmHg with 25.5 degrees C temperature difference. Morning SBP increased by approximately 0.41 mmHg per 1 degree C decrease in atmospheric temperature. A weaker correlation with temperature was observed for morning diastolic, evening systolic and DBP [74].

Seasonal changes in daily variations of blood pressure have been rarely studied in hemodialyzed patients. Takenata and others studied thirty hypertensive patients with end-stage renal diseases [87]. Home blood pressure measurements were performed at least for 1 week in each season. Morning and evening SBPs showed seasonal changes with the highest blood pressure in winter (162±18 and 135±22 mmHg in morning and evening). Morning DBP also showed seasonal changes with the highest blood pressure in fall (78±8 mmHg). Morning-evening differences in SBP and DBP were the greatest in winter (28±21 and 10±9 mmHg in SBP and DBP) and the smallest in summer (16±12 and 6±5 mmHg). Average blood pressure and variations of blood pressure were the largest in winter [87].

Because of the increasing use of heating systems, the seasonal variation in blood pressure levels may be smaller now than observed in earlier studies, especially in colder seasons when more heat is used. Hozawa and collaborators used continuous measurements of home blood pressure data to track seasonal variations of blood pressure and analyzed the relation between outside temperature and blood pressure values [88]. Blood pressure levels were lowest in the warmest months. A clear inverse association between temperature and blood pressure values was evident only in periods when outside temperatures were above 10°C. When the outside temperature was ≥ 10°C, 1°C increment of outside temperature corresponded to 0.40 and 0.28 mmHg decrease of SBP and DBP, whereas the corresponding values were 0.06 and 0.01 mmHg when the outside temperature was <10°C. In conclusion, only in warmer seasons an inverse association between outside temperature and blood pressure was observed [88].

Another study examined normotensive women and found biphasic seasonal variation in self-recorded blood pressure measured at home, environmental temperature and daytime length but no apparent seasonal variation in body weight and blood pressure measured in the office. The longest daytime length preceded and the highest environmental temperature lagged behind the lowest level of blood pressure. Conversely the shortest daytime length preceded the lowest outdoor and indoor temperature values [89].

Seasonal differences in daytime but not in night-time blood pressure means been reported [19,90]. For example, Goodwin and others reported 5–10 mmHg diurnal SBP and DBP within-participant variations between summer and winter, with a peak in winter, in elderly but not in young participants [17]. Employing a between-participant comparison approach, different studies showed differences between summer and winter in SBP and DBP means [91,83,86].

Not long ago, Pérez-Lloret and collaborators working in our laboratory, studied 2-month to 12-month infradian rhythms in the mean awake and asleep SBP and DBP in humans [16]. We studied an urban (Buenos Aires) sample of patients presenting for the evaluation of possible hypertension. The potential correlation with fluctuations in meteorological variables was also explored [16]. One thousand six hundred and eighty nine participants underwent

24-h ambulatory blood pressure monitoring during different periods of the year. Mean daily temperature, humidity, barometric pressure and wind velocity recordings for the same time span and geographical location were obtained considering that those challenges to energy homeostasis affect metabolic and cardiovascular functioning [92].

Awake SBP and DBP means were lower in summer and spring as compared with autumn and winter, whereas asleep SBP and DBP showed no seasonal differences. As a result, a higher proportion of participants were diagnosed as hypertensive in winter and as non-dippers in summer [16].

The mean awake SBP and DBP exhibited 12-month (Figure 6) and 3-month infradian rhythms. Overall rhythms showed a zenith in winter (July in the south hemisphere), a nadir in summer and a nadir-zenith difference of 6.2 ± 1.6 mmHg (SBP) and 4.2 ± 1.5 mmHg (DBP) [16].

The mean asleep SBP showed a 3-month rhythm with a nadir-zenith difference of 1.3 ± 1.9 mmHg (Figure 7). The mean asleep DBP exhibited 12-month and 3-month rhythms (Figure 7). The fitted overall rhythm had a zenith in summer (January), a nadir in winter. A nadir-zenith difference of 3.1 ± 1.4 mmHg accounted for 43% of total variability [16].

The amplitude of the 24-h SBP and DBP rhythms displayed 12-month, 6-month and 3-month periodicity. The 24-hour DBP rhythm amplitude also showed a 2-month rhythm (Figure 8). The overall rhythms of the asleep SBP and DBP fall had a zenith in winter, a nadir in summer. Nadir-zenith differences of 4.6 ± 0.9 and 6.8 ± 1.0 respectively explained 75% and 82% of total variability [16].

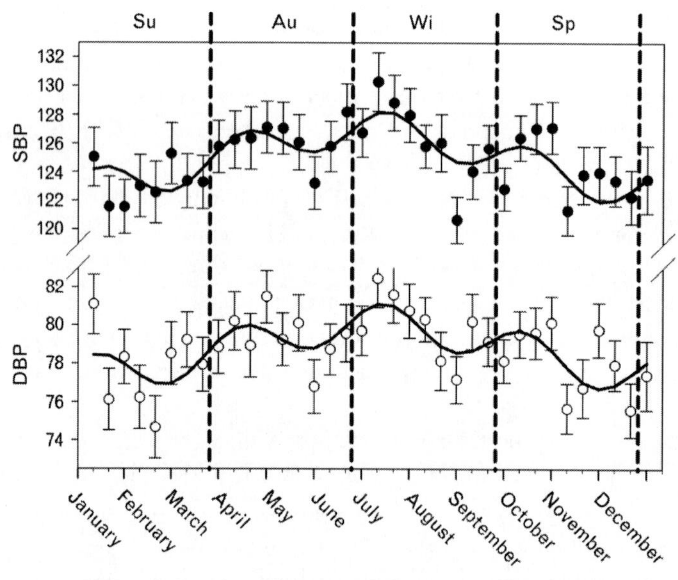

Age-adjusted and gender-adjusted mean awake systolic blood pressure (SBP) and diastolic blood pressure (DBP) during the year. The curves represent the overall fitted rhythms, which result from the superimposition of the significant rhythms identified by Fourier analysis. Su, summer; Au, autumn; Wi, winter; Sp, spring. Data shown as mean ± SEM.

Figure 6. Taken from Pérez-Lloret S et al. [16].

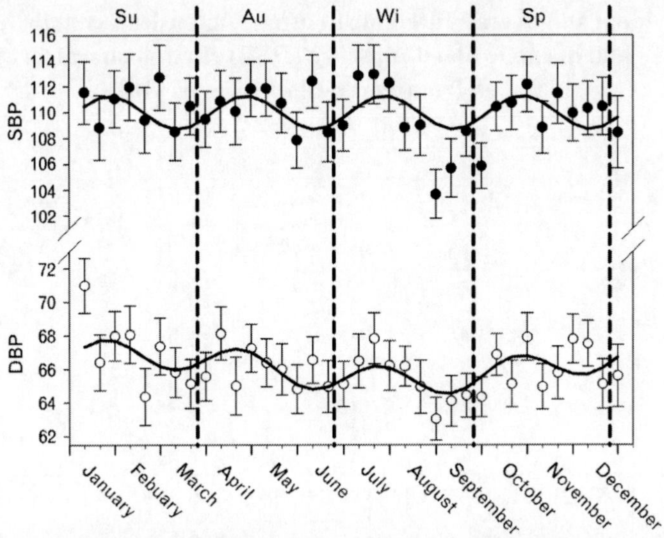

Age-adjusted and gender-adjusted mean asleep systolic blood pressure (SBP) and diastolic blood pressure (DBP) during the year. The curves represent the overall fitted rhythms, which result from the superimposition of the significant rhythms identified by Fourier analysis. Su, summer; Au, autumn; Wi, winter; Sp, spring. Data shown as mean ± SEM.

Figure 7. Taken from Pérez-Lloret S et al. [16].

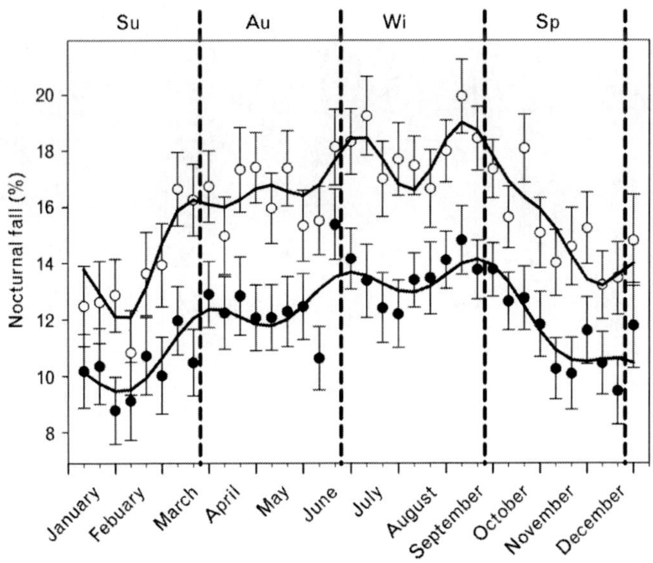

Age-adjusted and gender-adjusted mean systolic blood pressure (●) and diastolic blood pressure (○) nocturnal fall (percentage of awake values) during the year. The curves represent the overall fitted rhythms, which result from the superimposition of the significant rhythms identified by Fourier analysis. Su, summer; Au, autumn; Wi, winter; Sp, spring. Data shown as mean ± SEM.

Figure 8. Taken from Pérez-Lloret S et al. [16].

Table 1. Individual and overall fitted mean awake and asleep systolic blood pressure (SBP) and diastolic blood pressure (DBP) rhythm characteristics. Taken from Pérez-Lloret S et al. [16]

	SBP rhythms			DBP rhythms		
	Trough–peak difference	Time to peak*	R^2 (*P* value)	Trough–peak difference	Time to peak*	R^2 (*P* value)
Awake means (mmHg)						
12 months	4.0	7.0	39% (< 0.001)	2.6	7.0	27% (< 0.001)
3 months	2.6	0.8	8% (0.02)	2.0	0.7	5% (0.04)
Overall rhythm	6.2	7.3	55% (< 0.001)	4.4	7.3	45% (< 0.001)
Asleep means (mmHg)						
12 months	–	–	–	1.6	3.8	15% (< 0.01)
3 months	2.6	0.7	19% (0.02)	1.8	0.8	4% (0.03)
Overall rhythm	–	–	–	1.6	1.3	31% (< 0.02)
Nocturnal fall (%)						
12 months	3.4	6.9	60% (< 0.001)	4.6	6.7	64% (< 0.001)
6 months	1.0	2.9	2% (0.05)	1.6	3.1	5% (0.04)
3 months	1.4	2.9	6% (0.03)	1.4	2.9	4% (0.04)
2 months	–	–	–	1.2	0.3	4% (0.04)
Overall rhythm	4.6	7.6	75% (< 0.001)	6.8	7.3	82% (< 0.001)

* Times to peak are expressed as the month number starting from January (month number 1).

In relation with infradian meteorological rhythms, 12-month, 6-month, 4-month, 3-month and 2-month rhythms in average daily temperature and relative humidity were observed [16]. As far as barometric pressure and wind velocity are concerned, 12 and 6 months and 12 and 3 months could be fitted, respectively [16]. Tables 1 and 2 show that times to peak of the 12-month and 3-month blood pressure rhythms overlapped with the time to trough of the respective temperature and wind velocity rhythms and with the times to peak of the 12-month and 3-month humidity rhythms as well [16].

Table 2. Fitted mean temperature, humidity, wind velocity and barometric pressure rhythm characteristics. Taken from Pérez-Lloret S et al. [16]

Rhythm	Trough–peak difference	Time to peak–time to trough	R^2 (*P* value)
Temperature (°C)			
12 months	13.4	0.5–6.5	96% (< 0.001)
6 months	1.0	2.0–5.0	2% (0.01)
4 months	0.6	3.5–0.5	1% (0.01)
3 months	0.6	2.0–0.5	1% (0.01)
2 months	0.4	1.1–0.1	1% (0.01)
Humidity (%)			
12 months	14.2	5.1–11.1	75% (< 0.001)
6 months	2.0	4.0–1.0	1% (< 0.02)
4 months	2.0	1.9–3.9	1% (0.03)
3 months	1.2	0.8–2.3	1% (0.05)
2 months	1.0	1.9–0.9	1% (0.03)
Barometric pressure (Pa)			
12 months	16.4	4.5–10.5	12% (< 0.001)
6 months	8.4	0.7–3.7	1% (0.03)
Wind speed (km/h)			
12 months	3.6	10.7–4.7	54% (< 0.001)
3 months	0.4	2.5–1.0	1% (0.04)

Times to peak and times to troughs are expressed as month number starting from January (month number 1)

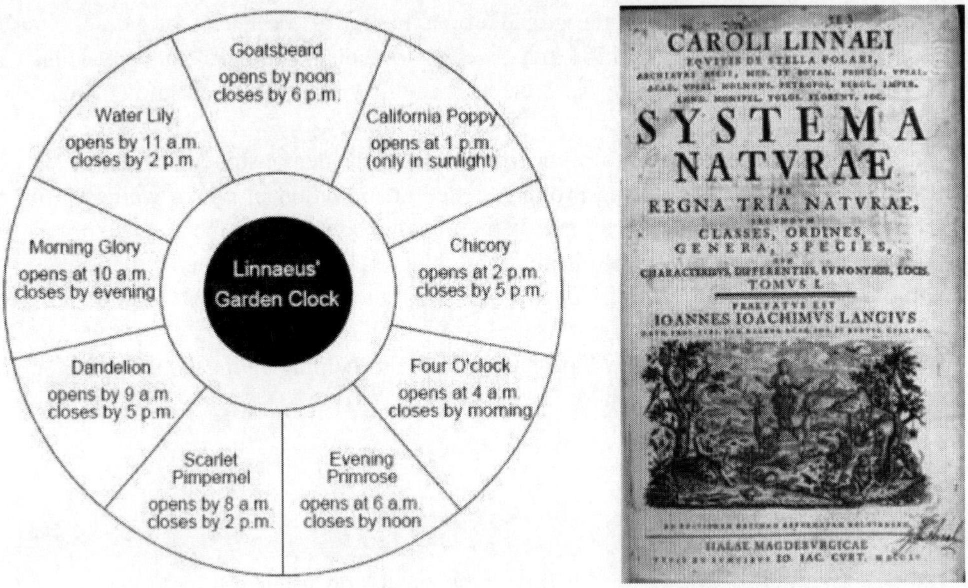

Figure 9. Left: Carolus Linneus' garden clock. Right: Cover of original Linneus' paper.

Awake SBP and DBP values were inversely associated with temperature related to the 12-month and 3-month rhythms and directly related to gender. Age was directly associated with the awake SBP and negatively with DBP values. Asleep SBP was inversely associated with the temperature value according to the 6-month rhythm and directly associated with age, gender and the relative humidity value according to the 3-month rhythm. Gender and age were identified as positive predictors of asleep DBP while temperature was a negative predictor asleep DBP according to the 12-month and 3-month rhythms. Moreover, we observed annual fluctuations in the mean awake SBP and DBP with zenith in winter and for the first time reported not only awake but also asleep blood pressure 3-month rhythms as well as a complex infradian pattern of blood pressure nocturnal fall [16].

Twelve-month and 3-month temperature variations [93,94] may account for the corresponding awake and asleep blood pressure variations [16]. Indeed, seasonal temperature, relative humidity and barometric pressure changes have been shown to influence the blood pressure in normotensive healthy participants [95], hemodialyzed patients [96,97] and essential hypertensive patients [98].

Chronobiological Patterns Express Chaos and Fractal Geometry

Historical Hits

The first acknowledged report of circadian periodicity bring us back to the IVth century BC when Androsthenes of Thasos, a geographer and ship captain serving under Alexander the Great, described the diurnal leaf movements of the tamarind, a tree commonly found in West Africa [99,100]. In 1729 Jean-Jacques d'Ortous de Mairan, a French scientist, first identified an endogenous clock dissociating the circadian oscillation of the leaves of Mimosa pudica from the environment [101]. In 1751 the Swedish botanist, zoologist and physician Carl Linneus used flower opening timings as a clock in the first ever published study of biological rhythms (Figure 9) [102].

Years later Patrick & Gilbert's pioneering experiment demonstrated the existence of a 24h cycle in sleepiness even during prolonged sleep deprivation in human beings [103]. In 1918, J.S. Szymanski showed that animals kept circadian behaviors in the absence of external cues [104]. In the late 1950s, the Romanian biologist Franz Halberg, one of the founders of chronobiology, coined the term "circadian". Not long ago, the first mammalian 'clock gene' was identified [105].

Bioclocks may represent an evolutionary advantage helping living beings to anticipate and cope with environmental demands.

Conclusion

Biologic rhythms are viewed as adaptive adjustments of our ancestors to cyclic changes in their environment during the 24-h day (ultradian), the month, and the year (infradian).

Clinical and experimental research and evidence-based medicine confirm the existence of circadian stage dependent diseases and events related to the cardiovascular system such as hypertension, heart attack, stroke, cardiac ischemia, sudden cardiac death, hypercholesterolemia, diabetes and others.

Both seasonal (infradian) and ultradian blood pressure fluctuations should be considered in the analysis, prevention and control of hypertension and other cardiovascular risk factors. Hypertensive patients with disrupted circadian blood pressure rhythms are at higher risk of morbid cardiovascular events and end-organ damage. Blood pressure cycles entail a crucial importance in management of hypertensive patients with end-stage renal diseases in particular.

Chronobiological and chronopharmacological studies are important experimental and clinical approaches to get a deeper insight into the physiological and pathophysiological regulation of the cardiovascular system including their rhythmic organization.

Matching drug release to the body's circadian rhythms is a fundamental strategy for selecting a new drug delivery system to increase the efficacy and safety of drugs by proportioning peak plasma concentrations during the 24 hours in synchrony with biological rhythm.

Overactivation of the renin-angiotensin system and a role of the renin-angiotensin system in blood pressure variability have been evidenced by experimental research studies. A tribute book will appear in 2014, a year marking the 75th anniversary of the discovery of angiotensin by Dr. Alberto C. Taquini, who founded our institute in 1944, and his coworkers.

Chronobiological Regulation of Blood Pressure

Traditionally the use of "Chaos theory" [non-linear complex systems' dynamics] has helped psychiatrists, in contraposition with determinism, to better understand neurobiological and neurochemical mechanisms underlying mental processes and the brain-mind connection [106-110].

This framework's formalism is suitable to study any domain where non-linear dynamics is *the* rule rather than the exception [111] and insofar it may contribute to broaden our comprehension of time-dependent cardiovascular behavior.

Blood pressure regulation comprises from cellular events up to endocrine influence. Blood pressure fluctuates within a given range, beyond which life is threatened. As blood pressure wave is restricted to a certain range in phase space and yet, the motion is never periodic, the properties of chaotic dynamics can be applied to blood pressure rhythms [112].

Fluctuations in cardiovascular data, as demonstrated in 24-hour ambulatory monitoring records of blood pressure can be examined from this perspective, applying spectral analysis.

The cardiovascular system may move between five kinds of behavior, each having a precise mathematical definition [107]:

1. Equilibrium describes a system at steady state
2. Periodicity describes a system with a simple rhythm, i.e., cycling frequency is set a priori.
3. Quasi-periodicity describes a more complex behavior: cycling with at least two frequencies whose ratio is not a rational number. Electrophysiological behaviors of the heart and the nervous system are examples of this.
4. Deterministic chaos: no particular rhythm is observed. The cardiovascular system adapts freely within imposed 'boundary conditions' preventing from collapse.
5. Random behavior: order breakdown, loss of coordination [chronos becomes caos].

Sharma has discussed the role of fractal structure and chaos in the cardiovascular system at the heart and vasculature, and at the cellular level along with the functional consequences of these phenomena, delineating a likely evolutionary origin of chaotic behavior and fractal structure [107].

The fractal exponent and the correlation dimension obtained from statistical treatment of data in mammals were reported and the convenience of these indexes for characterizing the irregularity of the signals was discussed [116]. The interdependence indexes between cardiac, respiratory and vascular signals may be conveniently used in physiological studies and clinical applications [116].

The cardiovascular system is a rich area for the study of dynamics, and it is a system in which clinical applications for chaos theory have already been found [112-114,116,131]. Fractal analysis of heart rate variability has allowed to predict sudden cardiac death in elderly subjects [117]. Practical applications of chaos theory enlightening the modulation of human ageing have been reported [115].

Cugini has discussed how intrinsical determination in biorhythms can break down into chaos depending on cycle stress limits, namely the limits in the oscillatory modulation [134]. Cugini and others studied 108 secondary hypertensives applying fractal mathematics to 24-h blood pressure data. The prevalence for a presumptive risk of hypertensive crisis was found in 11% of the patients regardless dipping condition or blood pressure variability (i.e., circadian rhythm conserved vs abolished). Presumptive risk was related to altered non-linear variability pattern in blood pressure, likely caused by neurovegetative mechanisms conferring chaos [disorder] to blood pressure rhythm. The same authors studied blood pressure circadian variation in 109 normotensives using the fractal interpolation and found presumptive risk in 12% of the subjects either dippers or non-dippers. Higher presumptive risk prevalence was observed in normotensives with disrupted circadian blood pressure rhythm (perturbations in the complex harmonic structure of blood pressure cycling) when compared to those with preserved circadian blood pressure cycle. Presumptive risk of hypertensive crisis was found in 14% of 380 patients with essential hypertension, independent on dipping condition, circadian periodicity or harmonic structure of the circadian blood pressure pattern. Neurovegetative mechanisms might account for non-linear chaotic variability in circadian blood pressure pattern [119-121,135-136].

Chronotherapeutics in Brief

Chronotherapeutics is an attractive goal in antihypertensive treatment and represents an advantage to conventional once-a-day drug administration helping the body to adapt to the changing needs. Chronobiological and chronopharmacological studies are important experimental and clinical ways to get a deeper insight into the physiological and pathophysiological regulation of the cardiovascular system including their rhythmic organization. Chronopharmacological studies comprise pharmacokinetic and pharmacodynamic studies, the combination of which aids in assessing the best time for drug administration [122]. At present the use of programmed chronotherapeutic drug delivery devices allows to match drug release to a given biological rhythm and match the body's changing needs at certain times of day or night in order to optimize therapeutic profile and to minimize side effects. Matching drug release to the body's circadian rhythms is a fundamental strategy for selecting a new drug delivery system to increase the efficacy and safety of drugs by rendering peak plasma concentrations during the 24 hours in synchrony with biological rhythm.

Chronopharmaceuticals for cardiovascular diseases have been extensively studied. Verapamil controlled-release tablets are by now successfully used to reduce the morning peak of both morbid and mortal cardiovascular events. Verapamil capsules (chronotherapeutic oral drug absorption system) are used for hypertension and angina [123-125]. Propranolol extended release capsules and graded-release diltiazem formulations are also used to treat hypertension [126,127].

Hermida and collaborators have extensively studied the benefits of proper modeling of the circadian BP profile by the timed administration of antihypertensive medication and have reported blood pressure reduction beyond the clinic-determined daytime or the ABPM-determined 24 h mean BP levels [13,128].

Conclusion

Biologic rhythms are viewed as adaptive adjustments of our ancestors to cyclic changes in their environment during the 24-h day (ultradian), the month, and the year (infradian).

Clinical and experimental research and evidence-based medicine confirm the existence of circadian stage dependent diseases and events related to the cardiovascular system such as hypertension, heart attack, stroke, cardiac ischemia, sudden cardiac death, hypercholesterolemia, diabetes and others.

Both seasonal (infradian) and ultradian blood pressure fluctuations should be considered in the analysis, prevention and control of hypertension and other cardiovascular risk factors. Hypertensive patients with disrupted circadian blood pressure rhythms are at higher risk of morbid cardiovascular events and end-organ damage. Blood pressure cycles entail a crucial importance in management of hypertensive patients with end-stage renal diseases in particular.

Chronobiological and chronopharmacological studies are important experimental and clinical approaches to get a deeper insight into the physiological and pathophysiological regulation of the cardiovascular system including their rhythmic organization.

Matching drug release to the body's circadian rhythms is a fundamental strategy for selecting a new drug delivery system to increase the efficacy and safety of drugs by proportioning peak plasma concentrations during the 24 hours in synchrony with biological rhythm.

Overactivation of the renin-angiotensin system and a role of the renin-angiotensin system in blood pressure variability have been evidenced by experimental research studies.

A tribute book will appear in 2014, a year marking the 75th anniversary of the discovery of angiotensin by Dr. Alberto C. Taquini, founder of our institute (1944) and his coworkers.

References

[1] Sharma, VK. Period responses to Zeitgeber signals stabilize circadian clocks during entrainment. *Chronobiol Int*, 2003,20, 389–404

[2] Manfredini, R; Manfredini, F; Malagoni, AM; et al. Chronobiology of Vascular Disorders,a “Seasonal” Link between Arterial and Venous Thrombotic Diseases?. *Journal of Coagulation Disorders*, 2010,2,61-67

[3] Ituarte; Philip, HG; Kamarck, TW; et al. Psychosocial mediators of racial differences in nighttime blood pressure dipping among normotensive adults. *Health Psychology*, 1999, 18,393-402

[4] Tokunaga, T; Kashiwagi, K; Tsumura, T; Taguchi, K; Tsukahara, S. Association between nocturnal blood pressure reduction and progression of visual field defect in patients with primary open-angle glaucoma or normal-tension glaucoma. *Jpn J Ophthalmol.*, 2004,48,380-5

[5] Sanchez, Gelós, DF; Otero-Losada, ME; Azzato, F; et al. Morning surge, pulsewave velocity, and autonomic function tests in elderly adults. *Blood Press Monit*, 2012,17, 103-9

[6] Sánchez-Gelós, D; Otero-Losada, ME; Grana, DR et al. Morning surge, pulse wave velocity and autonomic function tests in patients older than 65 years. Congress of the European Society of Cardiology. *Stockholm*, 2010,2703¨

[7] Kristal-Boneh, E; Harari, G; Green, MS. Seasonal change in 24-hour blood pressure and heart rate is greater among smokers than nonsmokers. *Hypertension*, 1997,30, 436–441

[8] Gupta, AK; Cornelissen, G; Greenway, FL; et al. Abnormalities in circadian blood pressure variability and endothelial function: pragmatic markers for adverse cardiometabolic profiles in asymptomatic obese adults. *Cardiovasc Diabetol*, 2010, 9,58

[9] Matteucci, E; Della, Bartola, L; Giampietro, O. Differences in circadian time structure of diastolic blood pressure between diabetes mellitus and essential hypertension. DiabetolMetabSyndr, 2012,4,51

[10] Matteucci, E; Giampietro, O. Circadian rhythm of blood pressure in diabetes mellitus:evidence, mechanisms and implications. *Curr Diabetes Rev*, 2012,8,355-61

[11] Hermida, RC; Chayán, L; Ayala, DE; Mojón, A; Domínguez, MJ; Fontao, MJ; Soler, R; Alonso, I; Fernández, JR. Association of metabolic syndrome and blood pressure nondipping profile in untreated hypertension. *Am J Hypertens.*, 2009,22, 307-13.

[12] Schmieder, RE; Bramlage, P; Schunkert, H. Chronobiology of blood pressure and chronopharmacotherapy of arterial hypertension. *Dtsch Med Wochenschr*, 2012, 137, 317-21

[13] Hermida, RC; Ayala, DE; Fernández, JR; Portaluppi, F; Fabbian, F; Smolensky, MH. Circadian rhythms in blood pressure regulation and optimization of hypertension treatment with ACE inhibitor and ARB medications. *Am J Hypertens*, 2011,24,383-91

[14] Otero-Losada, M; Grana, D; Perez, Lloret, S; Azzato, F; Milei, J. In: Circadian Rhythms: Biology, Cognition and Disorders. Eds: Luka Golovkin & Alexei Maliszkewicz. Chapter 15. Bio-Clocks & Cardiovascular Talk: Blood Pressure Meets Nature. ©Nova Science Publishers, Inc., 2011 (ISBN: 978-1-61324-858-4), 347 – 376

[15] Pérez-Lloret, S; Toblli, JE; Cardinali, DP; Malateste, JC; Milei, J. Nocturnal hypertension defined by fixed cut-off limits is a better predictor of left ventricular hypertrophy than non-dipping. *Int J Cardiol*, 2008, 127, 387-9

[16] Pérez-Lloret, S; Toblli, JE; Vigo, DE; et al. Infradian daytime and nighttime systolic and diastolic blood pressure rhythms in humans. *J Hypertens*, 2006, 24, 1273–1279

[17] Goodwin J, Pearce VR, Taylor RS; et al. Seasonal cold and circadian changes in blood pressure and physical activity in young and elderly people. *Age Ageing*, 2001, 30, 311–317

[18] Nakajima, J; Kawamura, M; Fujiwara, T; et al. Body height is a determinant of seasonal blood pressure variation in patients with essential hypertension. *Hypertens Res.*, 2000, 23, 587-92

[19] Brennan, PJ; Greenberg, G; Miall, WE; et al. Seasonal variation in arterial blood pressure. *Br Med J (Clin Res Ed)*, 1982, 285, 919–923

[20] Pittendrigh, CS. Circadian rhythms and the circadian organization of living systems. *Cold. Spr. Harb. Symp. Quant. Biol.* 1960, 25, 159–184

[21] Sharma, VK; Joshi, A. Clocks, genes, and evolution: the evolution of circadian organisation. In: Kumar, V, ed. Biological Clocks. New Delhi: Narosa Publishers and Berlin: Springer-Verlag., 2002, 5–23

[22] Moore, RY; Silver, R. Suprachiasmatic nucleus organization. *Chronobiol Int*, 1998, 15, 475–488

[23] Miller, JD. The SCN is comprised of a population of coupled oscillators. *Chronobiol Int*, 1998, 15, 489-511

[24] Rensing, L; Meyer-Grahle, U; Ruoff, P. Biological timing and clock metaphor: oscillatory and hourglass mechanisms. *Chronobiol Int*, 2001, 18, 329–369

[25] Shirakawa, T; Honma, S; Honma, K. Multiple oscillators in the suprachiasmatic nucleus. *Chronobiol Int*, 2001, 18, 371–387
[26] Smolensky, MH; Haus, E. Circadian rhythms and clinical medicine with applications to hypertension. *Am J Hypertens*, 2001, 14,280S-290S
[27] Wever, RA. The Circadian System of Man. Results of Experiments Under Temporal Isolation, New York, Springer-Verlag, 1979
[28] Rea, MA. Photic entrainment of circadian rhythms in rodents. *Chronobiol Int*, 1998, 15, 395– 424
[29] Hastings, MH; Duffield, GE; Smith, JD; et al. Entrainment of the circadian system of mammals by nonphotic cues. *Chronobiol Int*, 1998, 15, 425– 445
[30] Reinberg, A. Chronobiological field studies of oil refinery shift workers. *Chronobiologia*,1979,6, 1–119
[31] Arendt, J; Deacon, S.Treatment of circadian rhythm disorders—melatonin. *Chronobiol Int*, 1987,14, 185–204
[32] Ashkenazi, IE; Reinberg, AE; Motohashi, Y. Interindividual differences in the flexibility of human temporal organization: pertinence to jet lag and shiftwork. *Chronobiol Int*, 1997, 14, 99–11
[33] Devdhawala, MG; Seth, AK. Current status of chronotherapeutic drug delivery system: An overview. *J. Chem. Pharm. Res*, 2010,2, 312-328
[34] Guo, Y-F; Stein, PK. Circadian rhythm in the cardiovascular system: chronocardiology. *Am Heart J*, 2003,145, 779-86
[35] White WB [ed]. Blood pressure monitoring in cardiovascular medicine and therapeutics, Totowa, NJ, Humana Press, Inc., 2001
[36] Elliott, WJ. Circadian variation in the timing of stroke onset. A meta-analysis. *Stroke*, 1998, 29,992-6
[37] Ludka, O; Spinar, J; Pozdísek, Z; et al. Is there circadian variation of big endothelin and NT-proBNP in patients with severe congestive heart failure? *Vnitr Lek.*, 2010,56, 488-93
[38] Verdecchia, P; Angeli, F; Gattobigio, R. Clinical usefulness of ambulatory blood pressure monitoring. *J Am SocNephrol*, 15, Suppl 1, S30–S33, 2004
[39] White, WB. Ambulatory blood-pressure monitoring in clinical practice. *N Engl J Med*, 2003,348,2377–2378
[40] Lemmer, B; Mattes, A; Bohm, M; et al. Circadian blood pressure variation in transgenic hypertensive rats. Hypertension, 1993,22,97–101
[41] Witte, K; Lemmer B. Development of inverse circadian blood pressure pattern in transgenic hypertensive TGR[mREN2]27 rats. *Chronobiol Int*, 1999,16,293–303
[42] Baltatu, O; Janssen, BJ; Bricca, G; et al. Alterations in blood pressure and heart rate variability in transgenic rats with low brain angiotensinogen. *Hypertension,* 2001, 37,408–413
[43] Baltatu, O; Silva, JAJr; Ganten, D; et al. The brain renin-angiotensin system modulates angiotensin II-induced hypertension and cardiac hypertrophy. *Hypertension,* 2000,35,409–412
[44] Bader, M; Peters, J; Baltatu, O; et al. Tissue renin-angiotensin systems: new insights from experimental animal models in hypertension research. *J Mol Med*, 2001, 9,76–102
[45] Baltatu, O; Lippoldt, A; Hansson, A; et al. Local renin-angiotensin system in the pineal gland. *Brain Res Mol Brain Res*, 1998, 54, 237–242

[46] Bell-Pedersen, D; Cassone, VM; Earnest, DJ; et al. Circadian rhythms from multiple oscillators: lessons from diverse organisms. *Nat Rev Genet*, 2005,6,544–556

[47] Campos, LA; Plehm, R; Cipolla-Neto, J; et al. Altered circadian rhythm reentrainment to light phase shifts in rats with low levels of brain angiotensinogen. *Am J Physiol Regul Integr Comp Physiol*, 2006,290,R1122–R1127

[48] Campos, LA; Couto, AS; Iliescu, R; et al. Differential regulation of central vasopressin receptors in transgenic rats with low brain angiotensinogen. *Regul Pept*, 2004,119,177–182

[49] Baltatu, O; Afeche, SC; Jose, dos, Santos, SH; et al. Locally synthesized angiotensin modulates pineal melatonin generation. *J Neurochem*, 2002, 80, 328–334

[50] Mutoh, T; Shibata, S; Korf, HW; et al. Melatonin modulates the light-induced sympathoexcitation and vagal suppression with participation of the suprachiasmatic nucleus in mice. *J Physiol*, 2003,547,317–332

[51] Briaud, SA; Zhang, BL;Sannajust, F. Continuous light exposure and sympathectomy suppress circadian rhythm of blood pressure in rats. *J Cardiovasc Pharmacol Ther*, 2004,9,97–105

[52] Minamisava, K; Tochikubo, O; Ishii, M. Systemic hemodynamics during sleep in young or middle-aged and elderly patients. *Hypertension,* 1994,23, 167-73

[53] Lurbe, A; Redon, J; Pascual, JM; et al. Altered blood pressure during sleep in normotensive subjects with type I diabetes. *Hypertension,*1993,21,227-35

[54] Liu, M; Takahashi, H; Morita, Y; et al. Non-dipping is a potent predictor of cardiovascular mortality and is associated with autonomic dysfunction in haemodialysis patients. *Nephrol Dial Transplant*, 2003,*18*,563-9

[55] Amar, J; Vernier, I; Rossignol, E; et al. Nocturnal blood pressure and 24-hour pulse pressure are potent indicators of mortality in hemodialysis patients. *Kidney Int*, 2000,57,2485-91

[56] Tonbul, Z; Altintepe, L; Sozlu, C; et al. Ambulatory blood pressure monitoring in haemodialysis and continuous peritoneal dialysis [CAPD] patients. *J Hum Hypertens*, 2002, 16,585-9

[57] Shoda, J; Nakamoto, H; Okada, H; et al. Impact of introduction of continuous peritoneal dialysis on blood presure: analysis of 24-hour ambulatory blood pressure. *Adv Perit Dial*, 2000,16,97-101

[58] Covic, A; Goldsmith, DJ. Ambulatory blood pressure measurement in renal patient. *Curr Hypertens Rep*, 2002, 4,369-76

[59] Baranowicz-Gaszczyk, I; Jóźwiak, L; Bednarek-Skublewska, A; et al. Diurnal rhythm of blood pressure, heart rate and adrenergic activity in patients with normotension treated with continuous ambulatory peritoneal dialysis and haemodialysis. *Rocz Akad Med Bialymst.*, 2005,50,252-6

[60] Halberg, F; Cornelissen, G; Katinas, G; et al. International BIOCOS Group. Chronobiology's progress: season's appreciations, 2004-2005. Time, frequency, phase, variable, individual, age- and site-specific chronomics. *J Appl Biomed*, 2006,4,1–38

[61] Otsuka, K; Cornélissen, G; Halberg, F; et al. Excessive circadian amplitude of blood pressure increases risk of ischaemic stroke and nephropathy. *J Med Eng Technol*, 1997, 21,23–30

[62] Gupta, AK; Greenway, FL; Cornelissen, G; Pan, W; Halberg, F. Prediabetes is associated with abnormal circadian blood pressure variability. *J Hum Hypertens*, 2008,22,627-33

[63] Portaluppi, F; Smolensky, MH. Time-dependent structure and control of arterial blood pressure. *Ann NY Acad Sci*, 1996,783, 1–342

[64] Baumgart, P. Circadian rhythm of blood pressure: internal and external time triggers. *ChronobiolInt*, 1991,8,444-50

[65] Portaluppi, F; Montanari, L; Ferini, M; et al. Altered circadian rhythms of blood pressure and heart rate in non-hemodialysis chronic renal failure. *Chronobiol Int*, 1990,7, 321–327

[66] Portaluppi, F; Smolensky, MH. Circadian rhythm and environmental determinants of blood pressure regulation in normal and hypertensive conditions, in White WB [ed]: Blood pressure monitoring in cardiovascular medicine and therapeutics, Totowa, NJ, Humana Press, 2001, 79–138

[67] Pickering, TG.Ambulatory Monitoring and Blood Pressure Variability, London, Science Press, 1991

[68] Carrington, M; Walsh, M; Stambas, T; et al. The influence of sleep onset on the diurnal variation in cardiac activity and cardiac control. *J Sleep Res*, 2003,12, 213-21

[69] Iellamo, F; Placidi, F; Marciani, MG; et al. Baroreflex buffering of sympathetic activation during sleep: evidence from autonomic assessment of sleep macroarchitecture and microarchitecture. *Hypertension,* 2004,43, 814-9

[70] Lip, GY; Tan, EK; Lau, CK; et al. Diurnal variation in stroke onset in atrial fibrillation. *Stroke*, 2001, 32,1443-8

[71] Zhang, XW; Tan, ZJ; Li, YL; et al. A study on yearly and daily circadian rhythm of cardiovascular events. *Zhonghua Nei Ke Za Zhi*, 2009,48,818-20

[72] Pérez-Lloret, S; Toblli, JE; Cardinali, DP; et al. Gender differences in age-related increase of asleep blood pressure. *Arch Gerontol Geriatr.*, 2010,50, 319-22

[73] Sinha, P; Taneja, DK; Singh, NP; et al. Seasonal variation in prevalence of hypertension: Implications for interpretation. *Indian J Public Health.*, 2010,54,7-10

[74] Iwabu, A; Konishi, K; Tokutake, H; et al. Inverse correlation between seasonal changes in home blood pressure and atmospheric temperature in treated-hypertensive patients. *Clin Exp Hypertens.*, 2010,32,221-6

[75] Verdon, F; Boudry, JF; Chuat, M; et al. Seasonal blood pressure variations in hypertensive patients. *Schweiz Med Wochenschr.*, 1993, 123, 2363-2369

[76] Arntz, HR; Muller-Nordhorn, J; Willich SN. Cold Monday mornings prove dangerous: epidemiology of sudden cardiac death. *Curr Opin Crit Care*, 2001, 7, 139–144

[77] vanRossum, CT; Shipley, MJ; Hemingway, H; et al. Seasonal variation in cause-specific mortality: are there high-risk groups? 25-year follow-up of civil servants from the first Whitehall study. *Int J Epidemiol*, 2001, 30, 1109–1116

[78] Boulay, F; Berthier, F; Sisteron, O; et al. Seasonal variation in chronic heart failure hospitalizations and mortality in France. *Circulation*, 1999,100, 280–286

[79] Goodwin, J; Pearce, VR; Taylor, RS; et al. Seasonal cold and circadian changes in blood pressure and physical activity in young and elderly people. *Age Ageing*, 2001, 30, 311–317

[80] Kristal-Boneh, E; Harari, G; Green, MS; et al. Body mass index is associated with differential seasonal change in ambulatory blood pressure levels. *American Journal of Hypertension,* 1996,9,1179-1185

[81] Kristal-Boneh, E; Harari, G; Green, MS; et al. Summer–winter variation in 24 h ambulatory blood pressure. *Blood Press Monit*, 1996,1, 87–94

[82] Minami, J; Ishimitsu, T; Kawano, Y; et al. Seasonal variations in office and home blood pressures in hypertensive patients treated with antihypertensive drugs. *Blood Press Monit*, 1998, 3, 101–106

[83] Sega, R; Trocino, G; Lanzarotti, A; et al. Alterations of cardiac structure in patients with isolated office, ambulatory, or home hypertension. Data from the general population (Pressione Arteriose Monitorate E Loro Associazioni [PAMELA] Study). *Circulation*, 2001, 104, 1385-92

[84] Minami, J; Kawano, Y; Ishimitsu, T; et al. Seasonal variations in office, home and 24 h ambulatory blood pressure in patients with essential hypertension. *J Hypertens*, 1996: 14, 1421–1425

[85] Fujiwara, T; Kawamura, M; Nakajima, J; et al. Seasonal differences in diurnal blood pressure of hypertensive patients living in a stable environmental temperature. *J Hypertens*, 1995,13, 1747–1752

[86] Modesti, PA; Morabito, M; Bertolozzi, I; et al. Weather-related changes in 24-hour blood pressure profile: effects of age and implications for hypertension management.*Hypertension,* 2006,47, 155–161

[87] Takenaka, T; Kojima, E; Sueyoshi, K; et al. Seasonal variations of daily changes in blood pressure among hypertensive patients with end-stage renal diseases. *Clin Exp Hypertens*., 2010,32,227-33

[88] Hozawa, A; Kuriyama, S; Shimazu, T; et al. Seasonal Variation in Home Blood Pressure Measurements and Relation to Outside Temperature in Japan. *Clin Exp Hypertens*., 2011,33,153-8

[89] Imai, Y; Munakata, M; Tsuji, I; et al. Seasonal variation in blood pressure in normotensive women studied by home measurements. *Clin Sci (Lond)*., 1996,90, 55-60

[90] Hata, T; Ogihara, T; Maruyama, A; et al. The seasonal variation of blood pressure in patients with essential hypertension. *Clin Exp Hypertens A*., 1982,4, 341-354

[91] Sega, R; Cesana, G; Bombelli, M; et al. Seasonal variations in home and ambulatory blood pressure in the PAMELA population. PressioneArterioseMonitorate e Loro Associazioni. *J Hypertens*., 1998, 16, 1585–1592

[92] Chambers, JB; Williams, TD; Nakamura, A; et al. Cardiovascular and metabolic responses of hypertensive and normotensive rats to one week of cold exposure. *Am J Physiol Regul Integr Comp Physiol*, 2000,279, R1486–R1494

[93] Wilks DS. Time series: harmonic analysis. In: Wilks DS, editor. Statistical methods in the atmospheric sciences: an introduction. London: AcademicPress Ltd., 1995. 333–337

[94] Burroughs, WJ. Instrumental records: Shorter term cycles. In: Burroughs WJ, editor. Weather cycles: real or imaginary?.Cambridge: Cambridge UniversityPress, 1992. 58–59

[95] Jansen, PM; Leineweber, MJ; Thien T. The effect of a change in ambient temperature on blood pressure in normotensives. *J Hum Hypertens*, 2001, 15, 113-117

[96] Argani, H; Javanshir, MR. Seasonal variations of blood pressure in hemodialysis and renal transplant recipients. *Transplant Proc*, 2004,36, 148–149

[97] Tozawa, M; Iseki, K; Iseki, C; et al. Seasonal blood pressure and body weight variation in patients on chronic hemodialysis. *Am J Nephrol*, 1999,19, 660–667

[98] Jehn, M; Appel, LJ; Sacks, FM; et al. The effect of ambient temperature and barometric pressure on ambulatory blood pressure variability. *Am J Hypertens*, 2002, 15, 941–945

[99] Bretzl, H. BotanischeForschungen des Alexanderzuges. B.G. Teubner, *Leipzig*, 1903, 120-132

[100] Bretzl, H. BotanischeForschungen des Alexanderzuges. Leipzig: Teubner. Ed.: Galeni De SantitateTuenda. Leipzig, Verlag, Von BG Teubner, 1903

[101] De, MairanJJO. ObservationBotanique. Histoire de l'AcademieRoyale des Sciences, Paris, 1729,35-36

[102] Linnaeus, C. Systemanaturae per regna trianaturae:secundum classes, ordines, genera, species, cum characteribus, differentiis, synonymis, locis. 10th edition. Ed.: HolmiaeLaurentiiSalvii. 1758. 873 pages.

[103] Patrick, GTW; Gilbert, JA. Studies from the Psychological Laboratory of the University of Iowa. Ontheeffects of loss of sleep. *Psychological Review*, 1896,3,469-483

[104] Szymanski, JS. Versucheüber die Wirkung der Faktoren, die alsAntriebzum ErlerneneinerHandlungdienenkönnen. *Pflügers Archivfür die Gesamte Physiologie des Menschen und der Tiere*, 1918,171,374-385

[105] Vitaterna, MH; King, DP; Chang, AM; et al. Mutagenesis and mapping of a mouse gene, Clock, essential for circadian behavior. *Science*, 1994,264,719–725

[106] Fell J, Röschke J, Beckmann P. Deterministic chaos and the first positive Lyapunov exponent: a nonlinear analysis of the human electroencephalogram during sleep. *Biol Cybern*. 1993;69:139-46

[107] Sharma VK. Deterministic chaos and fractal complexity in the dynamics of cardiovascular behavior: perspectives on a new frontier. *Open Cardiovasc Med J*. 2009; 3:110-23

[108] Bob P. Chaos, brain and divided consciousness. *Acta Univ Carol Med Monogr*. 2007; 153: 9-80

[109] Korn H, Faure P. Is there chaos in the brain? II. Experimental evidence and related models. *C R Biol*. 2003; 326:787-840

[110] Wang X, Meng J, Tan G et al. Research on the relation of EEG signal chaos characteristics with high-level intelligence activity of human brain. *Nonlinear Biomed Phys*. 2010;4:2

[111] Pezard L, Nandrino JL. Dynamic paradigm in psychopathology: "chaos theory", from physics to psychiatry. *Encephale*. 2001;27:260-8

[112] Wagner CD, Nafz B, Persson PB. Chaos in blood pressure control. *Cardiovasc Res*. 1996; 31:380-7

[113] Perkiömäki JS, Mäkikallio TH, Huikuri HV. Fractal and complexity measures of heart rate variability. *Clin Exp Hypertens*. 2005; 27:149-58

[114] Huikuri HV, Perkiömäki JS, Maestri R et al. Clinical impact of evaluation of cardiovascular control by novel methods of heart rate dynamics. *Philos Transact A Math Phys Eng Sci*. 2009; 367:1223-38

[115] Kyriazis M. Practical applications of chaos theory to the modulation of human ageing: nature prefers chaos to regularity. *Biogerontology*. 2003; 4:75–90

[116] González JJ, Pereda E. Applications of fractal and non-linear time series analysis to the study of short-term cardiovascular control. *Curr Vasc Pharmacol.* 2004: 149-62

[117] Mäkikallio TH, Huikuri HV, Mäkikallio A, Sourander LB, Mitrani RD, Castellanos A, Myerburg RJ. Prediction of sudden cardiac death by fractal analysis of heart rate variability in elderly subjects. *J Am Coll Cardiol.* 2001; 37: 1395-402

[118] Huikuri HV, Mäkikallio TH. Heart rate variability in ischemic heart disease. *Auton Neurosci.* 2001; 90: 95-101

[119] Cugini P, De Rosa R, Coda S et al. Determination of the "presumptive risk" of hypertensive crisis with fractal interpolation of 24-hour arterial pressure. II: study with secondary hypertensive patients. *Clin Ter.* 2001; 152:165-9 [a]

[120] Cugini P, De Rosa R, Coda S et al. Identification of "presumptive risk" of hypertension crises with fractal interpolation of the 24-hour arterial pressure. III: study of normotensive subjects. *Clin Ter.* 2001; 152:225-9 [b]

[121] Cugini P, De Rosa R, Coda S et al. Individualization of the "presumptive risk" of hypertensive crisis using fractals interpolation of the 24-hour arterial pressure. Study of patients with essential hypertension. *Clin Ter.* 2001; 152:95-9 [c]

[122] Kalantzi LE, Karavas E, Koutris EX et al. Recent advances in oral pulsatile drug delivery. *Recent Pat Drug Deliv Formul.* 2009; 3:49-63

[123] Smith DH, Neutel JM, Weber MA. A new chronotherapeutic oral drug absorption system for verapamil optimizes blood pressure control in the morning. *Am J Hypertens.* 2001; 14:14-9

[124] White WB, Sica DA, Calhoun D et al. Preventing increases in early-morning blood pressure, heart rate, and the rate-pressure product with controlled onset extended release verapamil at bedtime versus enalapril, losartan, and placebo on arising. *Am Heart J.* 2002; 144:657-65

[125] Prisant LM, Black HR, Messerli F et al. Chrono: a community-based hypertension trial of a chronotherapeutic formulation of verapamil. *Am J Ther.* 2002; 9:476-83

[126] White WB, Lacourciere Y, Gana T et al. Effects of graded-release diltiazem versus ramipril, dosed at bedtime, on early morning blood pressure, heart rate, and the rate-pressure product. *Am Heart J.* 2004; 148:628-34

[127] Milei J, Schere D, Heguilen R et al. Trough to peak ratio with Diltiazem (300 mg sustained-release hydrophilic matrix tablet). Short and long-term treatment. *Intercont Cardiol* 2002; 11:69-72

[128] Hermida RC. Ambulatory blood pressure monitoring in the prediction of cardiovascular events and effects of chronotherapy: rationale and design of the MAPEC study. *Chronobiol Int.* 2007; 24: 749-75

[129] Pikkujämsä SM, Mäkikallio TH, Airaksinen KE, Huikuri HV. Determinants and interindividual variation of R-R interval dynamics in healthy middle-aged subjects. *Am J Physiol Heart Circ Physiol.* 2001; 280: H1400-6

[130] Mäkikallio TH, Huikuri HV, Hintze U, Videbaek J, Mitrani RD, Castellanos A, Myerburg RJ, Møller M; DIAMOND Study Group (Danish Investigations of Arrhythmia and Mortality ON Dofetilide). Fractal analysis and time- and frequency-domain measures of heart rate variability as predictors of mortality in patients with heart failure. *Am J Cardiol.* 2001; 87:178-82

[131] Delyukov A, Gorgo Y, Cornélissen G, Otsuka K, Halberg F. Infradian, notably circaseptan testable feedsidewards among chronomes of the ECG and air temperature and pressure. *Biomed Pharmacother*. 2001; 55:84s-92s

[132] Delyukov A, Gorgo Y, Cornélissen G, Otsuka K, Halberg F. Natural environmental associations in a 50-day human electrocardiogram. Int J Biometeorol. 2001; 45:90-9.

[133] Kyriazis M. Practical applications of chaos theory to the modulation of human ageing: nature prefers chaos to regularity. *Biogerontology*. 2003; 4:75-90

[134] Cugini P. From Chronos to Chaos: from the determinism of circadian rhythm of arterial pressure to the undeterminism of hypertensive crises. *Recenti Prog Med*. 1998; 89:188-99

[135] Cugini P, De Rosa R, Pellegrino AM, De Laurentis T, Fontana S, Petrangeli CM, Leone G, Cellitti R, Marsili D, Scardia C, Menghetti E, Tamura K. Age-related trend for blood pressure circadian rhythm in normotensive healthy subjects: estimates provided by the clinospectror method. *Clin Ter*. 2000; 151:405-10

[136] Cugini P, De Rosa R, De Laurentis T, Tamura K. Age-related trend in circadian rhythm of electrocardiographic sinusal R-R intervals in clinically healthy subjects. *Clin Ter*. 2002; 153:93-7

In: Recent Advances in Cardiology
Editors: José Milei and Giuseppe Ambrosio
ISBN: 978-1-63117-282-3

Chapter 10

Fetal, Pediatric Cardiology and Adult Congenital Heart Disease: Insights in the New Millennium

Paolo Guccione[1], Maddalena Milioni[2] and Stefania Troiani[2]
[1]Staff Member. Department of Pediatric Cardiology and Cardiac Surgery, Bambino Gesù Children's Hospital, Roma
[2]Unità di Terapia Intensiva Neonatale Pediatria (UTIN), Cardiologia Pediatrica Ospedale "S. Maria della Misericordia," Perugia, Italy

Abstract

Over the last few decades, Paediatric Cardiology has made enormous progress. This has resulted in earlier and more accurate diagnosis, with consequent improvement of patients' quality of life (Qol), from birth into adult life.

This chapter reviews some major advances in the assessment and diagnosis of fetal and paediatric heart disease. We will also discuss clinical and management issues of a specific population of patients called "GUCH", i.e., Grown-Up with Congenital Heart disease, namely adults with congenital heart disease (CHD) who have become a fast growing group, as a consequence of the advances in cardiac surgery and intensive care in the 1970s and 80s, which have allowed a larger number of children with CHD to survive into adulthood.

Introduction

Congenital heart diseases (CHD) are the most common among severe congenital abnormalities found in live births varying between 4 and 10 per 1000 live births [1]. A rise in incidence of CHD has been observed; this is likely a multifactorial phenomenon: a true rise in the number of newborns with CHD may be due to changing birth prevalence rates related to increasing maternal age, or exposure to medications during the first trimester of pregnancy.

At the same time, though, the substantial improvement in detection of CHD secondary to the introduction of cardiac ultrasound in the 1980s may have contributed to this finding.

Improvements in surgical techniques have also occurred, and this greater survival to adulthood has resulted in a shift in mortality beyond 18 years of age.

Finally, the increased ability to diagnose congenital heart disease *before* birth, during pregnancy, has allowed to treat certain conditions during fetal life (e.g., fetal treatment of arrhythmias, valvuloplasty), and most importantly to plan delivery in referral centers staffed by highly trained specialists and linked to neonatal intensive care units.

Insights into Fetal Cardiology

(Troiani S, Milioni M)

Prenatal diagnosis of CHD is one of the most important achievements of modern Paediatric Cardiology, as it has resulted in substantial reduction of perinatal mortality and optimization of obstetric and neonatal care. In the last few years the close collaboration between obstetricians and paediatric cardiologists has resulted in a better knowledge of anatomy and pathophysiology of fetal heart; at the same time, advances in echocardiographic technologies have allowed a comprehensive evaluation of fetal cardiovascular system encompassing both structural and functional assessment.

Finally, the continuous development of echocardiographic techniques has made possible to perform pharmacological and surgical cardiac interventions during fetal life, which can improve survival when a fetus is at high risk for prenatal or neonatal death.

Table 1. Fetal and maternal risk factors for congenital heart disease

Fetal factors	Increased nuchal translucency Suspected cardiac abnormalities at obstetrical ultrasound check Oligohydramnios or Polyhydramnios Hydrops Extracardiac abnormalities Abnormal fetal karyotype Fetal cardiac arrhythmias non-specific ultrasound diagnostic markers – e.g. echogenic cardiac foci, intrauterine growth restriction
Maternal factors	Family history/of Maternal CHD (Congenital heart disease) Diabetes mellitus Autoimmune antibodies (Anti-RO SSA, Anti-La SSB) Drugs and teratogens– e.g. Phenytoin, Carbamazepine, Lithium carbonate, Valproic acid

Fetal Echocardiography

At least half of all CHD should be detectable before birth because of their serious nature. However, if examination of the fetal heart is limited to traditional high risk groups, only about

10-20% of babies born with congenital heart disease will be identified [Table 1]. In this respect, an essential contribution in detecting fetal cardiac defects came with the widespread introduction of four-chamber view screening during the routine mid-trimester echocardiographic scan [2].

The most common indications for performing a fetal echocardiogram are maternal factors, especially a family history history of CHD, a maternal history of metabolic disease (diabetes mellitus, phenylchetonuria), maternal infections (Parvovirus, Rubella, Coxsackie), and maternal exposure to teratogens.

Several studies have also demonstrated that the first-trimester screening for aneuploidies by measurement of fetal nuchal translucency (NT) can identify another important high-risk group [3]. Other obvious indications are fetal extracardiac anomalies, fetal arrhythmias, and abnormal fetal karyotype.

Timing

In 2006 The International Society of Ultrasound in Obstetrics and Gynecology (ISUOG) published practice guidelines for cardiac screening examination during the second trimester of pregnancy [4]. The guidelines state that a fetal cardiac examination should be optimally performed between 18 and 22 weeks' menstrual age, even though some abnormalities can be identified during the late first and early second trimesters of pregnancy, particularly when increased nuchal translucency is detected.

Imaging Techniques

Fetal heart abnormalities can be evaluated using several imaging modalities [Table 2], although the examination should be tailored for specific cardiac alterations.

Table 2. Echocardiographic techniques for evaluation of fetal heart

Echocardiographic methods	Specific findings
Two-Dimensional (2-D) ultrasonography	Anatomic features (laterality, situs, ,cardiac connections, other abnormalities)
M-mode	Cardiac rhythm, mobile structures (e.g., valves), shortening fraction, long-axis evaluation
M-mode or Doppler	Cardiac function
Conventional Doppler	Fetal cardiac function parameters (E/A ratio, outflow tracts, myocardial performance index)
Tissue Doppler ultrasonography	Fetal myocardial global performance
Speckle Tracking ultrasonography	Fetal myocardial global performance
3-D and 4-D ultrasonography	High definition anatomical features and myocardial global performance

Two Dimensional Echocardiography

A complete two-dimensional (2-D) fetal echocardiography examination should evaluate: the main anatomical structures, such as cardiac axis and situs, atrial and ventricular morphology, interventicular and atrial septa, foramen ovale, the possible presence of pericardial effusions, venous-atrial, atrioventricular and ventriculo-arterial connections of the heart, size and relationship of left and right ventricular outflow tracts, and finally the atrioventricular and semilunar valves.

The basic cardiac screening examination generally starts with a four-chamber view of the fetal heart. In experienced hands, up to 60% of CHD can be diagnosed with this simple and easy technique when performed with careful standardization. However, several studies have demonstrated that a four-chamber view has certain limitations in detecting anomalies involving the ventricular outflow tracts and/or the great arteries [5]. In order to reduce false-negative rates, the ISUOG consensus statement published in 2008 suggested to introduce also arterial outflow tracts scanning, three vessels and trachea view, and an assessment of pulmonary venous return [6].

Motion Mode or M-Mode and Conventional Doppler

M-mode ultrasonography is applied to the evaluation of the motion of cardiac structures, specifically focused on the septa, free walls and valves. The most important application of M-mode is the assessment of fetal rhythm in order to detect fetal arrhythmias such as supraventricular tachycardia, atrial flutter and fetal heart block.

Conventional Doppler evaluation is useful for functional assessment of fetal heart and it might provide important information on the hemodynamics and cardiovascular adaptation to different perinatal complications. Cardiologists have 3 conventional pulsed-Doppler parameters available to estimate fetal cardiac function: the E/A waveforms, the outflow tracts flow, and the myocardial performance index (MPI). The E/A ratio represents the relationship between the maximum velocities of the E and A waveforms of ventricular filling, and therefore it partially reflects cardiac preload, whereas the outflow tracts reflect the cardiac after load, and both are usually evaluated together. The MPI is considered a marker of global cardiac function and it can be calculated either by estimating the total isovolumetric time (TIV) over the ET (ejection time), or by estimating the individual isovolumetric contraction (ICT) and relaxation (IRT) times over the ET.

Tissue Doppler and Speckle Tracking Techniques

Tissue Doppler Imaging (TDI) represents a more sensitive tool than standard methods to detect the presence of cardiac dysfunction. The use of C-TDI has some limitations in fetal life, due to the fetal position, fetal movements, and a high frame rate. Despite these limitations, due to its higher sensitivity, TDI is indeed a useful method to detect cardiac dysfunction alone or in combination with conventional Doppler. "Speckle tracking" is a non-Doppler ultrasound method using offline analysis of standard four-chamber and short axis views of the heart. This angle-independent method can measure both myocardial strain and strain rate, and it has the potential to assess detailed components of myocardial function, such as torsion and twist. Strain is a measure of tissue deformation in response to an applied force and may be described as a percentage of the original dimension, whereas strain rate represents the speed of deformation. This ultrasound technique offers the unique possibility of performing complex measurements of myocardial function offline, on routinely obtained echocardiographic images, and it is being developed as a useful clinical tool to study the consequences of congenital heart disease on myocardial function.

3D - 4D Ultrasound Method

Three-dimensional (3D) and four-dimensional (4D) applications in fetal ultrasound scanning have made impressive strides in the past two decades. Recent technological developments of motion-gated cardiac scanning allow almost real-time 3D/4D examination of the heart. Examining the fetal heart in motion is an important component of assessing cardiac structure and function. When displaying 3D information as moving images, the principal options are 3D cine-looping and 4D real-time imaging. The feasibility and reproducibility of these imaging technologies for 3D/4D fetal echocardiography has been demonstrated. Future research will clarify how these techniques are best utilized for fetal cardiac screening programs and for detailed evaluation of congenital cardiac disease. Among the most attractive aspects of 3D/4D scanning is the potential for digital archiving and sharing of examination data over a network.

Fetal Cardiac Intervention

Improved knowledge of the pathophysiology of CHD and of fetal echocardiography, with better understanding of the natural history of cardiovascular diseases, prompted in the last decades the possibility to develop strategies to prevent or correct the evolution of secondary disease before birth.

The primary aim of any form of fetal cardiac intervention (FCI) is to favorably modify the pathophysiology of an abnormal developing heart, so that to improve fetal and postnatal outcomes without risks to the maternal health. Since the first pharmacological intervention in 1975 of propranolol administration to the mother of a fetus with ventricular tachycardia [7], fetal echocardiography has acquired great importance in monitoring abnormalities and cardiac function both before and after intervention.

To minimize the risk for the mother and (with respect to surgical interventions) the risk of abortion, most of these interventions are usually performed during second and third trimester. Nowadays, pharmacological FCI is commonly used to treat fetal tachyarrhythmias, bradycardia, and fetal hydrops.

Closed fetal cardiac surgery was first performed in 1989 with a percutaneous balloon aortic valvuloplastic [8], and since then it has been performed to treat hypoplastic left heart syndrome and pulmonary atresia. Open fetal cardiac surgery has developed later, together with the study of extracorporeal circulatory bypass, as it is necessary for such a surgery (see below).

Pharmacological Fetal Cardiac Intervention

Persistence of fetal tachyarrhythmias or bradyarrhythmias may lead to heart failure and intrauterine death. Nowadays, fetal supraventricular tachyarrhythmias are classified as long and short V-A (ventricular-atrial, corresponding with electrophysiological long and short R-P) tachycardias, atrial flutter, or junctional ectopic tachycardia.

The most common fetal tachyarrhythmia is fetal supraventricular tachycardia, most often secondary to atrioventricular (AV) reentry or atrial flutter.

Ventricular tachycardia, which accounts only for 1-2% of all fetal tachyarrhythmias may occur isolated or in association with long QT syndrome, fetal cardiomyopathy, or cardiac tumors, and is typically suspected when there is a fast ventricular rate and a slower atrial rate with V-A dissociation.

As far as treatment of fetal supraventricular tachycardia is concerned, over the years many antiarrhythmic agents have been used; even though digoxin has still a role, other agents have been introduced more recently, including sotalol, amiodarone, and flecainide.

Transplacental therapy is usually effective in nonhydropic fetuses, but its outcomes remain suboptimal, with an overall fetal death rate of 10% of cases and an even higher percentage in fetuses with hydrops [9-10].

Indications for therapy may depend on fetal age and disease severity. When hydrops is present, pharmacological FCI may help to support delivery and postnatal treatment. In preterm fetuses, sustained tachycardia should probably be treated regardless of cardiac dysfunction or hydrops, because these sequelae can develop rapidly. As for intermittent tachycardia, treatment is generally not necessary, unless hydrops or cardiac dysfunction is evident. Transplacental delivery of certain drugs is impaired in the setting of hydrops, and supraventricular tachycardia may be refractory for other reasons as well. In such circumstances, intravascular administration and/or oral agents with better placental uptake kinetics may be indicated.

Direct administration, usually by percutaneous umbilical venous injection, carries the risks of cordocentesis and it is usually reserved for severe refractory cases. Fetal bradycardia may be caused by sinus node dysfunction, long-QT syndrome, AV block, or fetal distress with acidosis.

The most common fetal bradyarrhythmia and the primary indication for FCI is high-grade AV block. The potential consequences of fetal AV block are cardiomyopathy and hydrops. In the fetus, AV block generally occurs in association with either maternal autoimmune disease, or malformation syndromes such as heterotaxy or L-loop transposition of the great arteries. Autoimmune fetal AV block can be treated with maternal administration of dexamethasone and/or sympathomimetic agents. Although transplacental dexamethasone may prevent the progression of first-degree block to second- or third-degree block, several recent multicenter studies found that it does not reverse high-grade block and it is associated with higher risk of premature birth and growth restriction [11-12].

Sympathomimetic agents may increase heart rate in fetuses with bradycardia due to AV block or sinus node dysfunction, but they do not restore AV synchrony. We should finally consider that while pharmacological fetal cardiac interventions are well established in the management of fetal arrhythmias and heart block, there is definitely room for further improvement.

Surgical Fetal Cardiac Intervention

"Closed fetal cardiac interventions" consist primarily of percutaneous interventions in which a needle is used to gain uterine and fetal access without opening the uterus. Typically, this intervention is performed using a percutaneous ultrasound-guided approach under maternal anesthesia; in a minority of cases, laparotomy without hysterotomy is used to facilitate fetal access. The most common closed FCI procedure is aortic valvuloplasty and the primary indication for fetal aortic valvuloplasty is to modify the *in utero* natural history of midgestation fetal aortic stenosis (AS), which may evolve into hypoplastic left heart syndrome (HLHS).

HLHS is a rare congenital heart defect in which the left ventricle of the heart is severely underdeveloped. Some patients with HLHS are diagnosed during the second trimester with valvular AS and a normal-sized or dilated left ventricle (LV), evolving to HLHS over the course of gestation. The purpose of fetal aortic valvuloplasty is to decrease LV afterload and promote flow through the left heart, in order to prevent progressive left heart dysfunction and hypoplasia over the subsequent course of gestation and, in the process, prevent evolution to HLHS [13].

Approximately 5–19% of HLHS cases have also an intact or highly restrictive atrial septum that prevents oxygenated pulmonary venous blood from reaching the aorta, resulting in left atrium hypertension with pulmonary venous congestion [14]. Fetal left atrium hypertension may cause lung injury resulting in edema, lymphangiectasia, muscularized pulmonary veins and elevated pulmonary vascular resistance. A fetal intervention aimed at decompressing the fetal left atrium by balloon atrial septoplasty/septostomy (BAS), or laser atrial septotomy and stenting, may prevent the perinatal hypoxemia and acidosis generally associated with HLHS with intact or highly restrictive atrial septum. If left atrial decompression is achieved in early gestation, adverse pulmonary venous remodelling may also be prevented.

Another indication for surgical cardiac interventions is pulmonary atresia with evolving hypoplastic right heart: a fetal pulmonary valvuloplasty may in fact promote right heart growth and functional development increasing the chance of a biventricular circulation after birth.

However, although technical success is possible for fetal aortic and pulmonary valvulopasty and atrial septoplasty, we are far from routine application of these techniques. Looking forward, continuous advances in the understanding of natural history, patient selection for intervention, and myocardial response to invasive fetal interventions will undoubtedly lead to refinement of the procedures.

Insights into Pediatric Cardiology

In this chapter we focus on pulmonary hypertension and hybrid cardiac surgery, two of the most innovative fields of pediatric cardiology. With respect to pulmonary hypertension, in the last decade insights into pharmakocinetics and pharmacodinamics have lead to development of several new molecules, which have been added to previous and well known drugs used to treat pulmonary hypertension in children and newborns. At the same time, new surgical techniques have been developed in order to minimize the risk for newborns and small children using less invasive approaches to heart defect correction, with better outcomes in terms of survival rate and quality of life.

Pulmonary Hypertension

(Milioni M, Troiani S)

Pulmonary hypertension (PH) is defined as a mean pulmonary artery pressure (PAP) of ≥25 mmHg at rest. Several well-known pathological conditions may cause pulmonary hypertension in neonates and children, but adequate knowledge of the pathophysiological mechanisms for most forms of PH is still lacking. From a hemodynamic standpoint, the morbidity and mortality associated with PH are related to increased right-ventricular after load. Over time, compensatory mechanisms tend to fail, leading to right-heart failure and death. The most recent classification of PH was presented by an international group of experts during the 4th World Symposium on PH held in 2008 in Dana Point, California [Table 3], and published in 2009 by Simonneau G et al. [15].

In the neonatal population, persistent pulmonary hypertension of the newborn (PPHN) is one of the most frequent and critical disease due to increased pulmonary blood pressure. The incidence of PPHN is approximately 2 per 1,000 live births [16].

PPHN can be a primary disorder of the fetal pulmonary circulation, or it can be secondary to pathologic processes that impair transition from fetal to neonatal circulation, such as meconium aspiration or surfactant deficiency, or abnormalities of lung development, such as congenital diaphragmatic hernia.

There can be antenatal, perinatal, and postnatal risk factors associated with PPNH: together with lung and heart structural disease, such as pulmonary hypoplasia and congenital heart defects, and pulmonary parenchimal disease, such as pneumonia and meconium aspiration, perinatal risk conditions as asphyxia, fetal distress, placenta abruption and intrauterine growth restriction are associated with an increased incidence of PPHN.

The pathophysiology of PH is multifactorial, complex, and still not completely understood. In 2011, Fineman published an inclusive review of PH etiology, clinical manifestations, pathophysiological principles, and current and future therapies [17].

Over the past three decades, several research groups has discovered many different particular mechanisms of PH: increased *pulmonary vascular resistance* (PVR) and decreased compliance in *pulmonary arterial hypertension* (PAH) related to increased pulmonary vascular reactivity; sustained pulmonary vasoconstriction; vascular remodeling; and luminal obstruction due to in situ thrombosis and/or obstructive neointimal and plexiform lesions.

It is now appreciated that increased pulmonary vasoconstriction in PH is mainly mediated by altered endothelial function, where endogenous vasodilators, such as *nitric oxide* and *prostacyclin* (PGI2), are decreased while endogenous vasoconstrictors, such as *ET-1 and serotonin* (5-HT), are increased. Accordingly the majority of approved and emerging PH therapies are targeted to modulating endothelial-derived factors and/or their signal pathways.

Table 3. The most recent classification of PH presented by an international group of experts during the 4th World Symposium on PH held in 2008 in Dana Point, California

1. Pulmonary arterial hypertension (PAH)	1.1. Idiopathic PAH 1.2. Heritable 1.2.1. Bone morphogenetic protein receptor type 2(BMPR28) 1.2.2. Activin receptor-like kinase type 1(ALK1), endoglin (with or without hereditary hemorrhagic telangiectasia) 1.2.3. Unknown 1.3. Drug- and toxin-induced 1.4. Associated with 1.4.1. Connective tissue diseases 1.4.2. HIV infection (human immunodeficiency virus) 1.4.3. Portal hypertension 1.4.4. Congenital heart diseases 1.4.5. Schistosomiasis 1.4.6. Chronic hemolytic anemia 1.5 Persistent pulmonary hypertension of the newborn (PPNH)
1'. Pulmonary veno-occlusive disease (PVOD) and/or pulmonary capillary hemangiomatosis (PCH)	
2. Pulmonary hypertension owing to left heart disease	2.1. Systolic dysfunction 2.2. Diastolic dysfunction 2.3. Valvular disease
3. Pulmonary hypertension owing to lung diseases and/or hypoxia	3.1. Chronic obstructive pulmonary disease 3.2. Interstitial lung disease 3.3. Other pulmonary diseases with mixed restrictive and obstructive pattern 3.4. Sleep-disordered breathing 3.5. Alveolar hypoventilation disorders 3.6. Chronic exposure to high altitude 3.7. Developmental abnormalities
4. Chronic thromboembolic pulmonary hypertension (CTEPH)	
5. Pulmonary hypertension with unclear multifactorial mechanisms	5.1. Hematologic disorders: myeloproliferative disorders, splenectomy 5.2. Systemic disorders: sarcoidosis, pulmonary Langerhans cell histiocytosis:lymphangioleiomyomatosis, neurofibromatosis, vasculitis 5.3. Metabolic disorders: glycogen storage disease, Gaucher disease, thyroid disorders 5.4. Others: tumoral obstruction, fibrosing mediastinitis, chronic renal failure on dialysis

The most widely used PH therapies alter one of the three main endothelial signal transmission cascades: *nitric oxide/cyclic guanosine monophosphate* (NO-cGMP), *prostaglandin I2, and endothelin-1.*

INO (*inhaled nitric oxide*) is the best studied and most widely used agent for acute selective pulmonary vasodilation. INO is FDA-approved only for neonates with hypoxemic respiratory failure, but it is frequently used off-label to treat other forms of PH, and for diagnostic purposes.

Sildenafil is a phosphodiesterase-5 inhibitor that increases NO-cGMP signaling pathways and induces pulmonary vascular relaxation by inhibiting the degradation of cGMP. Despite limited data, the use of *sildenafil* in infants and children with PH after cardiac surgery is increasing.

L-arginine is decreased in neonates with PPHN and adults and children with PH related to various diseases. Like INO and *sildenafil*, *L-arginine* enhances the NO-cGMP cascade.

Despite the many recent advances in therapy, *prostanoids*, such as intravenous *prostaglandin I2* (epoprostenol), remain the best-proven and most effective therapy for chronic PH.

Treprostinil is another *prostaglandin I2* analog that has recently been approved for intravenous administration. There are no data available to compare the efficacy of intravenous *epoprostenol* to *treprostinil*. To achieve selective pulmonary vascular relaxation, various investigations have focused on delivering *prostanoids* through inhalation. *Iloprost* and *trepronistil* are *prostaglandin I2* analogs that are FDA-approved for inhalation.

Recent data suggest that *iloprost* reduces pulmonary vascular resistance as much as does INO, but at a lower cost. Newer drugs are aimed at inhibiting *endothelin-1* and *endothelin-A*, which are signaling pathways that, when inhibited, induce a vasodilation.

Other prospective drugs are currently being tested in patients with PH, including endothelial-based therapies that use infusions of endothelial progenitor cells, *superoxide dismutase*, *vasoactive intestinal peptide*, *adrenomedullin*, calcium-channel blockers, and anticoagulant therapies, which may show promise for patients with PH. *Statins* and several chemotherapic drugs used to treat leukemia are also now being used in patients with PH, to counteract pulmonary vascular remodeling.

Since no single drug or drug combination entirely revert symptoms of increased pulmonary vascular resistance in patients with PH, the main goal is to support the right ventricle function, by reducing right-ventricular afterload, to optimize right-ventricular blood volume, to increase right-ventricular contractility, and to maintain systemic vascular resistance with proper volume loading and inotropic support.

Atrial *septostomy* is an open or close surgical intervention for managing chronic PH, and has been advocated to decompress the right ventricle by promoting right-to-left shunting. Isolated lung transplantation, as opposed to heart-lung transplantation, is now a viable option for some children with end-staged PH.

Over the past several decades, fundamental advances in pulmonary vascular biology have been translated from research purpose into effective therapies that have improved the quality of life and prolonged survival for newborns, infants, and children with PH.

Hybrid Paediatric Cardiac Surgery

(Guccione P)

Surgical and medical treatment of congenital heart disease has made remarkable progresses over the past 60 years. Corrective surgery for many intracardiac defects began in the 1950s, with the introduction of the cardiopulmonary bypass pump; this technology allowed delicate intracardiac surgical procedures to be performed, even on small infants. Over the last two decades, complex surgical repair of congenital heart defects have been performed in ever younger and smaller infants. Currently, even low-birth-weight neonates benefit from successful complex intracardiac procedures. At the same time, less invasive catheter-based techniques evolved, so that many simple congenital cardiac lesions can now be successfully treated with intravascular trans-catheter procedures rather than through surgical interventions. This approach obviates the need of cardiopulmonary bypass with its inherent risks and, obviously, eliminates the surgical incision. Common congenital heart defect as secundum atrial septal defect and patent ductus arteriosus, and even neonatal severe pulmonary valve stenosis, can now be successfully addressed in the cardiac catheterization laboratory. Since the introduction in the clinical practice of atrial septostomy by Raskhind and Miller in 1966, the number of therapeutic transcatheter procedures performed in the cardiac catheterization laboratory has dramatically increased, reaching now 75% of all procedures performed.

Hybrid pediatric cardiac surgery is a new and emerging field that spans across different disciplines and combines skills and techniques traditionally used by pediatric cardiac surgeons and interventional pediatric cardiologists into, ideally, a single procedure.

A close collaboration between pediatric cardiologists, cardiac surgeons, and intensive care pediatricians is pivotal in the management of difficult lesions, such as tetralogy of Fallot with pulmonary atresia and other complex congenital heart defects. Until the introduction of hybrid approach, the procedures were mostly done in sequence between the cardiac catheterization laboratory and the operation room, or viceversa. Figure 1 illustrates the treatment of a patient with pulmonary atresia, ventricular septal defect and severely hypoplastic left pulmonary artery.

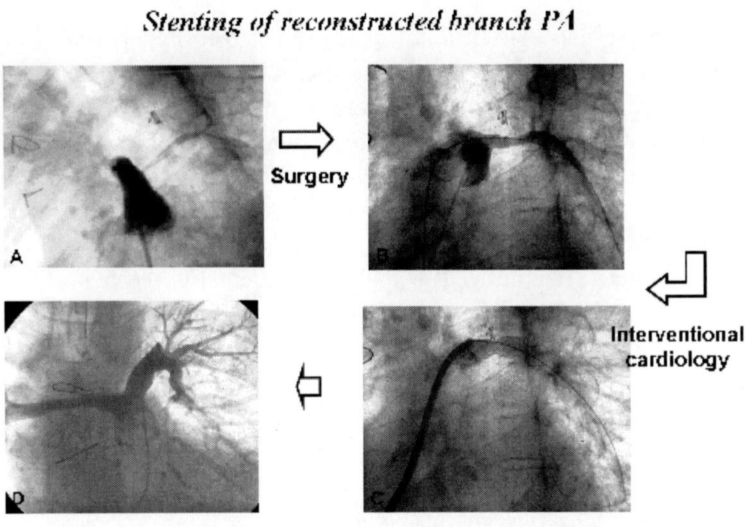

Figure 1. Staged reconstruction of the left pulmonary artery in a patient affected by pulmonary atresia and ventricular septal defect after palliative surgery. A: pulmonary angiogram with stop-flow of the right pulmonary artery. The left pulmonary artery is severely hypoplastic; B: the left pulmonary artery after surgical plastic. The increased diameter of the vessel allows subsequent transcatheter interventional procedure. C) an endovascular stent is positioned in the left pulmonary artery and subsequently dilated to a normal diameter (D).

In the sequence, first the surgeon performs the plastic of the vessel and subsequently the interventional cardiologist normalizes the dimensions of the left pulmonary artery with an endovascular stent.

The aim of hybrid pediatric cardiac surgery is to reduce the rate of therapeutic interventions in children by decreasing their numbers or their invasiveness, or to increase their effectiveness by opening new therapeutic possibilities.

The key difference with conventional surgery is the extensive use of intraoperative imaging techniques. Thus, hybrid techniques are especially useful in the following two scenarios: (1) when surgery or catheter-based interventions alone do not achieve a satisfactory result, and (2) when the combination of the two approaches results in less invasiveness and less trauma to the patient.

The evolution toward hybrid procedures goes along with the development of devices and techniques of real-time imaging, such as transesophageal echocardiography used to visualize the beating heart, as opposed to imaging an arrested flaccid heart as it occurs during extracorporeal circulation. In the end, setting up a truly hybrid operation room to perform both surgery and catheterization at the same table has become a reality.

The following hybrid procedures will be discussed:

- Hybrid Stage I Palliation for hypoplastic left heart syndrome (HLHS);
- Periventricular device closure of muscular ventricular septal defect (VSD);

Hybrid Stage I Palliation for Hypoplastic Left Heart Syndrome (HLHs)

HLHS actually represent a spectrum of disease related to hypoplasia or atresia of left-sided cardiac structures and ductus dependent systemic flow. If untreated, this lesion is usually fatal within the first weeks of life. Surgery usually involves the 3-staged Norwood procedure, which ultimately results in a 2-chamber heart in which the right ventricle functions as the systemic ventricle. Treatment has developed from the original Norwood procedure employing a systemic artery–pulmonary artery shunt [18], or right ventricle–pulmonary artery valveless conduit, as described by Sano [19].

A less-invasive alternative, utilized in high-risk patients, is the hybrid procedure [20]. The hybrid treatment of HLHS includes 3 major points: 1) placement of surgical bilateral pulmonary artery bands via a median sternotomy off cardiopulmonary bypass; 2) maintenance of ductal patency for systemic supply by deploying a stent into the ductus arteriosus through a surgically-placed sheath in the main pulmonary artery above the pulmonary valve; 3) decompression of left atrium enlarging a restrictive inter-atrial communication with balloon septostomy, balloon dilatation of the inter-atrial septum or by deploying a stent in the inter-atrial septum (Figure 2).

Bacha et al. [21] reported their hybrid stage I experience in 14 high-risk newborns with in-hospital survival of 78.5% in this high-risk group. Galantowicz et al. [22] reported their intermediate results in 40 patients, 36 of whom had undergone comprehensive stage II procedure while 15 went on to Fontan completion with a 82.5% overall survival.

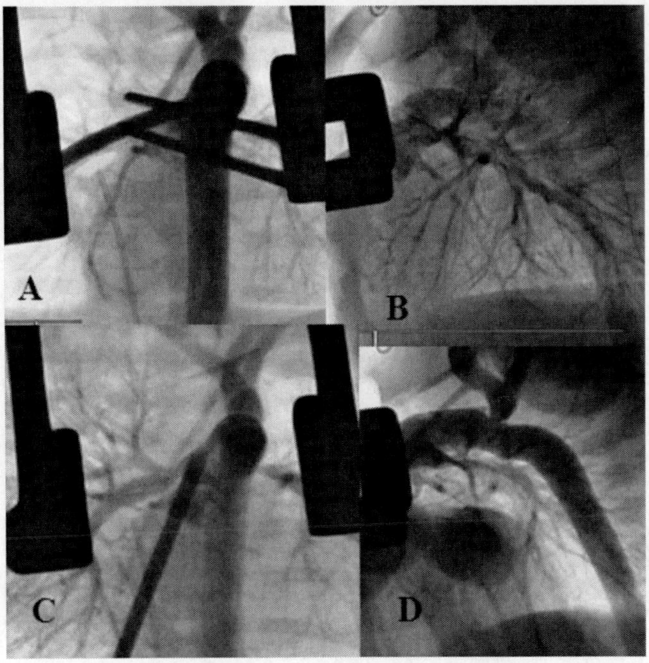

Figure 2. Single-stage hybrid approach for palliation of Hypoplastic Left Heart Syndrome. Selective bilateral pulmonary artery bands was realized bilaterally via median stenotomy (A and B). Ductal stenting (C and D) is realized anterogradly through a 7F sheat introduced in the main pulmonary artery.

Despite mathematical models predict increased ventricular workload and vulnerability of coronary perfusion in HLHS patients treated with hybrid procedure compared to those treated with Norwood procedure [23-24], hospital mortality and hospital stay are significantly lower in the hybrid group. Long term results are similar between the two strategies of treatment after the second stage. Survival after stage II palliation and subsequent Fontan completion is reported to be equivalent between the groups. The hybrid group had a higher pulmonary artery reintervention rate and smaller PA size. However, both strategies achieved adequate physiology for Fontan completion. Certainly, evolution of the hybrid strategy requires refinement to provide optimal pulmonary artery growth [25].

Finally, studies have demonstrated that in a subset of patients with left ventricle hypoplasia the ventricle is capable of postnatal growth. Consequently, identification of the specific flow mechanism of ventricular hypoplasia might induce -in a subset of hybrid palliated HLHS patients- post-natal left ventricular growth, thus allowing or at least facilitating the selection of patients for a 1- versus 2-ventricle repair.

Periventricular Device Closure of Muscular Ventricular Septal Defect (VSD)

Recently, surgical results for multiple muscular ventricular septal defects (muscVSDs) have improved in terms of hospital survival [26-27], but the need for right ventriculotomy is still frequent, particularly in low-weight patients. Indeed, palliative procedures such as pulmonary artery banding are often not effective. During cardiopulmonary bypass, since the heart is arrested and flaccid, some muscular VSDs cannot be found despite accurate searching by extensive resection of muscular trabeculations. This problem underlines the advantages of a technique that instead allows VSD closure without circulatory arrest and extracorporeal circulation, although the interventional approach is limited in low-weight patients by vascular access problems. The safety of periventricular puncture and device delivery has been validated in animal experiments [28].

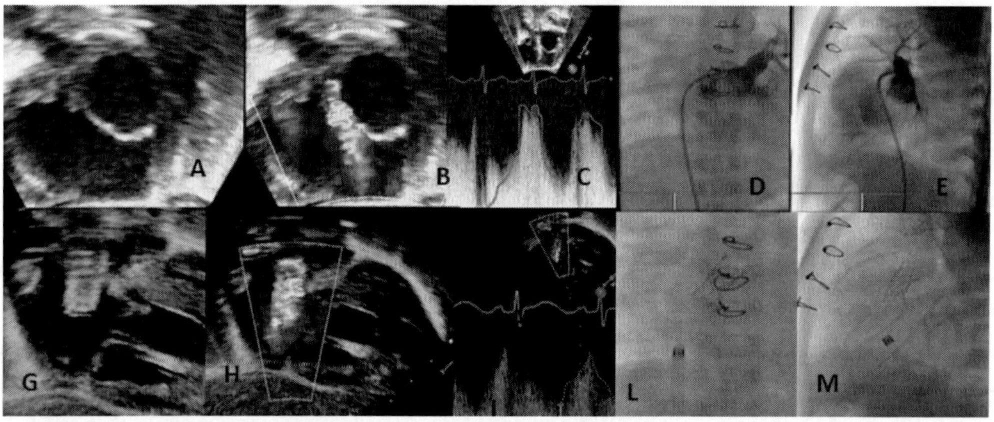

Figure 3. Echocardiograaphic images of restrictive interatrial communication in a patient affected by hypoplastic left heart syndrome, mitral atresia, aortic-atresia variant.

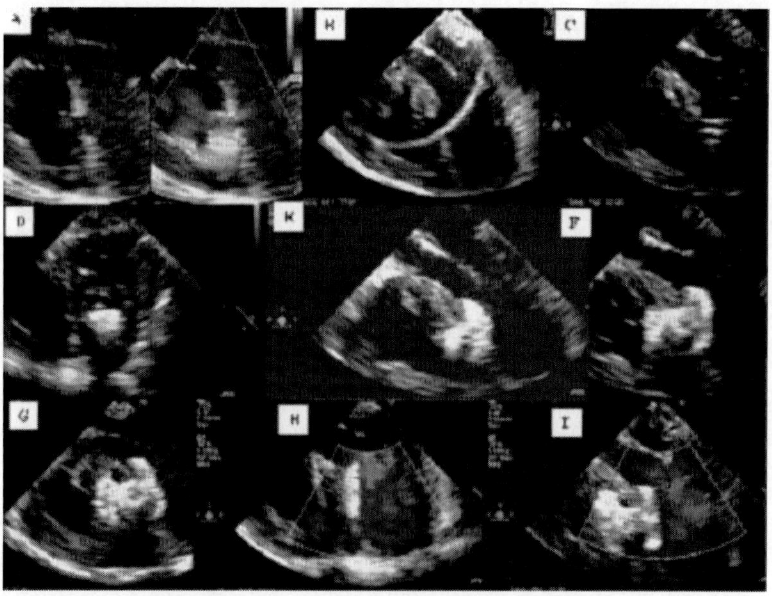

Figure 4. Periventricular device closure of muscular ventricular septal defect. A) Trans-esophageal echocardiography four-chamber view shows unrestrictive mid-muscular ventricular septal defect; B) the guidewire and the sheat (C) cross the ventricular septal defect; D) the left disk of the device is opened in the left ventricle and it is positioned over the left face of the ventricular septum (E and F); H: the device is still attached to the cable; I): the position is considered satisfactory and the device is released, thus obtaining complete closure of the ventricular septal defect.

Currently, this approach is proposed for children weighing less than 5 kg. There are no absolute contraindications to this technique. Under continuous trans-esophageal echocardiography (TEE) guidance and via median sternotomy, the best location for right ventricular free wall puncture is chosen. The puncture must be perpendicular to the VSD. The right ventricle is punctured using an 18G needle, and an 0.035-inch short guide wire is passed through the VSD in the left ventricle. Then, an introducer sheath with a dilator is positioned over the guidewire in the left ventricular cavity. The dilatator is then removed, and properly sized device (usually 1-2 mm larger than the size of VSD at end diastole) is chosen; the device utilized is usually the Amplatzer muscular VSD device. The device is positioned through the VSD and then it is released only when a safe and satisfactory position is achieved (Figure 3-4)

Hybrid therapy is an alternative approach for dealing with congenital heart disease and a great opportunity for surgical and medical teams to think and plan together, thus overcoming the limitations of the usual surgical or interventional procedure.

Insights into GUCH Cardiology

(Guccione P)

Since the inception of cardiac operations in the 1940s and 1950s, our knowledge about congenital heart disease and our ability to treat affected children have greatly improved. Despite many limitations, the best available evidence suggests that the prevalence of CHD in adults is now approximately 3,000 per million (AHJ), which means 0.3% of the general population. Considering that the reported incidence of CHD in newborns is reported at 0.8 % [28], about one out of three patient with CHD who were born more than 20 years ago now reaches adulthood. The great advancement in pediatric cardiovascular medicine and surgery supports the expectation of an increasing number of adult patients with congenital heart disease in the near future.

Detailed information about patients with ventricular septal defect (VSD), aortic stenosis (AS), and pulmonary stenosis (PS), has been obtained through two studies that reported on the natural history of such patients. Reported birth prevalence and survival to adulthood in case of "severe" CHD dramatically improved when we compare patients who were born before 1959, between 1960 and 1979, and after 1980. None of the patients born with transposition of the great arteries born before 1959 reached the adult age [29], while 75 % of those with the same defect born after 1980 became adult [30]. In case of pulmonary atresia the difference is less marked, with no survival to adulthood for patients born before 1959, and only 44% for those who were born after 1980 [31-32]. In case of less severe lesions, such as Tetralogy of Fallot, survival to adulthood increased form 20% to 79% for those born before 1959 and after 1979, respectively; even more marked is the improvement, from 15% to 95%, in case of patients with complex ventricular septal defect [31, 33-35]. Moller and Andreson (JACC 2013) reported the outcome of a cohort of 1,000 consecutive children with 43 to 54-year follow up. Of these, 362 died, 130 as adults, of whom 67 died from a cardiac cause. Importantly, they found that survival curve was in the normal range for simple lesions as ventricular septal defect, pulmonary valve stenosis, atrial septal defect, or patent ductus arteriosus.

Opotowsky et al. [36] reported the trends in hospitalizations for adults with ACHD in the U.S. These authors used nationally representative data from 1998 to 2005 to identify patients older than 18 years admitted to an acute care hospital with an International Classification of Diseases-9th Revision code designating a CHD diagnosis. National estimates of hospitalizations and total hospital charges per year were calculated. The number of hospital admissions for ACHD in the U.S. more than doubled between 1998 and 2005, from 35,992 in 1998 to 72,656 in 2005. Mean hospital charges per hospitalization increased by 127%, and the estimated total national charges for these hospitalizations increased by 357% from $691 million in 1998 to $3.16 billion in 2005. Verheugt et al. [37] reported on all hospital admissions from 2001 to 2006 of 5,798 adult patients with congenital heart disease (with a mean age of 39 years) from the Dutch national registry. Admission rate in these patients was high and exceeded by 2 to 3 fold that of the general Dutch population.

Conclusion

Because of the increasing number of adults living with congenital heart disease there is now wide consensus about the importance of ensuring an adequate standard of care. The hurdles of a successful transition from a pediatric to an adult health care setting, typically needed during adolescence and young adult period, reduces the availability of care for these patients. On the one hand, most adult cardiologists have little training or clinical experience in the diagnosis and management of congenital heart disease. On the other hand, pediatric cardiologists have little general medical training, and are ill-suited to comprehensive management of adults. As the population of adults with congenital heart disease increases, there will be additional need for specialists with training in both congenital cardiac disease and adult medicine to manage and coordinate care for these patients.

References

[1] Hoffman, JI; Kaplan, S. The incidence of congenital heart disease. *J. Am. Coll. Cardiol.* 2002;39:1890 –900.

[2] Campbell, M. Natural history of cyanotic malformations and comparison of all common cardiac malformations. *Br. Heart J.* 1972; 34:3-8.

[3] Moons, P; Bovijn, L; Budts, W; et al. Temporal trends in survival to adulthood among patients born with congenital heart disease from 1970 to 1992 in Belgium. *Circulation* 2010;122:2264-72.

[4] Samánek, M. Children with congenital heart disease: probability of natural survival. *Pediatr Cardiol* 1992;13:152-8.

[5] Leonard, H; Derrick, G; O'Sullivan, J; et al. Natural and unnatural history of pulmonary atresia. *Heart* 2000;84:499-503.

[6] Bertranou, EG; Blackstone, EH; Hazelrig, JB; et al. Life expectancy without surgery in tetralogy of Fallot. *Am. J. Cardiol* 1978;42:458-66.

[7] Frontera-Izquierdo, P; Cabezuelo-Huerta, G. Natural and modified history of isolated ventricular septal defect: a 17-year study. *Pediatr. Cardiol.* 1992;13:193-7

[8] Campbell, M. Natural history of cyanotic malformations and comparison of all common cardiac malformations. *Br. Heart J.* 1972; 34:3-8.

[9] Opotowsky, AR; Siddiqi, OK; Webb, GD. Trends in hospitalizations for adults with congenital heart disease in the U.S. *J. Am. Coll. Cardiol.* 2009;54:460 –7.

[10] Verheugt, CL; Uiterwaal, CSPM; van der Velde, ET; et al. The emerging burden of hospital admissions of adults with congenital heart disease. *Heart* 2010;96:872– 8.

[11] Norwood, WI; Lang, P; Castaneda, AR; et al. Experience with operations for hypoplastic left heart syndrome. *J Thorac Cardiovasc Surg* 1981;82:511-9.

[12] Sano, S; Ishino, K; Kawada, M; et al. Right ventricle-pulmonary artery shunt in first-stage palliation of hypoplastic left heart syndrome. *Operat Tech Thorac Cardiovasc Surg: a comparative atlas* 2005;10:141-51.

[13] Gibbs, JL; Wren, C; Watterson, KG; et al. Stenting of the arterial duct combined with banding of the pulmonary arteries and atrial septectomy or septostomy: a new approach to palliation for hypoplastic left heart syndrome. *Br Heart* J 1993;699:551-5.

[14] Bacha, EA; Daves, S; Hardin, J; et al. Single-ventricle palliation for high risk neonates: The emergence of an alternative hybrid stage I strategy. *J Thorac Cardiovasc Surg* 2006;131:163-71.

[15] Galantowicz, M; Cheatham, JP; Phillips, A; et al. Hybrid approach for hypoplastic left heart syndrome: Intermediate results after the learning curve. *Ann Thorac Surg* 2008;85:2063-71.

[16] Maher, KO; Pizarro, C; Gidding, SS; et al. Hemodynamic profile after the Norwood procedure with right ventricle to pulmonary artery conduit. *Circulation* 2003;108: 782-4.

[17] Baker, CE; Corsini, C; Cosentino, D; et al. For the Modeling of Congenital Hearts Alliance (MOCHA) Investigators. Effects of pulmonary artery banding and retrograde aortic arch obstruction on the hybrid palliation of hypoplastic left heart syndrome. *J Thorac Cardiovasc Surg* 2013 Feb 20).

[18] Baba, K; Kotani, Y; Chetan, D; et al. Hybrid versus Norwood strategies for single-ventricle palliation. *Circulation* 2012;126(11 Suppl 1):S123-31.

[19] Kitagawa, T; Durham, LA III; Mosca, RS; et al: Techniques and results in the management of multiple ventricular septal defects. *J Thorac Cardiovasc Surg* 1998;115:848-856.

[20] Myhre, U; Duncan, BW; Mee, RBB; et al. Apical right ventriculotomy for closure of apical ventricular septal defects. *Ann Thorac Surg* 2004;78:204-208.

[21] Amin, Z; Berry, JM; Foker, JE; et al. Intraoperative closure of muscular ventriocular septal defect in a canine model and application of the technique in a baby. *J Thorac Cardiovasc Surg* 1998;115:1374-1376.

[22] Marelli, AJ; Mackie, AS; Ionescu-Ittu, R et al. Congenital Heart Disease in the General Population Changing Prevalence and Age Distribution. *Circulation* 2007;115:163-172.

[23] Persico, N; Moratalla, J; Lombardi, CM; et al. Fetal echocardiography at 11-13 weeks by transabdominal high-frequency ultrasound. *Ultrasound Obstet Gynecol* 2011;37:296-301.

[24] Makrydimas, G; Sotiriadis, A; Ioannidis, JP. Screening performance of first-trimester nuchal translucency for major cardiac defects:a meta-analysis. *Am. J. Obstet. Gynecol.* 2008;31:256-260.

[25] International Society of Ultrasound in Obstetrics ang Gynecology (ISUOG). Cardiac screening guidelines of the fetus: guidelines for permirming the "basic" and "extended basic" cardiac scan. *Ultrasound Obstet. Gynecol.* 2006;27;107-113.

[26] Lee, W; Allan, W; Carvalho, JS; et al. ISUOG consensus statement: what constitutes a fetal echocardiogram? *Ultrasound Obstet. Gynecol.* 2008;32:239-242.

[27] Vinals, F; Heredia, F; and Giuliano, A. The role of the three vessels and trachea view (3VT) in the diagnosis of congenital heart defects. *Ultrasound Obstet. Gynecol.* 2003; 22: 358–367.

[28] Eibschitz, I; Abinader, EG; Klein, A; et al. Intrauterine diagnosis and control of fetal ventricular arrhythmia during labor. *Am. J. Obstet. Gynecol.* 1975;122:597– 600.

[29] Carpenter, R; Strasburger, JF; Garson, A; et al. Fetal ventricular pacing for hydrops secondary to complete atrioventricular block. *J. Am. Coll. Cardiol.* 1986;8:1434 –1436.

[30] Van den Heuvel, F; Bink-Boelkens, MT; du Marchie Sarvaas, GJ; et al. Drug management of fetal tachyarrhythmias: are we ready for a systematic and evidence-based approach? *Pacing Clin. Electrophysiol.* 2008;31(suppl 1):S54 –S57.

[31] Strasburger, JF; Cuneo, BF; Michon, MM; et al. Amiodarone therapy for drug-refractory fetal tachycardia. *Circulation* 2004;109:375–379.

[32] Friedman, DM; Kim, MY; Copel, JA; et al. Prospective evaluation of fetuses with autoimmune-associated congenital heart block followed in the PR Interval and Dexamethasone Evaluation (PRIDE) Study. *Am. J. Cardiol.* 2009;103:1102–1106.

[33] Maeno, Y; Himeno, W; Saito, A; et al. Clinical course of fetal congenital atrioventricular block in the Japanese population: a multicentre experience. *Heart* 2005;91:1075–1079.

[34] Mäkikallio, K; McElhinney, DB; Levine, JC; et al. Fetal Aortic Valve Stenosis and the Evolution of Hypoplastic Left Heart Syndrome. Patient Selection for Fetal Intervention. *Circulation* 2006;113:1401-1405.

[35] Rychik, J; Rome, JJ; Collins, MH; et al. The hypoplastic left heart syndrome with intact atrial septum: atrial morphology, pulmonary vascular histopathology and outcome. *J. Am. Coll. Cardiol.* 1999;34:554–60.

[36] Simonneau, G; Robbins, IM; Beghetti, M et al. Updated clinical classification of pulmonary hypertension. *J. Am. Coll. Cardiol.* 2009;54(1 Suppl):S43-S54.

[37] Steinhorn, RH. Neonatal Pulmonary Hypertension. *Pediatr Crit. Care Med.* 2010;11(2 Suppl): S79–S84.

[38] Oishi, P; Datar, SA; Fineman, JR. Advances in the Management of Paediatric Pulmonary Hypertension. *Respir. Care* 2011;56(9):1314 –1339.

In: Recent Advances in Cardiology
Editors: José Milei and Giuseppe Ambrosio

ISBN: 978-1-63117-282-3

Chapter 11

Percutaneous Cryoablation of Cardiac Arrhythmias

Jorge González-Zuelgaray[1,2,*]***, Fernando de Valais***[1]***, Claudio Muratore***[1]***, América Pérez***[3] ***and Ariel Szyszko***[3]

[1]Sanatorio de la Trinidad San Isidro, Buenos Aires, Argentina
[2]Instituto de Investigaciones Cardiológicas "Prof. Dr. Alberto C. Taquini," University of Buenos Aires, Argentina
[3]Fundación PRONETAC
(Programa de Estudio y Tratamiento de las Arritmias Cardíacas), Buenos Aires, Argentina

Abstract

Catheter ablation of cardiac arrhythmias has become an accepted therapeutic tool. After a relatively short initial period with direct current (with significant limitations), radiofrequency ablation became the almost universal source of energy. In the last decade, cryoablation (employed in different types of surgery with significant success) appeared as an attractive option due to a favorable risk-benefit ratio.

Cryoablation lesions are clearly demarcated and do not disrupt the architecture of cardiac or vascular structures compared with radiofrequency.

The previously mentioned advantages make cryoablation an attractive source of energy for arrhythmias as AV node reentry, AV reentry involving accessory pathways located in the vicinity of the AV node/His bundle area, atrial ectopic tachycardias close to the normal conduction system, junctional ectopic tachycardia, atrial flutter, tachyarrhythmias close to the sinus node, ventricular arrhythmias arising near the sinuses of Valsalva (with risk of damage to the coronary circulation by radiofrequency) and bundle branch reentry. The value for atrial fibrillation therapy has not yet been established conclusively, although cryoablation also seems an attractive option.

* Address for reprints: Jorge Gonzalez-Zuelgaray MD, PhD. FAX: +5411-4801-7446. E-mail: arritmias@arritmias.org.ar.

Introduction

The possibility of a curative approach for cardiac arrhythmias started with cryosurgery of accessory pathways and was later followed by direct current ablation of the AV node and certain locations of accessory connections. The former required open heart surgery with its risks and the latter was not devoid of serious complications including cardiac tamponade as a consequence of the barotrauma caused by the emission of energy.

The aforementioned limitations were greatly eliminated after the introduction of radiofrequency ablation in 1991. As the risk-benefit ratio was truly attractive, and after the understanding of the mechanism of different arrhythmias evolved dramatically as a process of "learning by burning", it became the accepted approach for percutaneous treatment.

Unfortunately, radiofrequency is not free of shortcomings as the emission of energy is accompanied by an "all or none" phenomenon. This creates the risk of irreversible collateral damage to nearby structures like the AV node, the sinus node and the coronary circulation. Approximately 0.5-2% of radiofrequency ablations of the slow AV nodal pathway with the aim of treating AV node reentry may cause complete AV block with necessity of a permanent pacemaker. The same is true (with even higher risk) for accessory connections in the proximity of the normal conduction system, and for other substrates. [1]

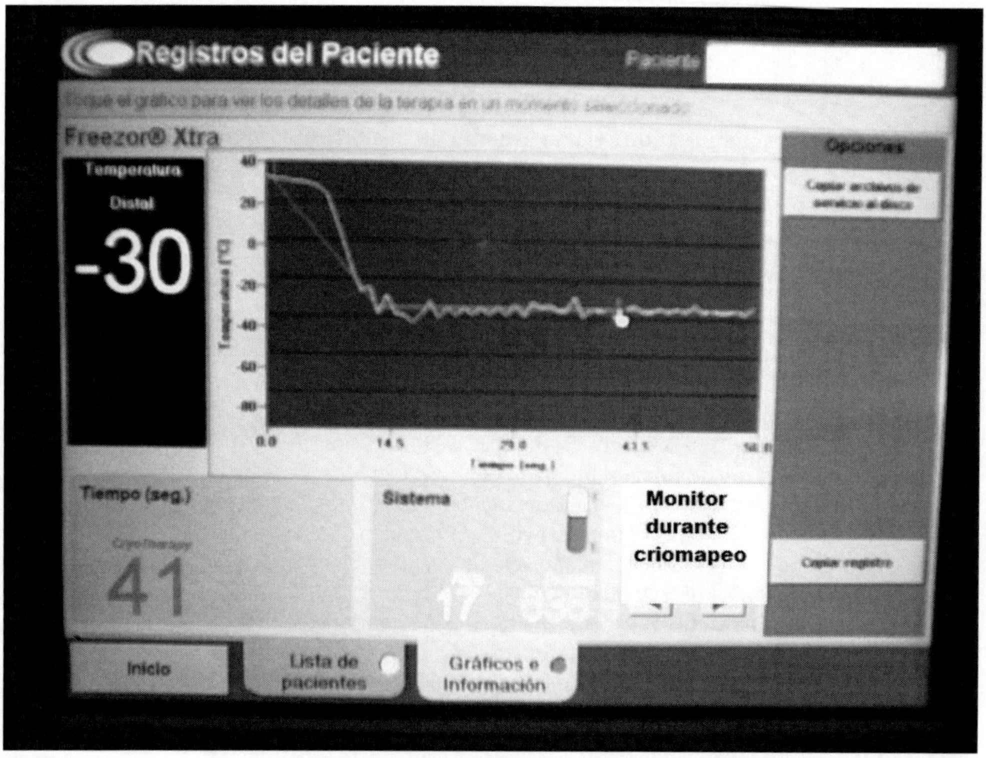

Figure 1. The screen of the cryoconsole shows the temperature curve until the cryomapping value of -30 ºC was achieved.

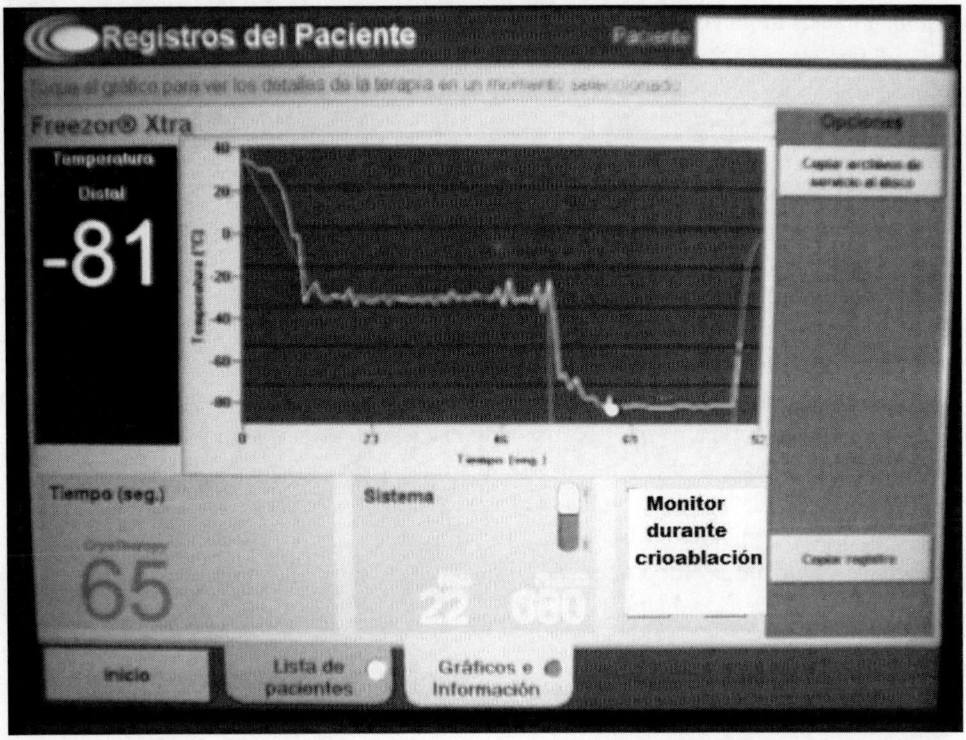

Figure 2. The cryoablation value of -81 °C has been reached and permanent damage is being produced.

The evolution of technology has allowed better manipulation of catheters as well as an expansion of the indications, including pulmonary vein isolation in patients with atrial fibrillation.

Our experience is the first in South America and we shall delineate the criteria for selection of patients, our results and some clinically relevant technical considerations.

AV Node Reentry

The crucial advantage of percutaneous cryoablation of the slow pathway resides in the significantly lower risk of complete AV block. [2-5] However, the approach is different as, characteristically, the absence of thermal injury does not provoke junctional tachycardia at the sites of the effective lesion. The absence of this junctional rhythm which during radiofrequency indicates the existence of an effective lesion converts this method in a time-consuming approach requiring more radiation time. To solve this limitation, we carried out a prospective investigation to validate a parameter for selecting the area considered adequate for cryomapping.

In 34 consecutive patients (25 females, age 38.7 ± 6.3 years) with typical AV node reentry, the distance (in mm) from the point with the most proximal His deflection to the location of the effective cryolesion (analyzed in 30° right anterior and 45° left anterior oblique views) was plotted against the magnitude of the "jump" (difference in H1-H2 before and after change of antegrade conduction from the fast to the slow pathway during programmed atrial stimulation). According to the magnitude of the jump, cryomapping was initially attempted in each of three areas of the triangle of Koch as follows: a) for a "jump" duration ≥ 150 msec, the lesion was created at the posterior zone (closer to the coronary sinus os); b) for a "jump" duration of 100-149 msec, at the medial zone; and c) for a duration of 50-99 msec, at the anterior zone (closer to the compact AV node) (Figure 3).

There was a good correlation between the magnitude of the "jump" and the distance from the area of the most proximal His deflection to the site of the effective cryolesion (r-Pearson-0.64; $p < 0.001$). The number of cryomapping attempts preceding the effective cryolesion was 5.6 ± 2.9, with a total radiation time of 11.3 ± 3.1 minutes. Figure 4 shows the close location between the site of the cryoablation catheter and the compact AV node in a patient with a jump of 73 msec. After a follow-up of 41.4 ± 7.9 months, there was one recurrence (2.9%).

We arrived at the conclusion that, in the absence of junctional rhythm to suggest the adequate location of the catheter as occurs with cryoenergy, the magnitude of the "jump" of the H1-H2 during programmed atrial stimulation in patients with AV nodal reentrant tachycardia helps to identify the correct site for cryomapping.

Regarding the endpoint for the procedure, it is more stringent compared with radiofrequency ablation as the complete elimination of the “jump” is necessary to predict long-term success after cryoablation.

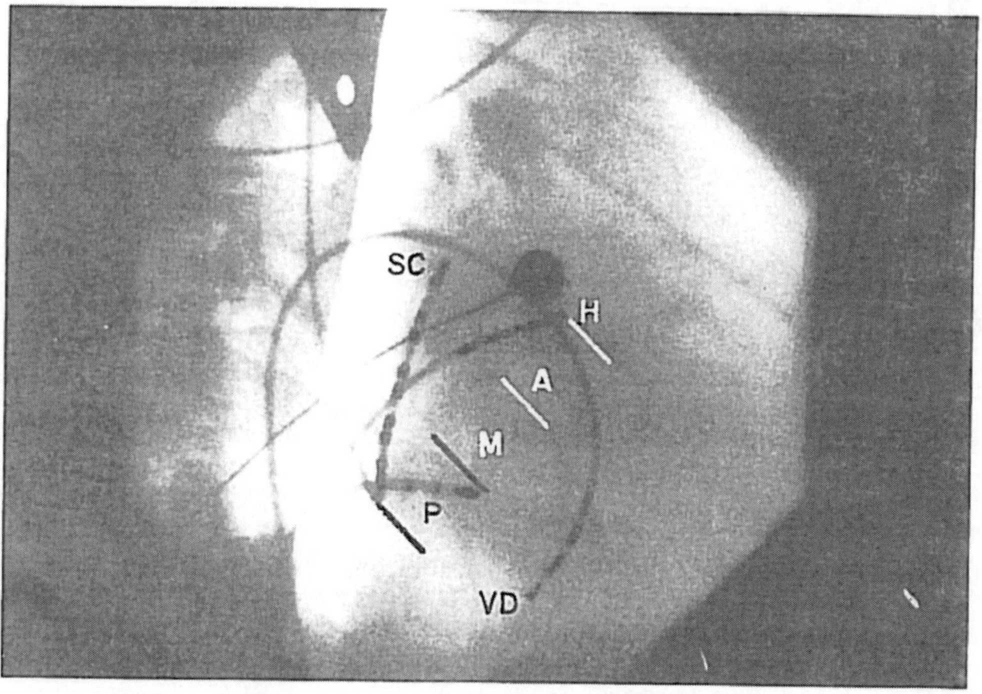

Figure 3. Fluoroscopic view in right anterior oblique position, showing the division of the triangle of Koch in three zones (posterior -P, medial –M- and anterior -A).

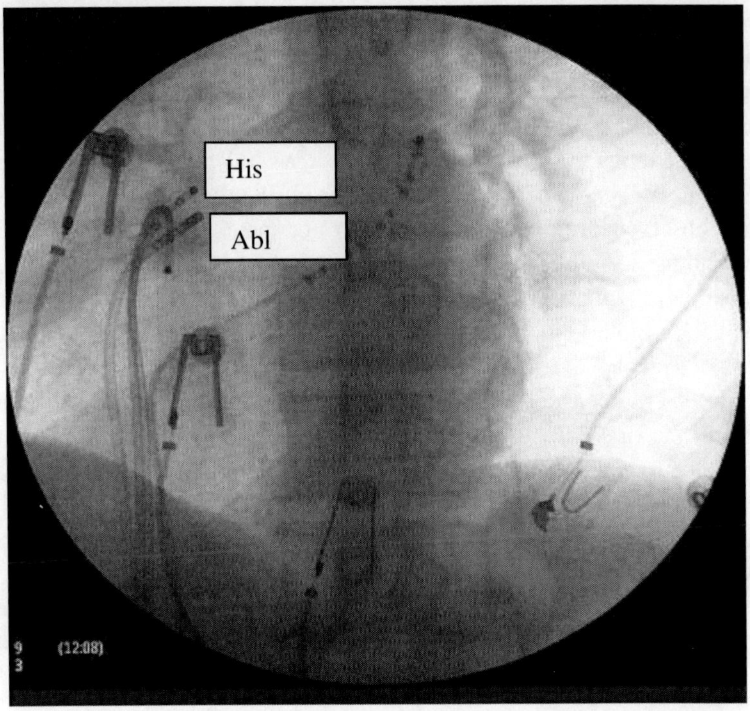

Figure 4. In a left anterior oblique view, the cryoablation catheter (Abl) is located close to the zone where the His bundle electrogram is recorded (His).

Atrioventricular Reentry

Accessory pathways close to the compact AV node or the bundle of His were initially estimated to represent 5% of the total population with either concealed or manifest connections. However, radiofrequency ablation is indicated earlier and even in asymptomatic individuals both by adult and pediatric electrophysiologists. As a result, left or right sided connections (which offer the best results with radiofrequency) are progressively less frequently encountered and septal pathways (closer to the normal conduction system) constitute a growing population for ablation. This location has the serious risk of damage of the His bundle and, more easily, the compact AV node (which is not protected by the fibrous trigone as happens with the bundle of His). [6] Figure 5 shows the electrocardiogram pre and post-cryoablation of a parahisian accessory connection in a professional runner and figure 6 depicts the intracardiac electrograms, with a clearly identifiable His bundle deflection in the site of the effective lesion.

We had excellent results with the ablation of parahisian pathways (109 out of 123 cryoablations were successful – 88.6%), with some important points to consider:

1) In pediatric patients, careful catheter manipulation is of utmost importance, as the pathways are prone to be eliminated traumatically more likely than during radiofrequency ablation probably due to a more subendocardial location compared with adults and because of the stiffer characteristic of the cryoablation catheter

(although they have recently become softer). The transient disappearance of the pathway (both antegradely and retrogradely) is usually accompanied by a failure of the procedure as there is no endpoint to demonstrate the effect of the lesion.

2) The safety lesion, consisting of 240 seconds of emission of cryoenergy after the first successful attempt, is clearly valuable to increase the long-term success.
3) A close monitoring is of utmost importance during the emission of cryoenergy as the effects observed during cryomapping do not match completely with the effect of cryoablation at -80ºC. We have seen persistence of normal conduction during cryomapping with later transient complete or advanced AV block during cryoablation (although both were completely reversible after the interruption of energy delivery).
4) The aforementioned considerations also apply when considering the extra (safety) lesion, as the first 240 seconds at -80ºC may show therapeutic effect with preserved AV conduction, and the extra lesion may cause complete or advanced AV block (also completely reversible after the interruption of the emission of cryoenergy).
5) It is noteworthy that the effect of cryoablation has a reproducible "decrescendo" effect, as the damage of the AV conduction system clearly declines within the first 10 minutes. This behavior is opposite to what is seen with radiofrequency, in which the trend is to an expansion of the lesions, with a persistent effect of damage.

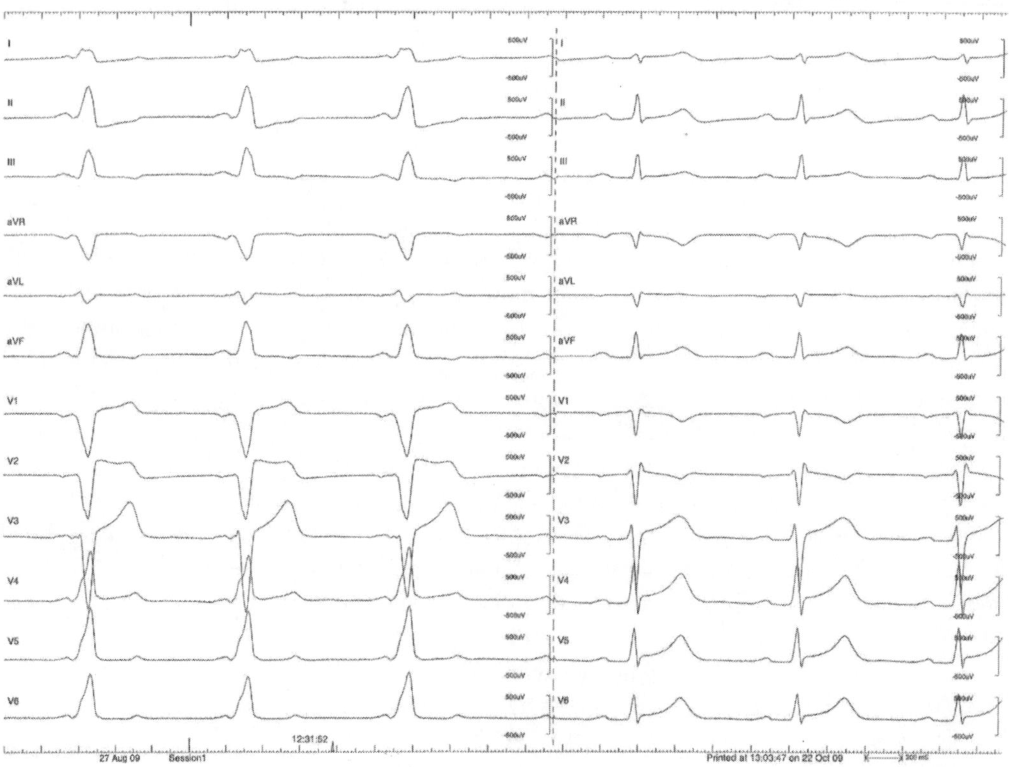

Figure 5. Electrocardiogram pre (left) and post-cryoablation (right) of a parahisian accessory pathway.

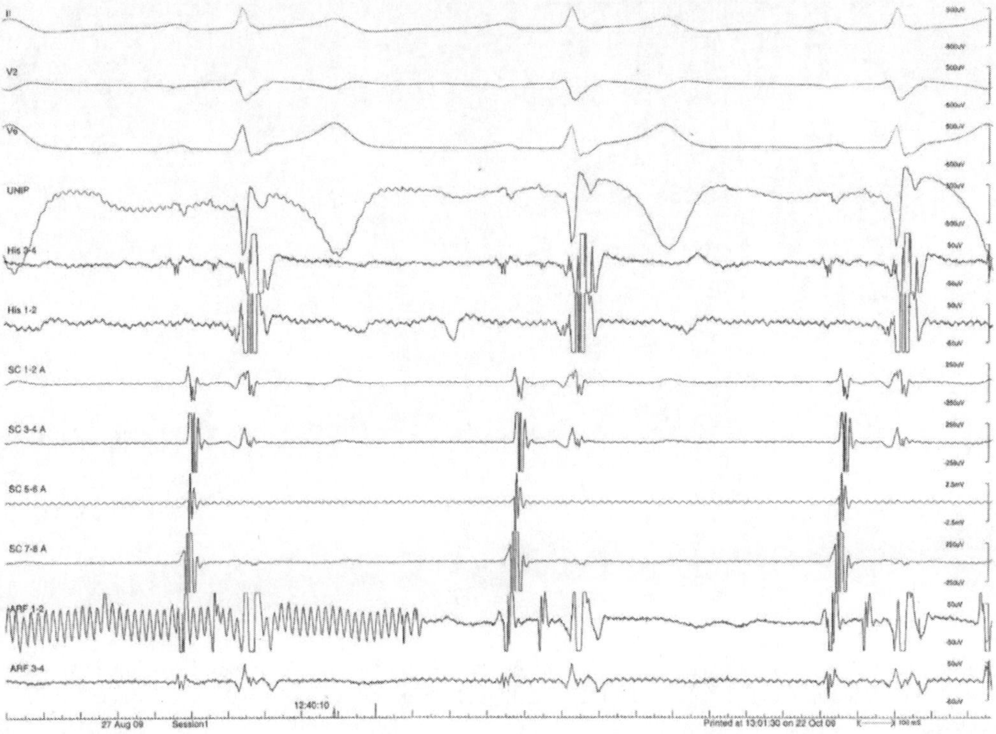

Figure 6. In the same patient whose ECG is shown in figure 5, the His bundle electrogram is clearly recorded by the ablation catheter, with persistence of normal AV conduction and absence of preexcitation at the end of cryoenergy delivery.

Junctional Ectopic Tachycardia (JET)

This arrhythmia is characterized by narrow QRS complexes frequently with AV dissociation (Figure 7). It is more prevalent (although not exclusive) in the pediatric population, tends to be permanent or incessant and in some cases may cause deterioration of the systolic function (tachycardiomyopathy). The response to antiarrhythmic medications is frequently discouraging, with the additional limitation of serious side effects of amiodarone, which is relatively more effective. As JET arises in the immediate vicinity of the normal conduction system, the risk of complete or high grade AV block associated with radiofrequency energy is particularly elevated. [7]

We have performed cryoablation of a JET in 7 patients (one of them with depressed left ventricular ejection fraction). In 5 cases the method was successful acutely with one recurrence in the long-term follow-up, and the ejection fraction normalized in the mentioned case (in which the arrhythmia was abolished by cryoablation at the left atrial septum after advancing the catheter through a patent foramen ovalis).

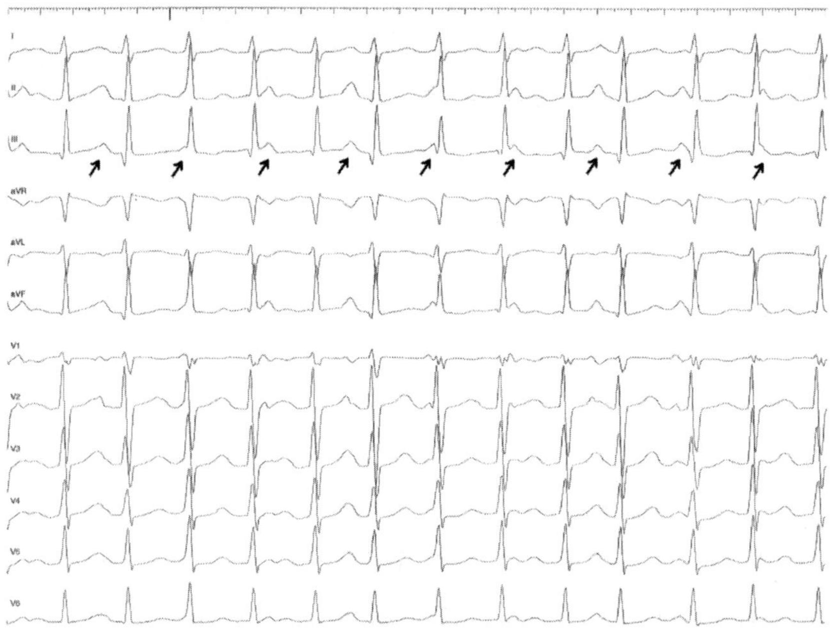

Figure 7. Junctional ectopic tachycardia. The arrows correspond to sinus P waves dissociated from the ventricular activity, with the exception of the fourth and seventh P waves, which are conducted to the ventricles.

Long-Term Efficacy

Although cryoablation is considered a safe source of energy-especially for substrates near critical structures as the conduction system-, there has been some controversy regarding the risk of recurrences after an initially successful procedure.

To analyze the long-term effectiveness of catheter cryoablation, we analyzed this important aspect in all patients with a successful catheter cryoablation performed between August 2007 and July 2012. They were periodically controlled at the Arrhythmia Clinic or contacted through telephonic interviews, mails or calls to their referring physycians. In all cases, after a safe initial cryomapping attempt, two cryolesions were created at -80°C with a brief interval in-between.

One hundred and seventy-three patients were included, aged 28.3 ± 10.6 years (range 9-66): 102 were females and 71 males. The substrates were: manifest parahisian accessory pathways in 109 cases, AV node reentry in 47, focal atrial tachycardia with origin near the compact AV node/His bundle in 12, and junctional ectopic tachycardia in 5 patients. Follow-up lasted 12-71 months (mean 37.6 ± 12.4).

Clinically significant remodeling was seen only in one patient with AV node reentry (prolonged PR interval between days 3 and 20 post-ablation).

There were 6 recurrences of parahisian accessory pathways from a total of 109 patients (5.5%), 2 recurrences of AV node reentry from a population of 47 patients (4.2%), one recurrence of a junctional ectopic tachycardia from a total of 5 patients and no recurrences after cryoablation of a focal atrial tachycardia. This represents 9 recurrences in 173 patients

(5.2%), which is not different from our experience and the published reports worldwide following radiofrequency catheter ablation.

In conclusion, catheter cryoablation is accompanied by persistent effectiveness following an initially successful procedure.

Cryoablation of Atrial Fibrillation

The introduction of a balloon cryocatheter to ablate the circumference of the pulmonary vein ostia created much expectation and is considered an attractive option against the classical isolation of the pulmonary veins by means of radiofrequency energy. The theoretical advantages reside mainly in the reduction of the risk of pulmonary vein stenosis (based on the lack of effect on the architecture of the cardiac structures) and in the lower likelihood of atrioesophageal fistulization (which is a very infrequent but usually mortal complication). [8-11]

We are awaiting long-term results from experiences which are being carried out in different centers.

Conclusion

Percutaneous catheter cryoablation is expanding steadily as the results are encouraging both at the short and long-term. The main advantage lies on safety (which is essential, especially in the case of arrhythmias which are not life-threatening). Reducing the risk of a permanent pacemaker in children or in relatively young patients is an absolute priority, as well as the reduction in the risk of damage to the coronary circulation (as may happen during ablation of tachycardias arising in the sinuses of Valsalva). [12] Also, tachycardias near the sinus node can be safely eliminated with cryoablation with much lower risk of deterioration of sinus node automaticity.

Cryoablation undoubtedly has been incorporated in the armamentarium of the curative therapy of cardiac arrhythmias.

References

[1] Akdeniz C, Ergul Y, Kiplapinar N, Tuzcu V. Catheter ablation of drug resistant supraventricular tachycardia in neonates and infants. *Cardiol. J.* 2013; 20:241-6.

[2] Cokkinakis C, Avramidis D, Alexopoulos C, Kirvassilis G, Papagiannis J. Cryoablation of atrioventricular nodal reentrant tachycardia in children and adolescents: improved long-term outcomes with increasing experience. *Hellenic J. Cardiol.* 2013; 54:186-91.

[3] Hoffmann BA, Brachmann J, Andresen D, Eckardt L, Hoffmann E, Kuck KH, Schumacher B, Spitzer SG, Schirdewahn P, Tebbenjohanns J, Horack M, Senges J, Salukhe TV, Rostock T, Willems S. Ablation of atrioventricular nodal reentrant tachycardia in the elderly: results from the German Ablation Registry. *Heart Rhythm* 2011; 8:981-7.

[4] Peyrol M, Sbragia P, Uhry S, Boccara G, Dolla E, Quatre A, Guenoun M, Lévy S, Paganelli F. Slow pathway elimination for atrioventricular nodal reentrant tachycardia with the 8-mm tip cryoablation catheter: an 18-month follow-up study. *J. Interv. Card. Electrophysiol.* 2013; 37:105-9.

[5] Eckhardt LL, Leal M, Hollis Z, Tanega J, Alberte C. Cryoablation for AVNRT: importance of ablation endpoint criteria. *J. Cardiovasc. Electrophysiol.* 2012; 23:729-34.

[6] Bastani H, Insulander P, Schwieler J, Tabrizi F, Braunschweig F, Kennebäck G, Drca N, Jensen-Urstad M. Cryoablation of superoparaseptal and septal accessory pathways: a single centre experience. *Europace* 2010; 12:972-7.

[7] Eizmendi I, Almendral J, Hadid C, Ortiz M. Successful catheter cryoablation of Hisian ectopy using 2 new diagnostic criteria based on unipolar and bipolar recordings of the His electrogram. *J. Cardiovasc. Electrophysiol.* 2012; 23:325-9.

[8] Packer DL, Kowal RC, Wheelan KR, Irwin JM, Champagne J, Guerra PG, Dubuc M, Reddy V, Nelson L, Holcomb RG, Lehmann JW, Ruskin JN; STOP AF Cryoablation Investigators. Cryoballoon ablation of pulmonary veins for paroxysmal atrial fibrillation: first results of the North American Arctic Front (STOP AF) pivotal trial. *J. Am. Coll. Cardiol.* 2013; 61:1713-23.

[9] Ernst S. Cryoballoon pulmonary vein isolation: is it really all so "simple"? *J. Am. Coll. Cardiol.* 2013; 61:1724-5.

[10] Stöckigt F, Schrickel JW, Andrié R, Lickfett L. Atrioesophageal fistula after cryoballoon pulmonary vein isolation. *J. Cardiovasc. Electrophysiol.* 2012; 23:1254-7.

[11] Mandell J, Amico F, Parekh S, Snow J, Germano J, Cohen TJ. Early experience with the cryoablation balloon procedure for the treatment of atrial fibrillation by an experienced radiofrequency catheter ablation center. *J. Invasive Cardiol.* 2013; 25:288-92.

[12] Di Biase L, Al-Ahamad A, Santangeli P, Hsia HH, Sanchez J, Bai R, Bailey S, Horton R, Gallinghouse GJ, Burkhardt DJ, Lakkireddy D, Yang Y, Badhwar N, Scheinman M, Tung R, Dello Russo A, Pelargonio G, Casella M, Tomassoni G, Shivkumar K, Natale A. Safety and outcomes of cryoablation for ventricular tachyarrhythmias: results from a multicenter experience. *Heart Rhythm* 2011; 8:968-74.

Editors' Contact Information

Dr. José Milei
Instituto de Investigaciones Cardiologicas
ININCA.UBA.CONICET
Director, Marcelo T. de Alvear 2270 CPAAJ,
Buenos Aires, Argentina
Phone/Fax: +54+11 45083836
ininca@fmed.uba.ar

Dr. Giuseppe Ambrosio
Cardiologia e Fisiopatologia Cardiovascolare
Ospedale S.M. della Misericordia
S. Andrea delle Fratte, 06131 Perugia, Italy
Tel: +39 0755271509; Fax: +39 0755271244
giuseppe.ambrosio@ospedale.perugia.it

Index

A

B

C

D

E

F

N

O

P

Q

R

S

T

U

V

W

X

Y

Z